617.514 CAP

Cranial, Craniofacial and Skull Base Surgery

Paolo Cappabianca · Luigi Califano
Giorgio Iaconetta
Editors

Cranial, Craniofacial and Skull Base Surgery

Foreword by
Michael L. J. Apuzzo

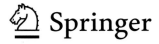

Editors

Paolo Cappabianca
Department of Neurological Sciences
Division of Neurosurgery
Università degli Studi di Napoli Federico II
Naples, Italy

Giorgio Iaconetta
Department of Neurological Sciences
Division of Neurosurgery
Università degli Studi di Napoli Federico II
Naples, Italy

Luigi Califano
Department of Head and Neck Surgery
Università degli Studi di Napoli Federico II
Naples, Italy

ISBN 978-88-470-1166-3

e-ISBN 978-88-470-1167-0

DOI 10.1007/978-88-470-1167-0

Springer Dordrecht Heidelberg London Milan New York

Library of Congress Control Number: 2009940679

9 8 7 6 5 4 3 2 1

Cover design: Simona Colombo, Milan, Italy

Typesetting and production: Scienzaperta S.r.l. Publishing Services, Novate Milanese (Milano), Italy
Printing and binding: Printer Trento S.r.l., Trento, Italy
Printed in Italy

Springer-Verlag Italia S.r.l, Via Decembrio 28, I-20137 Milano, Italy
Springer is part of Springer Science+Business Media (www.springer.com)

Foreword

The Fruits of Reinvention

Surgery related to the human head, its compartment and contents has been reinvented over the past 40 years. A number of instruments, most notably the sophisticated medical imaging device and the operating microscope, have principally fueled this evolution. Along the way, endoscopy and sophisticated navigation capabilities have added to the realization of a unique comprehension of normal and abnormal microanatomy permitting corridors and manipulations that allow novel strategies for surgery in these highly vital functional areas.

Cappabianca, Califano and Iaconetta have created a detailed and fully modern review of methods and strategies related to complex surgery and therapies associated with this robust reinvention. Technical innovations abound!

Distinguished practitioners of these unique developments in the history of surgical enterprise present these amazing technical exercises. The catalog of these approaches, instrumentation, techniques, strategies and manipulations is inspiring and stands as a testimony to the remarkable progress that we have witnessed in recent decades.

The presentation in truly "modern" and represents in many aspects pinnacles of operative achievement.

We must ask ourselves, what will be next?

Los Angeles, November 2009   *Michael L.J. Apuzzo, M.D., Ph.D (hon)*

Preface

We belong to a lucky and happy generation, living during a period of many dramatic, if not revolutionary, technical and technological innovations, such as the digital era, which have changed and improved our routine surgical practice, together with the quality and quantity of life of our patients.

Furthermore, the possibility of easily obtaining and exchanging information has facilitated cooperation among different specialties, thus favoring a real team-work attitude. No-man's land has become an area where many subjects have settled and produced new results.

Technologies and instruments previously used by a single group of specialists have been adopted and modified by others to perform the same kind of action in a different environment. Cross fertilizations have pushed the envelope towards the management and control of diseases that could not have been imagined a few years ago.

Previous paradigms have been demolished by conceptual and technical progress that has been determined by the exchange of knowledge. For patients, functional and even esthetic and/or cosmetic demands have taken over from the naked result of saving life by hazardous surgery.

Some surgeons have achieved innovations by novel approaches and others, at the same time, have refined established procedures taking advantage of recent technical advances. An example of both these conditions can be considered the recent advent of endoscopic endonasal skull-base surgery, introduced as an approach to the pituitary region, such that some tumors and/or pathological entities, once considered amenable only to open transcranial surgery, can now also be managed through this alternative option. Another example is the standardization and diffusion of operations to the cerebellopontine angle that are performed today with fixed coordinates and indications under adequate intraoperative neurophysiological and radiological monitoring.

Further progress can be expected to result from the ongoing experience of leading centers and contemporary teaching with modern facilities. At the same time, instrument development, perhaps robotics, will add a new impulse to the never-ending effort towards achieving perfect results.

The multiplicity of possible approaches and their refinement have led us to consider this an opportune time to collect presentations from different schools on various cranial, craniofacial, skull-base extended and small-size approaches. We asked individual specialists to produce a chapter on a single technique by providing anatomical images, that we have always considered the foundation of any surgical procedure, followed by operative images and explanatory text for each operation.

We hope readers, most importantly including young surgeons, will find our efforts useful in improving their expertise in and knowledge of the various techniques described.

Naples, November 2009   *Paolo Cappabianca*
                                                                                        Luigi Califano
                                                                                 Giorgio Iaconetta

Contents

Section I   Cranial Neurosurgery

Section II   Maxillofacial Surgery

Contributors

Julio Acero-Sanz Complutense University and Department of Oral and Maxillofacial Surgery, Gregorio Marañon University Hospital, Madrid, Spain

Andrea Battisti Division of Maxillofacial Surgery, "Sapienza" University of Rome, Italy

Evaristo Belli Maxillofacial Department, Sant'Andrea Hospital, "Sapienza" University of Rome, Italy

Ludwig Benes Klinik für Neurochirurgie, Baldingerstrasse, Marburg, Germany

Antonio Bernardo Department of Neurological Surgery, Weill Medical College of Cornell University, New York, NY, USA

Helmut Bertalanffy Department of Neurosurgery, University Hospital of Zurich, Switzerland

Federico Biglioli Department of Maxillo-Facial Surgery, San Paolo Hospital, University of Milan, Italy

Oliver Bozinov Department of Neurosurgery, University Hospital of Zurich, Switzerland

Roberto Brusati Department of Maxillo-Facial Surgery, San Paolo Hospital, University of Milan, Italy

Luigi Califano Department of Head and Neck Surgery, Università degli Studi di Napoli Federico II, Naples, Italy

Paolo Cappabianca Department of Neurological Sciences, Division of Neurosurgery, Università degli Studi di Napoli Federico II, Naples, Italy

Ricardo L. Carrau Department of Neurological Surgery and Department of Otolaryngology, University of Pittsburgh School of Medicine, Pittsburgh, PA, USA

Andrea Cassoni Division of Maxillofacial Surgery, "Sapienza" University of Rome, Italy

Luigi M. Cavallo Department of Neurological Sciences, Division of Neurosurgery, Università degli Studi di Napoli Federico II, Naples, Italy

Pasqualino Ciappetta Department of Neurological Sciences, University of Bari Medical School, Bari, Italy

Olga V. Corriero Department of Neurological Sciences, Division of Neurosurgery, Università degli Studi di Napoli Federico II, Naples, Italy

Aneela Darbar Centre for Minimally Invasive Neurosurgery, Prince of Wales Private Hospital, Randwick, New South Wales, Australia

Oreste de Divitiis Department of Neurological Sciences, Division of Neurosurgery, Università degli Studi di Napoli Federico II, Naples, Italy

Roberto Delfini Department of Neurological Sciences, Neurosurgery, "Sapienza" University of Rome, Italy

Matteo de Notaris Department of Neurological Sciences, Division of Neurosurgery, Università degli Studi di Napoli Federico II, Naples, Italy

Francesco S. De Ponte School of Maxillofacial Surgery, University Hospital G. Martino of Messina, Italy

Luc De Waele Department of Neurosurgery, Sint-Lucas Hospital, Ghent, Belgium

Alessandro Ducati Department of Neurosurgery, University of Torino, Italy

Ian F. Dunn Department of Neurosurgery, Brigham and Women's Hospital, Harvard Medical School, Boston, MA, USA

Pietro I. D'Urso Department of Neurological Sciences, University of Bari Medical School, Bari, Italy

Joaquim Enseñat Department of Neurosurgery, Hospital Clinic, Faculty of Medicine, Universitat de Barcelona, Spain

Felice Esposito Division of Neurosurgery and Division of Maxillo-Facial Surgery, Università degli Studi di Napoli Federico II, Naples, Italy

Isabella Esposito Department of Neurological Sciences, Division of Neurosurgery, Università degli Studi di Napoli Federico II, Naples, Italy

Enrique Ferrer Department of Neurosurgery, Hospital Clinic, Faculty of Medicine, Universitat de Barcelona, Spain

Takanori Fukushima Carolina Neuroscience Institute for Skull Base Surgery, Raleigh, NC, and Duke University, Durham, NC, and University of Morgantown, WV, USA

Renato J. Galzio Department of Health Sciences, University of L'Aquila, and Department of Neurosurgery, San Salvatore City Hospital, L'Aquila, Italy

Paul A. Gardner Department of Neurological Surgery, University of Pittsburgh School of Medicine, Pittsburgh, PA, USA

Paolo Gennaro Division of Maxillofacial Surgery, "Sapienza" University of Rome, Italy

Venelin M. Gerganov International Neuroscience Institute, Hannover, Germany

Rüdiger Gerlach Department of Neurosurgery, Johann Wolfgang Goethe University, Frankfurt am Main, Germany

Pankaj A. Gore Providence Brain Institute, Portland, OR, USA

Giovanni Grasso Department of Neurosurgery, University of Palermo, Italy

Giorgio Iaconetta Department of Neurological Sciences, Division of Neurosurgery, Università degli Studi di Napoli Federico II, Naples, Italy

Domenico G. Iacopino Department of Neurosurgery, University of Palermo, Italy

Giorgio Iannetti Division of Maxillofacial Surgery, "Sapienza" University of Rome, Italy

Christoph Kappus Klinik für Neurochirurgie, Baldingerstrasse, Marburg, Germany

Amin B. Kassam Department of Neurological Surgery and Department of Otolaryngology, University of Pittsburgh School of Medicine, Pittsburgh, PA, USA

Daniel F. Kelly Brain Tumor Center and Neuroscience Institute, John Wayne Cancer Institute at Saint John's Health Center, Santa Monica, CA, USA

Niklaus Krayenbühl Department of Neurosurgery, University Hospital of Zurich, Switzerland

Edward R. Laws Department of Neurosurgery, Brigham and Women's Hospital, Harvard Medical School, Boston, MA, USA

Andrew S. Little Centre for Minimally Invasive Neurosurgery, Prince of Wales Private Hospital, Randwick, New South Wales, Australia

Alice S. Magri Maxillofacial Surgery Section, Head and Neck Department, University Hospital of Parma, Italy

Dennis R. Malkasian Department of Neurosurgery, David Geffen School of Medicine, University of California at Los Angeles, CA, USA

Luciano Mastronardi Department of Neurosurgery, Sant'Andrea Hospital, "Sapienza" University of Rome, Italy

Pietro Mortini Department of Neurosurgery, University Vita e Salute, San Raffaele Hospital, Milan, Italy

Carlos Navarro-Vila Complutense University and Department of Oral and Maxillofacial Surgery, Gregorio Marañon University Hospital, Madrid, Spain

Angelo Pichierri Department of Neurological Sciences, Neurosurgery, "Sapienza" University of Rome, Italy

Pasquale Piombino Department of Maxillofacial Surgery, School of Medicine and Surgery, Università degli Studi di Napoli Federico II, Naples, Italy

Tito Poli Maxillofacial Surgery Section, Head and Neck Department, University Hospital of Parma, Italy

Alberto Prats Galino Department of Human Anatomy and Embryology, Faculty of Medicine, Universitat de Barcelona, Spain

Daniel M. Prevedello Department of Neurological Surgery, University of Pittsburgh School of Medicine, Pittsburgh, PA, USA

Alessandro Ricci Department of Neurosurgery, San Salvatore City Hospital, L'Aquila, Italy

Madjid Samii International Neuroscience Institute, Hannover, Germany

Volker Seifert Department of Neurosurgery, Johann Wolfgang Goethe University, Frankfurt am Main, Germany

Enrico Sesenna Maxillofacial Surgery Section, Head and Neck Department, University Hospital of Parma, Italy

Carl H. Snyderman Department of Neurological Surgery and Department of Otolaryngology, University of Pittsburgh School of Medicine, Pittsburgh, PA, USA

Domenico Solari Department of Neurosurgery, Università degli Studi di Napoli Federico II, Naples, Italy

Vita Stagno Department of Neurosurgery, Università degli Studi di Napoli Federico II, Naples, Italy

Philip E. Stieg Department of Neurological Surgery, Weill Medical College of Cornell University, and New York-Presbyterian Hospital, New York, NY, USA

Ulrich Sure Klinik für Neurochirurgie, Universitätsklinikum Essen, Germany

Oguzkan Sürücü Department of Neurosurgery, University Hospital of Zurich, Switzerland

Charles Teo Centre for Minimally Invasive Neurosurgery, Prince of Wales Private Hospital, Randwick, New South Wales, Australia

Francesco Tomasello Department of Neurosurgery, University of Messina, Italy

Manfred Tschabitscher Institute of Anatomy and Cell Biology, Medical University of Vienna, Austria

Valentino Valentini Division of Maxillofacial Surgery, "Sapienza" University of Rome, Italy

Introduction
Evolution of Techniques to Approach the Base of the Skull

Francesco Tomasello

History: The Past

The skull base is not only the dividing wall between the intracranial content and the facial compartment with the upper respiratory and digestive tracts, but it also allows the passage of vital neurovascular structures entering and exiting the brain. For this reason skull-base surgery is one of the most challenging areas of surgery.

Since the first successful attempts to remove a skull-base tumor at the end of the eighteenth century, surgeons coming from different disciplines have compared their skills in this area. Skull-base surgery was the first successful brain surgery procedure. Francesco Durante, a general surgeon born in Letojanni, Sicily, but working in Rome, removed an anterior cranial fossa meningioma using an original transpalatine approach. The patient was still alive and in good health 12 years after surgery [1]. It should be underlined that this pioneer of neurosurgery used a transoral, transpalatine approach presaging the multidisciplinary approach needed in modern skull-base surgery to fully manage complex skull-base lesions.

Another pioneer of surgery worthy of mention is Sir William Macewen who successfully removed a brain tumor over the right eye in a 14-year-old boy using general anesthesia with endotracheal intubation instead of tracheostomy [2]. In the last century, advances in skull-base surgery paralleled those of neurosurgery, and ENT, maxillofacial and plastic surgery. In 1907 Schloffer was the first to report successful removal of a pituitary tumor via a transnasal, transsphenoidal approach. His approach used a transfacial route with significant esthetic problems due to paranasal scarring [2]. Three years later Hirsch, an otorhinolayngologist, first described the endonasal transseptal approach to reach the sellar content with local anesthesia [3]. Subsequently Cushing modified this approach with a sublabial incision using general anesthesia. His results in 231 patients, operated upon between 1910 and 1925, showed a 5.6% mortality rate; however, he later abandoned this technique in favor of a transcranial route due to the high risk of CSF rhinorrhea, difficult in controlling hemorrhage and postoperative cerebral edema [2]. Dott, learning the transsphenoidal approach directly from Cushing, reported in 1956 no deaths in 80 consecutive patients.

The next milestones in the evolution of transnasal-transsphenoidal technique were reached with the routine use of two different technical adjuncts. Guiot, introducing the intraoperative radiofluoroscope, extended the approach to craniopharyngiomas, chordomas and parasellar lesions and, finally, Hardy from Montreal, Canada, proposed and diffused the use of the surgical microscope and dedicated instrumentation [4]. Thus, the evolution of the transphenoidal approach to the pituitary gland and its worldwide application involved three basic factors: first and most important, the pioneering efforts of giants of surgery working on their intuition and often against colleagues' skepticism; second, the progress of technology; and third, its application to routine procedures. This is the paradigm of the skull-base surgery. In the 1960s, House, an ENT surgeon, and Doyle, a neurosurgeon, began to remove acoustic neuromas through a middle fossa approach. This was one of the first skull-base teams to introduce the concept of a multidisciplinary approach [5].

F. Tomasello (✉)
Dept of Neurosurgery
University of Messina, Italy

P. Cappabianca et al. (eds.), *Cranial, Craniofacial and Skull Base Surgery.*
© Springer-Verlag Italia 2010

The history of skull-base surgery with its basic principles has to include a tribute to Gazi Yasargil. He popularized the pterional approach and demonstrated that with removal of the sphenoid wing and meticulous microneurosurgical technique many areas of the skull base could be reached without or with minimal brain retraction. Yasargil's lesson was applied to many approaches, and even today it represents the undisputed basic concept for any neurosurgeon dealing with skull-base lesions [6, 7]. The concept of "move the bone away and leave the brain alone" is the basis of modern skull-base surgery.

As in many fields of medicine, the widespread diffusion of knowledge, techniques and technologies drives surgeons through over-indication. It should not be considered as an absolute mistake, but as an unavoidable step in the continuous progress of science. This was the case in cavernous sinus surgery. In the 1980s and 1990s many neurosurgeons demonstrated the surgical anatomy of the cavernous sinus and many approaches to reach lesions within it. It seemed that the cavernous sinus, formerly considered a "no-man's land", became as accessible as any other part of the skull base and each lesion growing into or extending to it could be completely resected without significant morbidity [8–10]. However, during the last decade, the long-term evaluation of surgical results and the development of alternative techniques to manage lesions in this area generally reduced the enthusiasm of the proponents of the approach, limiting indications to the routine opening and exploration of the cavernous sinus [11, 12] (Fig. 1).

Chronicles: The Present

As with any innovation in the field of medicine, strategies for resection in skull-base surgery are first greeted with skepticism, then they diffuse with an enthusiastic underestimation of morbidity and mortality, to reach maturity with a better application to each specific case. It is hard to say if we are in the mature phase of skull-base surgery. Recent studies have demonstrated the

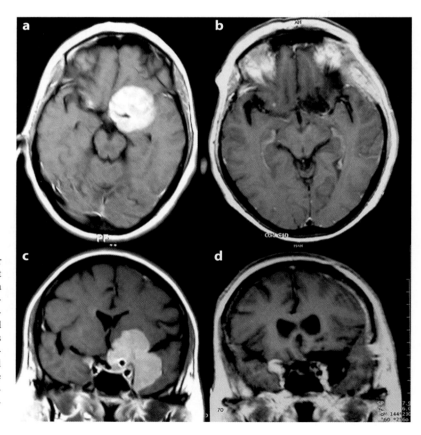

Fig. 1 T1-weighted MR imaging after contrast agent administration of a giant left sphenocavernous meningioma with a small contralateral clinoidal meningioma. **a, c** Preoperative axial and coronal images. **b, d** Postoperative axial and coronal images. The meningioma was completely resected except for the intracavernous portion via a left pterional craniotomy. Residual tumor within the cavernous sinus and the contralateral clinoidal meningioma did not show progression at the 3-year follow-up

prominent role of standard neurosurgical approaches, as the pterional or retrosigmoid, in the management of most skull-base lesions minimizing the need for a transfacial and transpetrosal route [7, 12, 13].

For many years neurosurgeons and neurotologists have discussed the best way to approach and resect acoustic neuromas. The introduction and widespread diffusion of MRI has allowed the diagnosis of small intracanalicular tumors, shifting the paradigm of management from simple tumor resection to facial nerve sparing and, finally, hearing preservation. Moreover, surgery is not the only treatment modality available to patients. Long-term results of radiosurgical series as primary treatment in these patients are now available: tumor control and preservation of the function of the cranial nerves are considered today at least comparable [14]. The discussion is still open, and no-one has the definitive answer. Modern radiosurgical techniques continue to gain a prominent role as primary treatment in many skull-base lesions and the apparently short-term morbidity should be measured in relation to long-term outcome, and both should be measured in terms of tumor control and new neurological deficits.

As outcome measures have increasingly become more sophisticated, surgeons analyzing their series cannot state that a patient had a good outcome just because no new neurological deficits occurred. Measures of quality of life as perceived by the patient and his relatives should be considered as the gold standard parameter to evaluate a treatment modality.

Neuronavigation is now a standard tool in a modern neurosurgical operating room. Its routine use in skull-base surgery can optimize the intraoperative time and make the surgeon confident in the identification of major skull-base vessels during bone dissection. How it modifies the outcome is matter of controversy. Technological advances have almost always anticipated major improvements in skull-base surgery. This was the case for endoscopy and its introduction into skull-base surgery. Neurosurgeons capitalized on the ENT sur-

geons' experience in endoscopic surgery of the paranasal sinuses [15]. Jho, Cappabianca, de Divitiis and Kassam were pioneers in this field [2, 16]. Jho and Carrau (the latter an ENT surgeon) reported the first surgical series of 50 patients harboring a sellar lesion operated on via an endoscopic endonasal approach [17]. In the last 10 years under the guidance of Naples and Pittsburgh centers, hundreds of endoscopic procedures in the sellar region have been performed all over the world. The use of a pure or assisted endoscopic technique to approach the sellar region is probably the most important conquest in contemporary skull-base surgery.

Vision of the Next Step: The Future

Recently the Naples and Pittsburgh groups have developed an extended endoscopic approach to anterior cranial fossa lesions such as tuberculum sellae and olfactory groove meningiomas. Criticism and limitations of the standard surgical technique obviously appeared greater in relation to the extended approach, in which untoward hemorrhage and CSF leakage are difficult to control [18–30]. If the endoscopic endonasal approach to the pituitary has to be considered a standard approach, its extension has to be validated in larger series.

Research and efforts should be directed toward the improvement of waterproof closure of the basal dura and the development of new instrumentation for dissection, better visualization, control of neurovascular structures and hemostasis. The use of intraoperative imaging and sonography, the development of a new dural substitute and sealants may improve the use of the endoscopic approach and make it accepted worldwide as the new frontier in skull-base surgery. Diffusion and acceptance of new outcome quality-of-life patient-oriented scales should better define the concept of minimally invasive surgery and its ability to obtain long-term tumor control.

References

1. Tomasello F, Germano A (2006) Francesco Durante: the history of intracranial meningiomas and beyond. Neurosurgery 59:389–396; discussion 389–396
2. Maroon JC (2005) Skull base surgery: past, present, and future trends. Neurosurg Focus 19:E1
3. Hirsch O (1910) Endonasal method of removal of hypophyseal tumors. With a report of two successful cases. JAMA 55:772–774
4. Hardy J (1967) Surgery of the pituitary gland, using the open trans-sphenoidal approach. Comparative study of 2 technical methods (in French). Ann Chir 21:1011–1022
5. House WF (1961) Surgical exposure of the internal auditory canal and its contents through the middle, cranial fossa. Laryngoscope 71:1363–1385
6. Yasargil MG (1999) A legacy of microneurosurgery: memoirs, lessons, and axioms. Neurosurgery 45:1025–1092
7. d'Avella D, Salpietro FM, Alafaci C, Tomasello F (1999) Giant olfactory meningiomas: the pterional approach and

its relevance for minimizing surgical morbidity. Skull Base Surg 9:23–31

8. Al-Mefty O, Smith RR (1988) Surgery of tumors invading the cavernous sinus. Surg Neurol 30:370–381

9. Dolenc V (1983) Direct microsurgical repair of intracavernous vascular lesions. J Neurosurg 58:824–831

10. Sekhar LN, Burgess J, Akin O (1987) Anatomical study of the cavernous sinus emphasizing operative approaches and related vascular and neural reconstruction. Neurosurgery 21:806–816

11. Abdel-Aziz KM, Froelich SC, Dagnew E et al (2004) Large sphenoid wing meningiomas involving the cavernous sinus: conservative surgical strategies for better functional outcomes. Neurosurgery 54:1375–1383; discussion 1383–1374

12. Tomasello F, de Divitiis O, Angileri FF et al (2003) Large sphenocavernous meningiomas: is there still a role for the intradural approach via the pterional-transsylvian route? Acta Neurochir (Wien) 145:273–282; discussion 282

13. Chang SW, Wu A, Gore P et al (2009) Quantitative comparison of Kawase's approach versus the retrosigmoid approach: implications for tumors involving both middle and posterior fossae. Neurosurgery 64:44–51; discussion 51–42

14. Tamura M, Carron R, Yomo S et al (2009) Hearing preservation after gamma knife radiosurgery for vestibular schwannomas presenting with high-level hearing. Neurosurgery 64:289–296; discussion 296

15. Stammberger H (1986) Endoscopic endonasal surgery – concepts in treatment of recurring rhinosinusitis. Part I. Anatomic and pathophysiologic considerations. Otolaryngol Head Neck Surg 94:143–147

16. Cappabianca P, Alfieri A, de Divitiis E (1998) Endoscopic endonasal transsphenoidal approach to the sella: towards functional endoscopic pituitary surgery (FEPS). Minim Invasive Neurosurg 41:66–73

17. Jho HD, Carrau RL (1997) Endoscopic endonasal transsphenoidal surgery: experience with 50 patients. J Neurosurg 87:44–51

18. Cappabianca P, Buonamassa S, Cavallo LM et al (2004) Neuroendoscopy: present and future applications. Clin Neurosurg 51:186–190

19. Cappabianca P, Cavallo LM, Esposito F et al (2008) Extended endoscopic endonasal approach to the midline skull base: the evolving role of transsphenoidal surgery. Adv Tech Stand Neurosurg 33:151–199

20. Cappabianca P, Decq P, Schroeder HW (2007) Future of endoscopy in neurosurgery. Surg Neurol 67:496–498

21. Cappabianca P, Kelly DF, Laws ER Jr (2008) Endoscopic transnasal versus open transcranial cranial base surgery: the need for a serene assessment. Neurosurgery 63:240–241; discussion 241–243

22. Cavallo LM, de Divitiis O, Aydin S et al (2008) Extended endoscopic endonasal transsphenoidal approach to the suprasellar area: anatomic considerations – part 1. Neurosurgery 62:1202–1212

23. de Divitiis E, Cavallo LM, Cappabianca P, Esposito F (2007) Extended endoscopic endonasal transsphenoidal approach for the removal of suprasellar tumors: Part 2. Neurosurgery 60:46–58; discussion 58–49

24. de Divitiis E, Cavallo LM, Esposito F et al (2008) Extended endoscopic transsphenoidal approach for tuberculum sellae meningiomas. Neurosurgery 62:1192–1201

25. de Divitiis E, Esposito F, Cappabianca P et al (2008) Tuberculum sellae meningiomas: high route or low route? A series of 51 consecutive cases. Neurosurgery 62:556–563; discussion 556–563

26. de Divitiis E, Esposito F, Cappabianca P et al (2008) Endoscopic transnasal resection of anterior cranial fossa meningiomas. Neurosurg Focus 25:E8

27. Fernandez-Miranda JC, Gardner PA, Prevedello DM, Kassam AB (2009) Expanded endonasal approach for olfactory groove meningioma. Acta Neurochir (Wien) 151:287–288; author reply 289–290

28. Gardner PA, Kassam AB, Thomas A et al (2008) Endoscopic endonasal resection of anterior cranial base meningiomas. Neurosurgery 63:36–52; discussion 52–34

29. Kanaan HA, Gardner PA, Yeaney G et al (2008) Expanded endoscopic endonasal resection of an olfactory schwannoma. J Neurosurg Pediatr 2:261–265

30. Kassam AB, Thomas A, Carrau RL et al (2008) Endoscopic reconstruction of the cranial base using a pedicled nasoseptal flap. Neurosurgery 63:ONS44–52; discussion ONS52–43

Instruments

1

Paolo Cappabianca, Felice Esposito, Luigi M. Cavallo
and Olga V. Corriero

1.1 Introduction

Among the determinants of the success of a surgical technique are an in-depth knowledge of the surgical anatomy, the combining of the expertise of the different professionals, and the availability of dedicated instruments and tools, which permit advances to take place in terms of expanding the indications, improving the results and reducing the complications.

Advances in surgical instrumentation, in hemostatic techniques and materials, and in image guidance systems, and, most importantly, collaboration between neurosurgeons and otolaryngologists/head and neck surgeons/maxillofacial surgeons, together with the contribution of new imaging devices and techniques, have resulted in recent dramatic changes in the practice of skull-base surgery, ultimately resulting in a movement toward less-invasive procedures, as in most fields of modern medicine.

If on one hand such technological advances push the development of new surgical techniques, the opposite is also true: the introduction of a novel surgical approach or technique often requires the design and refinement of new dedicated instruments and tools, contributing to the mutual relationships between surgeons and biomedical engineers and manufacturers.

Surgery of the skull base is amongst the most difficult, complex and, at the same time, rewarding experiences. Skull-base surgery does not just require the acquisition of perfect surgical skill: surgeons also need to acquire a thorough knowledge of anatomy, mastery of the pros and cons of all the materials and instruments to be used during the operation, the ability to share his/her peculiarities with others, versatility in choosing among the different approaches (transcranial, transfacial, combined transcranial–transfacial, etc.), and knowledge of the pros and cons of each one of them, etc [1, 2] .

This chapter focuses on one of these aspects: the possibilities and limitations of the main instruments and tools used during most of the surgical approaches described in the following chapters throughout the book.

1.2 Types of Instrument

There are two types of instrument in skull-base surgery: instruments with a single shaft and a functional tip (for example, hooks, dissectors, curettes, knives, etc), and those that fall within what the instrument manufacturers call the "forceps family" (for example bipolar forceps, tumor-holding forceps, biopsy rongeurs, vascular forceps, and scissors). Some approaches, e.g. the transsphenoidal approaches, performed under certain conditions such as endoscopy, demand dedicated instruments [11].

There are very different principles involved in handling and using these two groups of instruments. It is possible to hold the single-shaft instruments anywhere along the shaft. Where the instrument is grasped depends on the working depth, i.e. the distance between the tip of the index finger and the tissue plane being dissected. Instruments of the forceps group are very different. They are made with a definite area to grasp the

P. Cappabianca (✉)
Dept of Neurological Science, Division of Neurosurgery
Università degli Studi di Napoli Federico II, Naples, Italy

P. Cappabianca et al. (eds.), *Cranial, Craniofacial and Skull Base Surgery*.
© Springer-Verlag Italia 2010

instrument and to control the opening and closing action of the tips.

The design of microsurgical instruments should incorporate stability, flexibility, and mobility. Their use in microsurgery can be compared to that of a pencil during writing. The forearm is supported on a specifically designed rest. The hand is then free and relaxed and is supported at the surface edge of the wound by the fourth and fifth fingers. The instrument is grasped and controlled using the index and middle fingers, together with the thumb. From the opening of the dura until it has been closed by suturing, the operation is performed under the operating microscope and/or the endoscope. During this time the surgeon mainly uses the bipolar forceps and suction tip.

1.3 Microscope

Microsurgical techniques, which require the use of the operating microscope, are a key part of skull-base surgery and the acquisition of skill and proficiency in the use of the mobile operating microscope is the first step in microsurgery [3, 4].

The operating microscope, which as well as magnifying improves illumination and provides stereoscopic and telescopic vision, is the key instrument in the microsurgical treatment of intracranial lesions. The magnification, which is variable between ×3 and ×25, is ultimately derived from the optical relationship between the objective lens, the side of the binocular tubes, and the magnification of the eyepieces. Besides magnification, the unique characteristic of the microscope compared with the other surgical visualizing tools, such as the endoscope, is its most useful function, stereoscopic 3D vision. This function, coupled with the zoom capabilities of the optical system, brings the plane of the operative field closer to the observer, maintains the optical capacity of depth perception, and allows the surgeon to work bimanually.

The degree of illumination depends upon the light source used, on the degree of magnification (the greater the magnification, the less the passage of light), and on whether a beam splitter for the attachment of observation tubes and camera equipment is employed.

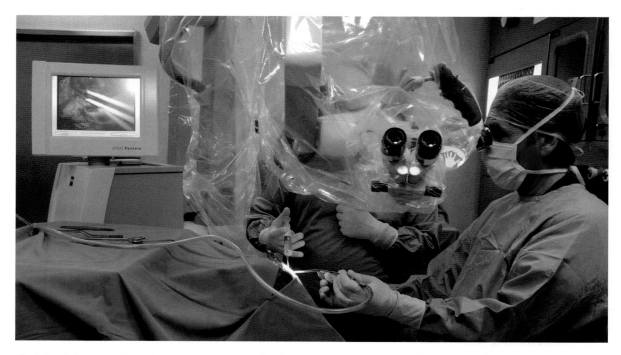

Fig. 1.1 Modern operating microscopes are no longer just instruments to provide a magnified image, but are rather fully integrated into the modern operating room and allow information to flow between all the other instruments, offering new horizons in improving the surgical workflow

The surgeon, acting through controls on the hand-pieces, can rotate, raise, translate, and lower the microscope optics and make fine adjustments to its position. The other face of the medal is that the use of the microscope entails an unavoidable restriction of movement, and also requires the surgeon to maintain a restricted postural position.

Latest generation microscopes (Fig. 1.1) represent a concentration of technology and advances. They are able to combine solutions for the basic requirements—illumination and magnification of the surgical field—with a variety of additional benefits including intraoperative fluorescence, integration with endoscopy and neuronavigation devices, integration of the entire digital video chain, integration into the hospital's information and communication infrastructure, and user-friendly solutions for the operating room staff.

1.4 Endoscope

The endoscope permits access to deep anatomic structures in a minimally invasive manner. It allows the visualization of deep, hidden structures in the brain and transmits clear and usable images to the surgeon. Its main characteristic and advantage is that it brings the eyes of the surgeon close to the relevant anatomy. In such a way it can increase the precision of the surgical action and permit the surgeon to differentiate tissues, so that selective removal of the lesion can be achieved [5-7]. Endoscopes are classified as either fiberoptic endoscopes (fiberscopes) or rod-lens endoscopes. Endoscopes specifically designed for neuroendoscopy can be classified into four types: (1) rigid fiberscopes, (2) rigid rod-lens endoscopes, (3) flexible endoscopes, and (4) steerable fiberscopes [5, 6, 8].

These different endoscopes have different diameters, lengths, optical quality, and number and diameter of working channels, all of which vary with size. The choice between them should be made on the basis of the surgical indication and personal preference of the surgeon. In general, for endoscopic skull-base surgery, the best endoscopes are rigid rod-lens scopes (Fig. 1.2). The main advantage is the better quality of vision than with the other type. It allows the surgeon to remain oriented because of the panoramic view and permits the other instruments to be inserted alongside it. Rod-lens endoscopes consist of three main parts: a mechanical shaft, glass fiber bundles for light illumination, and optics (objective, eyepiece, relay system). The angle of

view of the rod-lens ranges from 0° to 120°, according to the objective, but angled objectives of more than 30° are used only for diagnostic or visualizing purposes. The most frequently used angles are 0°, 30° and 45°. The 0° objective provides a frontal view of the surgical field and minimizes the risk of disorientation. It is used during the major part of the operation. The advantages of 30° is that this type of endoscope, through the rotation of the lens, increases the surface area of the field of view. Moreover, visualization of the instruments is improved as they converge toward the center of the image, while with the 0° objective the instruments remain in the periphery of the image.

The endoscope is usually used through a sheath, which is connected to a cleaning system. The irrigation system permits cleaning and defogging of the distal lens, thus avoiding the repeated insertion and removal of the endoscope from the nostril. Endoscopes used for endonasal skull-base surgery have no working channel (diagnostic endoscopes), and the other instruments are inserted either into the same nostril, slid alongside the sheath, or into the contralateral nostril. The diameter of rod-lens endoscopes varies between 1.9 and 10 mm, but for most surgical approaches to the skull base only endoscopes with a diameter of 4 mm are usually used. In some cases a 2.7-mm endoscope can be used. In skull-base surgery, such tools can be used freehand or fixed to a scope holder.

During the first step of the operation (the approach itself), it is better to use the endoscope freehand, so that the various instruments can be handled dynamically

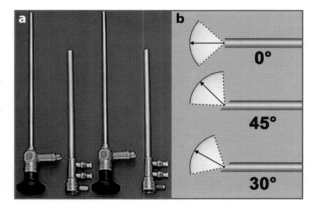

Fig. 1.2 Rigid rod-lens endoscopes **a**, without working channels, used in skull-base surgery. They allow the surgeon to remain oriented because of the panoramic view and allow other instruments to be inserted alongside. **b** The most frequently used objective angles are 0°, 30° and 45°

while creating the working space for the later steps in the procedure. In such a way, the surgeon can progressively gain a sense of depth by fixing in mind some surgical landmarks to guide orientation. A perfect knowledge of surgical anatomy does the rest. The endoscope can then either continue to be use free-hand or be fixed to a scope holder.

For the freehand technique, the scope is used in a dynamic fashion and the surgeon continuously receives feedback about the anatomy and depth of the operative field based on the in-and-out movements of the scope. If the option of a scope holder is chosen, a variety of systems exist. Variables include a steerable or extensible arm, and a rigid or jointed arm that can be straight, curved, or pneumatic. With such devices, the endoscope is fixed in a particular position, and the surgeon can use both hands to manipulate the surgical instrumentation. Another possibility is to have the endoscope held by an assistant. With this method the dynamic movements of the scope are preserved and, at the same time, the surgeon can simultaneously use two instruments either in the same nostril or in both nostrils.

1.4.1 Video Camera and Monitor

The endoscope is connected to a dedicated video camera, and the endoscopic images are projected onto a monitor placed in front of the surgeon [9]. Additional monitors can be placed in other locations in the operating room, as well as in hallways or adjacent rooms, to permit other members of the team to watch the surgery. Also such tools are being continuously improved to offer high-quality endoscopic images with tremendous visualization of the operative field, and of the lesion and its relationships with the surrounding anatomical structures.

Several types of endoscopic video camera are available, the most common of which utilize a CCD (charge-coupled device) sensor. Buttons located on the camera control the focus and the zoom. Optical zoom is preferable because it enlarges the image with the same number of pixels; the electronic zoom increases the size of each pixel, which degrades the definition of the image.

The video signals are usually brought to the monitor and to the recording devices in RGB, S-video, or composite video formats. Today, digital 3-CCD endoscope cameras (with three CCD sensors) are available, which produce the highest quality images. These cameras can be directly connected to video recorders for high-quality video reproduction [10].

The images produced by the endoscope camera are displayed on one or more monitors. These monitors need to have a high-resolution screen to support the signal quality arising from the camera. The monitors most commonly used in endoscopic surgery have a minimum horizontal resolution of 750 lines, in order to visualize all the details of the endoscopic images.

A further improvement in the resolution of both the video cameras and the monitors is represented by high-definition (HD) technology (Fig. 1.3), which offers the ultimate image quality and is ready for the 3-D endoscopes of the future. A full HD 16:9 flat monitor (1080p60) needs to be coupled to the HD camera in order to visualize the HD images.

1.4.2 Light Source

The endoscope transmits the cold light that arises from a source (Fig. 1.4a) inside the surgical field through a connecting cable made of a bundle of glass fibers that brings the light to the endoscope, virtually without dispersion of visible light (Fig. 1.4b). Furthermore, heat is poorly transmitted by glass fibers, thus the risk of burning the tissues is reduced [7].

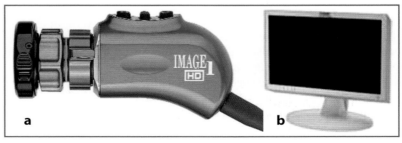

Fig. 1.3 High-definition (HD) cameras **a** offer the ultimate image quality. They require a full HD 16:9 flat monitor **b** in order to visualize the HD images

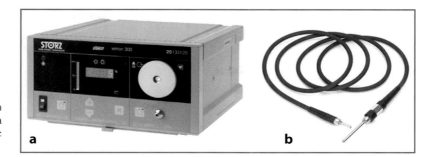

Fig. 1.4 Xenon-based light sources **a** bring cold light to the endoscope via a cable comprising a bundle of optic fibers **b**

1.4.3 Video Documentation

Several systems are available to document endoscopic surgical operations. Any one of a number of films or digital cameras, analog or digital VCRs, mass memory, CD- or DVD-based systems can store and even improve the images coming from the video camera. Such systems can be connected to dedicated devices and route the pictures and/or the videos for a complete digital exchange, for computer or video streaming or teleconferencing, for E-learning, or tele-counseling. Furthermore, it is possible for modern integrated operating rooms to share digital images and video by simply pressing a touch screen, which can even be done by the surgeon while operating.

1.5 Perforator and Craniotome

Craniotomy is one of the critical parts of the operation in that the surgeon is very much dependent on correct and reliable instrument function. Various perforators and craniotomes are available. Usually the different systems include a perforator (different size) craniotome, and a handpiece to attach round burrs, which are used to drill off bony structures such as the sphenoid wing, the prominence of the frontotemporal bone, the mastoid bone over the sigmoid sinuses, etc. Drilling with a burr might be performed under the operating mi-

croscope. The majority of craniotomies are made by first placing one burr hole, and then cutting the craniotomy with a craniotome. If the dura is not carefully dissected from the cranium before using the craniotome, there is a high risk that it will be torn. A selection of dissectors is necessary for adequate dural dissection. In particular, a flexible dural dissector is recommended, which is used after initially freeing the dura immediately around the burr hole with a rigid, conventional dissector. The flexible dissector is used to free the dura along the whole length of the proposed cutting line of the craniotomy.

1.6 High-Speed Microdrill

High-speed low-profile drills, either electric or pneumatic, may be very helpful for opening the bony structures to gain access to the dural space. A drill with forward and reverse rotation is preferred. The use of the drill should be planned so that the burr rotates away from critical structures. Only diamond burrs, and not cutting burrs, are used near important structures because only they can be used effectively in reverse. Drills for skull-base surgery should have some special characteristics. They should be low-profile and also long enough but not too bulky, so they can be easily used together with the possible combined use of the endoscope (Fig. 1.5). The combined use of such drills and

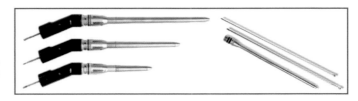

Fig. 1.5 Low-profile extra-long drills (Anspach Effort, Palm Beach Gardens, Florida, USA), easily used in combination with the endoscope

bone rongeurs has proven to be effective and time-saving during the extended approaches to the skull base, especially for access to restricted regions. It is important to find a good balance between the length of the tip and stability during fine drilling, as a too-long tip may vibrate dangerously. The high-speed drill is used to open the internal acoustic canal, optic canal, clivus and anterior and posterior clinoids, to remove the sphenoid wing, orbit indentation and petrous bone, and to open the foramen magnum.

A specifically designed endonasal transsphenoidal handpiece has recently been introduced for the ultrasonic bone curette (Sonopet, Miwatec, Tokyo, Japan), which is very low-profile and also quite safe since it works well and precisely in removing the bone structures but, at the same time, it respects the soft tissues, thus lowering the risk of injury to the neurovascular structures that may be close to the bone structure to be removed. For example, in endonasal skull-base surgery it has proven to be useful during the removal of the tuberculum sellae in cases of a prefixed chiasm, where it removes the tumor and leaves the soft tissues, such as the dura and, obviously, the chiasm beneath.

1.7 Bleeding Control

One of the most difficult problems is the control of bleeding.

Monopolar coagulation is easy because it can be simply performed with the use of monopolar sticks and it is usually quite effective. For hemostasis over larger areas, special ball-tipped attachments to the monopolar cable are very efficient. They are available in a variety of sizes with straight and curved shafts. Because of the heat produced when using this method, copious irrigation following each short phase of coagulation is recommended. Some monopolar electrodes incorporate a suction cannula to aspirate the smoke during coagulation, which maintains a clear surgical field. Monopolar coagulation must be avoided close to major neurovascular structures, in the intradural space or in proximity to nerve or vascular bony protuberances within the sphenoid sinus.

Bipolar forceps are the most adaptive and functional tool available to the neurosurgeon. They not only provide bipolar coagulation, but are also the main instrument of dissection. This feature makes them particularly suitable for opening arachnoid planes, separating membranes, grasping small amounts of tumor tissue from the normal brain parenchyma, and dissecting blood ves-

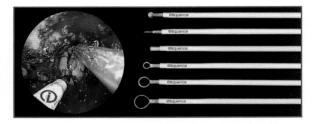

Fig. 1.6 Radiofrequency coagulating systems (Elliquence, Oceanside, NY, USA) have the advantage of minimal spatial heat dispersion, with a consequent minimal risk of heating injury to the neurovascular structures. They can also be used to debulk fibrous lesions

sels. The bipolar unit can be used to coagulate in areas where unipolar coagulation would be dangerous, for instance near neurovascular structures. In general, bipolar coagulation is preferable, either alone or in association with hemostatic agents. The use of the microsurgical bipolar forceps, developed for the microscope, is not feasible with the endoscope. Consequently, different endonasal bipolar forceps have been designed, with various diameters and lengths, that have proven to be quite effective in bipolar control of bleeding. New coagulating instruments, monopolar and bipolar, based on radiofrequency waves have also been proposed (Fig. 1.6). They have the advantage that the spatial heat dispersion is minimal, with a consequent minimal risk of heating injury to the neurovascular structures. Besides, the radiofrequency bipolar forceps do not need to be used with irrigation or to be cleaned every time.

1.8 Retraction Devices

Ideally, a brain retraction system should not compress the brain at all, but protect it. The injurious effects of retraction are directly related to the force of protective retraction and how long it is applied [12, 13]. Currently, the primary functions of retraction systems are to protect the brain, to provide gentle retraction during the initial stages of dissection, and to counteract gravity during the course of a tumor resection where the overlying cortex is tending to fall into the cavity. Today, most surgeons try to avoid the use of a retractor as much as possible and work with two instruments, mainly the suction tube which provides gentle traction after adequate room has been obtained by CSF outflow or tumor debulking.

1.9 MicroDoppler Probe

Prior to opening the dura mater and whenever the surgeon thinks it is appropriate (especially while working very close to vascular structures), it is of utmost importance to use the microDoppler probe to insonate the major arteries [14]. The use of such a device is recommended every time a sharp dissection is performed to minimize the risk of injury to either the carotid or the basilar artery or the other vascular structures that may be close to or even compressed by the lesion.

1.10 Neuronavigation System

Orientation is one of the most important factors in neurological surgery. Without proper orientation, the surgeon will waste time and sometimes do unnecessary harm to the brain. The rapid development of computer-assisted diagnostic imaging including CT, MRI , and angiography, has led to a great improvement in the diagnostic ability of neurosurgeons. These image data provide a neurosurgeon with accurate coordinates and size of a lesion and even a functional area mapping of individual cases. Some systems (image guided surgery systems or neuronavigators) correlate these data directly into the operating field.

The neuronavigator consists of a personal computer, a multijoint sensing arm and an image scanner. The three-dimensional coordinates of the arm tip are always monitored by the computer and are automatically translated into CT/MRI coordinates and finally displayed as a cursor on the CT/MRI images on the computer screen. The basic function of the navigator is to obtain the location of the arm tip within a surgical field and to translate it into CT/MRI coordinates. The patient's head should initially be related to the CT/MRI coordinates. The relationship is established using a set of fiducial points on the patient's head.

Intraoperatively, the location of the navigator tip is thereafter automatically converted into the CT/MRI coordinates and projected onto the corresponding CT/MRI slice on the computer screen represented by cross-shaped cursors. The system thus provides information on the location of the instruments in terms of the CT/MRI coordinates which guides the surgeon during the operation.

Neuronavigation systems also make it possible to avoid the use of fluoroscopy, thus avoiding unnecessary radiation exposure to the patient and the surgical team.

1.11 Intraoperative MRI

Despite many technical and instrumental advances, the extent of resection is often difficult to assess and is sometimes largely overestimated by the surgeon. This was demonstrated after introducing intraoperative MRI (iMRI) into the operating room. The implementation of iMRI in standard neurosurgical procedures has been widely appreciated due to the benefit of immediate tumor resection control. Besides the advantage of approaching a tumor without x-ray exposure of the patient and staff, the use of an iMRI integrated navigation system allows precise intraoperative tracking of residual tumor based on updated images acquired within minutes while surgery is paused. Thus remaining tumor can be removed by further navigation-guided resection. Intraoperative MRI systems differ with respect to scanner features (low field [15–18] or high field [19]) and their impact on the ergonomic workflow, which means either patient or scanner movement. Recently the first papers reporting the use of a 3-T iMRI [20, 21] have been published.

1.12 Tumor Enucleation

The best instrument for tumor enucleation is the suction apparatus. For slightly firmer tumors that are more resistant, the best technique is to grasp a portion of the tumor with ring-tipped forceps or a fork, or even a biopsy rongeur, and to apply gentle traction, while using dissectors in one hand to help free and finally lift away a portion of tumor. A selection of biopsy rongeurs in two different lengths (long and short) and with a variety of jaw sizes, is available. A large, rigid tumor can be excised with scissors, with the bipolar or monopolar loop attachment.

The loop for the monopolar electrode is available in a variety of sizes and permits rapid debulking of firm tumors. Furthermore, radiofrequency monopolar ball electrode technology (Elliquence, Oceanside, NY, USA), which uses radiofrequency power to vaporize the tumor thus obtaining an effect similar to that achieved with an ultrasonic aspirator system, is particularly useful for central debulking of a meningioma, particularly if it is of firm consistency, before starting the dissection of its capsule from the surrounding neurovascular structures (Fig. 1.6).

For the debulking of softly to moderately firm tumor, ultrasonic aspirator systems have proven to be helpful

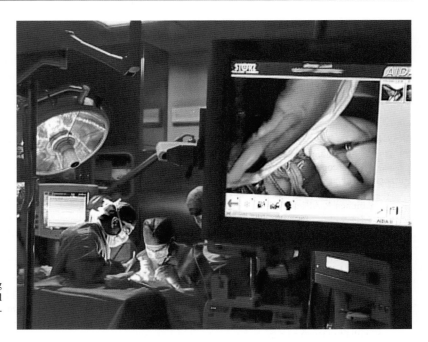

Fig. 1.7 Modern integrated operating room helps optimize teamwork and all the equipment is controlled via user-friendly interfaces

in open cranial surgery. The system relies on a titanium shaft that moves axially at ultrasonic speeds to emulsify tissue 1–2 mm from the tip. It supplies continuous irrigation and suction to aspirate the emulsified tissue.

1.13 Operating Room

The design of the operating room can itself be considered a surgical instrument. An integrated operating room helps to optimize teamwork and improve patient care [5, 22]. In the modern operating room, all the equipment is controlled via a user-friendly interface that provides a great sense of personal accomplishment among surgeons, anesthesiologists and nurses (Fig. 1.7).

The main characteristics of such a modern operating room are:

- Compartmentalization of sterile and nonsterile activities
- Fluidity of the workflow during the procedure
- Optimal access to the patient in case of emergency.

Thanks to communication technology the operating room may become a world surgical amphitheater: internet allows real-time, two-way transmission of digital encrypted data throughout the world.

During surgical procedures the archiving system is an efficient and cheap mechanism for storing and analyzing neurosurgical images. All patient data collected during surgery are transmitted and stored for future reference; they are easily accessible, confidential and protected from manipulation. These technological advances provide the best possible care to patients, ultimate ease and convenience to the surgical team, and excellent quality education and training to students, residents and visiting surgeons.

References

1. Cappabianca P (2006) Advice for a young neurosurgeon. Surg Neurol 65:35–37
2. Cappabianca P, Decq P, Schroeder HW (2007) Future of endoscopy in neurosurgery. Surg Neurol 67:496–498
3. Yasargil MG (1996) Instrumentation and equipment. In: Yasargil MG (ed) Microneurosurgery. Thieme, Stuttgart New York, pp 2–25
4. Yasargil MG (1996) Laboratory training. In: Yasargil MG (ed) Microneurosurgery. Thieme, Stuttgart New York, pp 26–27
5. Cappabianca P, Cavallo L, de Divitiis E (2008) Endoscopic pituitary and skull base surgery. Anatomy and surgery of the endoscopic endonasal approach. EndoPress, Tuttlingen
6. Cinalli G, Cappabianca P, de Falco R et al (2005) Current state and future development of intracranial neuroendoscopic surgery. Expert Rev Med Devices 2:351–373

7. Leonhard M, Cappabianca P, de Divitiis E (2003) The endoscope, endoscopic equipment and instrumentation. In: de Divitiis E, Cappabianca P (eds) Endoscopic endonasal transsphenoidal surgery. Springer, Vienna New York, pp 9–19

8. Cappabianca P, Cinalli G, Gangemi M et al (2008) Application of neuroendoscopy to intraventricular lesions. Neurosurgery 62 [Suppl 2]:575–597

9. Tasman AJ, Stammberger H (1998) Video-endoscope versus endoscope for paranasal sinus surgery: influence on stereoacuity. Am J Rhinol 12:389–392

10. Tasman AJ, Feldhusen F, Kolling GH, Hosemann W (1999) Video-endoscope versus endoscope for paranasal sinus surgery: influence on visual acuity and color discrimination. Am J Rhinol 13:7–10

11. Cappabianca P, Alfieri A, Thermes S et al (1999) Instruments for endoscopic endonasal transsphenoidal surgery. Neurosurgery 45:392–395; discussion 395–396

12. Wise BL (1994) A review of brain retraction and recommendations for minimizing intraoperative brain injury. Neurosurgery 35:172–173

13. Zhong J, Dujovny M, Perlin AR et al (2003) Brain retraction injury. Neurol Res 25:831–838

14. Dusick JR, Esposito F, Malkasian D, Kelly DF (2007) Avoidance of carotid artery injuries in transsphenoidal surgery with the Doppler probe and micro-hook blades. Neurosurgery 60:322–328; discussion 328–329

15. Black PM, Moriarty T, Alexander E 3rd et al (1997) Development and implementation of intraoperative magnetic resonance imaging and its neurosurgical applications. Neurosurgery 41:831–842; discussion 842–835

16. De Witte O, Makiese O, Wikler D et al (2005) Transsphenoidal approach with low field MRI for pituitary adenoma (in French). Neurochirurgie 51:577–583

17. Hadani M, Spiegelman R, Feldman Z et al (2001) Novel, compact, intraoperative magnetic resonance imaging-guided system for conventional neurosurgical operating rooms. Neurosurgery 48:799–807; discussion 807–799

18. Steinmeier R, Fahlbusch R, Ganslandt O et al (1998) Intraoperative magnetic resonance imaging with the magnetom open scanner: concepts, neurosurgical indications, and procedures: a preliminary report. Neurosurgery 43:739–747; discussion 747–738

19. Fahlbusch R, Keller B, Ganslandt O et al (2005) Transsphenoidal surgery in acromegaly investigated by intraoperative high-field magnetic resonance imaging. Eur J Endocrinol 153:239–248

20. Hall WA, Galicich W, Bergman T, Truwit CL (2006) 3-Tesla intraoperative MR imaging for neurosurgery. J Neurooncol 77:297–303

21. Pamir MN, Peker S, Ozek MM, Dincer A (2006) Intraoperative MR imaging: preliminary results with 3 tesla MR system. Acta Neurochir Suppl 98:97–100

22. Cappabianca P, Cavallo LM, Esposito F et al (2008) Extended endoscopic endonasal approach to the midline skull base: the evolving role of transsphenoidal surgery. Adv Tech Stand Neurosurg 33:151–199

Subfrontal Approaches

2

Oreste de Divitiis, Domenico G. Iacopino, Domenico Solari, Vita Stagno and Giovanni Grasso

2.1 Historical Background

Among the different transcranial approaches routinely used for the management of anterior cranial base lesions, the subfrontal approach is one of the most common and versatile surgical procedures, with the unilateral or bilateral alternative, according to the lesion's extension and size.

The unilateral subfrontal approach was described for the first time by Lewis in 1910 and afterwards, in its extradural variations, by McArthur [1] in 1912 and Frazier [2] in 1913. Krause [3] introduced, in 1914, the frontal osteoplastic flap in this an approach, later widely adopted following the contribution of Cushing [4].

It was not yet the 1940s when Tonnis described the first bifrontal craniotomy, a median frontoorbital approach with division of the anterior sagittal sinus and falx, and preservation of frontal brain tissue. Finally, Wilson [5] introduced in the 1971 the concept of keyhole surgery describing MacCarty's point for exposure of both the frontal fossa dura and periorbita. This is performed 1 cm behind the frontozygomatic suture and along the frontosphenoid suture. The "keyhole" in the subfrontal unilateral and bilateral approaches permits a choice of the correct limited craniotomy as a key characteristic for entering a particular intracranial space and for working with minimum trauma. Since that time, all patients with various anterior skull-base lesions have been surgically treated by means of the keyhole philosophy.

Indications for a subfrontal approach include the following:
1. Aneurysms
2. Giant suprasellar macroadenomas
3. Olfactory groove meningiomas
4. Tuberculum sellae meningiomas
5. Tumors of the third ventricle
6. Hypothalamic and chiasmatic gliomas
7. Craniopharyngiomas
8. Cerebrospinal fluid (CSF) fistulas.

2.2 Subfrontal Unilateral Approach

2.2.1 Positioning and Skin Incision

The patient is placed in the supine position on the operating table with the head fixed in a three-pin Mayfield headholder. The degree of head rotation depends on the site and size of the lesion. Lateral rotation not always necessary because most surgeons find orientation easier if the head is straight rather then turned. The patient's neck is retroflected, resulting in an angle of approximately 20° between the plane of the anterior cranial base and the vertical plane of the axis. This position allows the frontal lobe to fall away from the anterior cranial floor and facilitates good venous drainage during surgery. Fine adjustments of the patient's position are accomplished by tilting the operating table.

After a precise definition of the frontal anatomic landmarks (e.g., the orbital rim, supraorbital foramen, temporal line and zygomatic arch), the line of the incision is marked on the skin. Thereafter the skin is prepared with Betadine solution. The surgeon should be

O. de Divitiis (✉)
Dept of Neurological Science, Division of Neurosurgery
Università degli Studi di Napoli Federico II, Naples, Italy

P. Cappabianca et al. (eds.), *Cranial, Craniofacial and Skull Base Surgery*.
© Springer-Verlag Italia 2010

careful to make the incision while holding the knife in an oblique position in relation to the surface of the skin so that cutting is parallel to the pilose follicles;

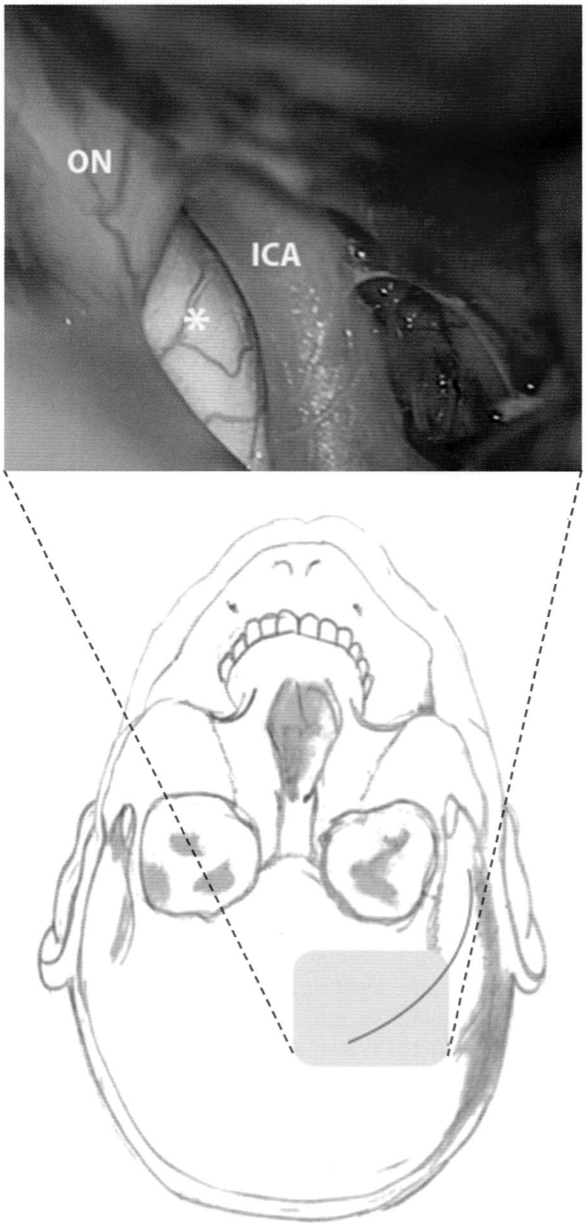

Fig. 2.1 Drawing showing the skin incision (*red line*), the craniotomy and the microsurgical intraoperative view of the subfrontal unilateral approach. This approach provides a wide intracranial exposure of the frontal lobe and easy access to the optic nerves, the chiasm, the carotid arteries and the anterior communicating complex

this avoids alopecia in the cicatrix and, consequently, a visible scar.

The skin incision, usually placed behind the hairline, begins less than 1 cm anteriorly to the tragus on the side of the craniotomy and extends medially in a curvilinear fashion above the superior temporal line, slightly crossing the midline by 1 or 2 cm (Fig. 2.1).

The incision should not be extended below the zygomatic arch to avoid injury to the branches of the facial nerve that could cross the surgical field. At this level usually the superficial temporal artery runs tortuously upward and forward to the forehead, supplying the muscles, integument and pericranium. Therefore, blunt vessel forceps are used to dissect the superficial temporal artery aiming to spare this vascularization. It is of the utmost importance to preserve the harvesting of the pericranium for the reconstruction phase.

Once the epidermis and dermis are incised and the subcutaneous tissue is encountered, a blunt vessel forceps are usual to dissect and preserve the superficial temporal artery. As the skin is reflected anteriorly along with the pericranium and retracted with temporary fishhooks, the galea will merge with the superficial layer of the temporalis fascia. At the supraorbital ridge, care should be taken to identify and preserve the supraorbital nerve and the supraorbital artery passing along the medial third of the superior orbital rim.

Upon retraction of the skin-aponeurosis flap, a semilunar incision is made through the pericranium under the frontozygomatic process, 0.5 cm superior to the temporal line and diagonally along the frontal lobe. At this point the pericranium is separated from the inferior surface of the frontozygomatic process and reflected.

Exposure and mobilization of the temporal muscle should be restricted to a minimum to prevent postoperative problems with chewing. Careful dissection and minimal retraction of the orbicular and frontal muscular layer are essential to avoid a postoperative periorbital hematoma. Before starting the craniotomy local hemostasis must be performed.

2.2.2 Craniotomy

The craniotomy is started using a high-speed drill, with the placement of a single frontobasal burr hole at MacCarty's point, posterior to the temporal line, just above the frontosphenoid suture or at the frontozygomatic point. This is the keyhole that represents an anatomic window that provides access to the anterior cranial base (Fig. 2.2a). A high-speed craniotome is then used to create the bone flap, which must extend anteriorly to the origin of the frontozygomatic process and parallel to the temporal line. The craniotome is directed from the first hole superiorly and describes a curve in the frontal area (Fig. 2.2b).

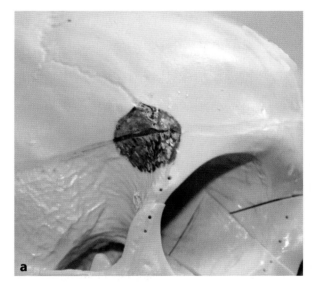

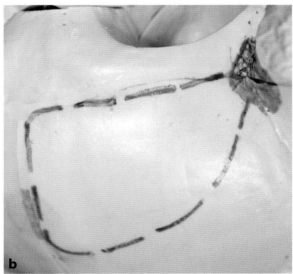

Fig. 2.2 Cranial model shows **a** the MacCarty's keyhole 1 cm behind the frontozygomatic suture and along the frontosphenoid suture, and **b** the unilateral subfrontal craniotomy extended anteriorly to the origin of the frontozygomatic process and parallel to the temporal line to create the bone flap

The limits are the supraorbital foramen medially and the sphenoid wing laterally. The lateral border of the frontal sinus has to be considered during craniotomy. Continuous irrigation during the drilling avoids thermal damage to the brain and allows more precise bone cutting. A hand-held retractors is used to provide the necessary soft-tissue retraction and exposure as the craniotome is turned around the flap. If dissection of the dura cannot be easily accomplished from a single burr hole, then a second burr hole can be made.

Usually the surgeon determines the numbers of burr holes to be made. Before removal of the bone flap, careful separation of the dura from the inner surface of the bone using a blunt dissector avoids laceration of the dura mater. An important next step is the drilling of the inner edge of the orbital roof protuberances with a high-speed drill (unroofing) to optimize the exposure to the anterior cranial fossa and the angle to reach the fronto-basal area.

2.2.3 Dural Incision and Intradural Dissection

Typically, the dura is opened in a C-shaped fashion, under the operating microscope, with its base toward the cranial base, parallel along the orbital floor. It is reflected anteriorly and anchored with stay sutures. A clearance of several millimeters should be allowed between the bone margin and the dural incision, to facilitate the final closure of the dura. When it is reflected, special attention should be paid in the proximity of the superior sagittal sinus. Elevation and retraction of the frontal lobe pole will subsequently expose the target area at the frontal base of the skull.

Different corridors can be used for the surgical maneuvers in tumor removal:
- The subchiasmatic corridor between the optic nerves and below the optic chiasm, suitable for lesions that enlarge the subchiasmatic area.
- The opticocarotid corridor between the optic nerve and carotid artery, chosen if the space between the carotid artery and the optic nerve is widened by parasellar extension of the tumor.
- Laterally to the carotid artery opening the oculomotor cistern, suitable for lesions with far lateral extension in the cavernous sinus.
- Translamina terminalis above the optic chiasm through the lamina terminalis [6], selected when the tumor extends into the third ventricle.

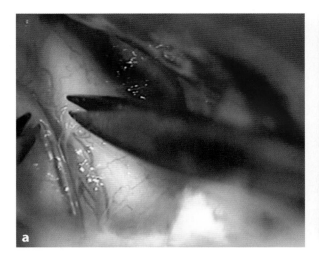
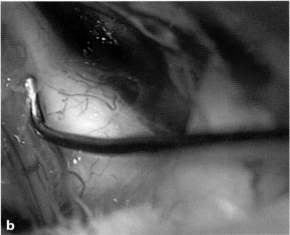

Fig. 2.3 Intraoperative microsurgical photograph showing dissection of the arachnoidal plane along the optic nerve performed with sharp (**a**) and blunt (**b**) dissection technique

After the dural opening the first important step to attempt some brain relaxation is the opening of the chiasmatic and carotid cisterns.

After releasing the CSF, the frontal lobe is retracted gently so that the basal cisterns can be opened carefully until the optic nerves, the chiasm, the A1 segment, and the anterior communicating artery are exposed and the olfactory nerve is identified and preserved. The arachnoid is slightly incised with an arachnoidal hook, or as an alternative, bipolar forceps could be used to make a hole in the arachnoid membrane [7]. It is important to follow the arachnoid plane using the microforceps and the suction tip to achieve a stepwise dissection until the lesion is reached (Fig. 2.3). During these surgical maneuvers, when a certain degree of brain retraction is needed, a self-retaining brain retractor attached to a flexible arm permits fine adjustment, preserving the normal tissue. Hemostasis must be accurately controlled during the intracranial procedure, and the intradural space should be filled with Ringer's solution at body temperature.

Sometimes the unilateral subfrontal approach could be used for some asymmetric midline lesions with the possibility of cutting the falx above the crista galli and saving the superior sagittal sinus to gain access also to the contralateral side (Fig. 2.4). In case of lesions such as meningiomas that involve the optic canal, a wider access could be gained by removal of the anterior clinoid that could be achieved via an extradural or intradural route. Furthermore, better visualization of the

optic nerve is achieved at this level by cutting the dural sheath longitudinally at its entrance in the canal.

After the lesion has been managed, the dural incision is sutured water-tight using continuous sutures. The bone flap is appositioned medially and frontally without bony distance to achieve the optimal cosmetic outcome and fixed with low-profile titanium plates and screws. After final verification of hemostasis, the galea

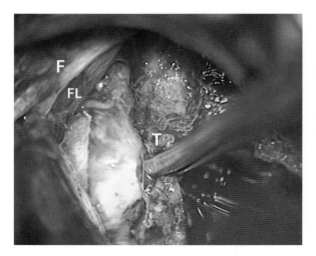

Fig. 2.4 Intraoperative microsurgical photograph showing contralateral extension of the tumor (*T*) dissected via a unilateral subfrontal approach. Note on the left side the falx cerebri (*F*) and the mesial surface of the left frontal lobe (*FL*)

with the subcutaneous layers are reapproximated with several interrupted absorbable sutures and the skin is closed with a Donati suture. At the end of the procedure the Mayfield pin headrest is removed and general anesthesia is reversed.

2.3 Subfrontal Bilateral Approach

2.3.1 Positioning and Skin Incision

The patient is carefully placed in a supine position, with the knees slightly flexed and the head with no lateral rotation, extended and fixed in a three-point Mayfield-Kees skeletal fixation headrest. This position allows the frontal lobe to fall away from the anterior cranial floor and facilitates venous drainage. Fine readjustments of the patient's position during surgery are accomplished by tilting the operating table by Trendelenburg or reverse Trendelenburg maneuvers. After a precise definition of the frontal anatomic landmarks (e.g., the orbital rim, supraorbital foramen, temporal line and zygomatic arch), the line of the incision is marked on the skin. Thereafter the skin is prepared with Betadine solution and the patient is draped in the usual sterile fashion.

A bicoronal skin incision, posterior to the frontal hair line, is performed, 13–15 cm from the orbital rim and 2 cm behind the coronal suture. It starts 0.5–1 cm anterior to the tragus of the ear and extends in a curvilinear fashion up to the opposite side (Fig. 2.5).

Care is taken not to go below the line of the zygomatic arch or too anterior to the tragus to avoid frontotemporal branches of the facial nerve and the superficial temporal artery. The flap is elevated in a single skin-aponeurosis layer and Raney's clips are applied to the full thickness of the scalp, including plastic drape in the jaws. Subsequently, it is retracted with temporary fishhooks, taking care to preserve the supraorbital nerve as it comes out from the supraorbital foramen. Careful dissection and minimal retraction of the orbicular and frontal muscular layer are essential to avoid a postoperative periorbital hematoma. Then the pericranium is taken up separately from the scalp flap. It can be incised behind the posterior edge of the incision and elevated off, between the temporal crest bilaterally, to the supraorbital margins, as far as the nasofrontal suture anteriorly (Fig. 2.6).

Because the frontal sinus is entered during a bilateral frontal craniotomy, at the end of the procedure the pericranium flap is useful during closure. Generally, the

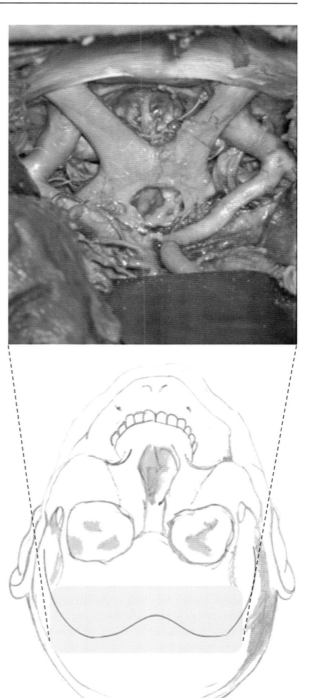

Fig. 2.5 Drawing showing the skin incision (*red line*), the craniotomy and the microsurgical anatomic view of the subfrontal bilateral route. This approach provides a wide symmetrical anterior cranial fossa exposure and easy access to the optic nerves, the chiasm, the carotid arteries and the anterior communicating arteries complex

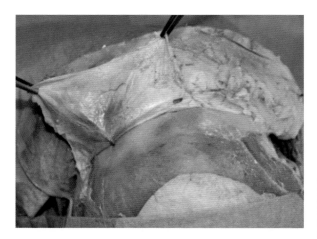

Fig. 2.6 Anatomical photograph showing the supraorbital nerve as it comes out from the supraorbital foramen, after the pericranium is taken up separately from the scalp flap and elevated off, between the temporal crest bilaterally, to the supraorbital margins anteriorly

temporalis muscle does not require elevation, although a small amount of dissection along the superior temporal line may be required sometimes to expose the keyhole for burr-hole placement. Exposure and mobilization of the temporal muscle should be restricted to a minimum to prevent postoperative problems with chewing.

2.3.2 Craniotomy

As general rule, two burr holes are placed at the Mac-Carty's keyhole bilaterally. These are positioned in the anterosuperior margin of the right temporalis muscle, immediately below the superior orbital ridge for cosmetic purposes. A third burr hole is placed near the longitudinal sinus, 4 cm beyond the nasofrontal suture, so that the dura at this level can be dissected from the bone more safely, thus avoiding sinus injuries (Fig. 2.7a).

The bone flap is realized with the craniotome, extending anteriorly as close as possible to the supraorbital ridge and posteriorly along the convexity of the frontal bone. The basal line of the craniotomy involves both tables of the frontal sinuses. The bone flap is detached from the subjacent dura with blunt elevators, with special caution over the sagittal sinus (Fig. 2.7b).

Once the frontal sinus has been entered, the mucosa should be stripped off before the dural opening (frontal sinus *cranialization*) and packed with antibiotic-soaked

absorbable gelatin sponge (Gelfoam). A flap of pericranial tissue from the back of the skin flap is turned down over the sinus and sewn to the adjacent dura. In some cases, as additional filling materials in this procedure, the galea capitis, the temporalis fascia, the tensor fascia lata muscle, or a synthetic or heterologous dural substitute could be used.

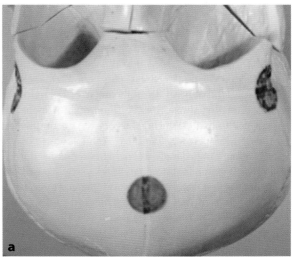

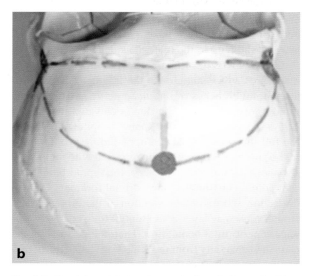

Fig. 2.7 Cranial model showing: **a** the burr holes at the Mac-Carty's keyhole bilaterally, while the third burr hole is near the longitudinal sinus, 4 cm beyond the nasofrontal suture, so that the dura at this level can be dissected from the inner bone more safely, thus avoiding sinus injury; **b** the bilateral subfrontal craniotomy extended anteriorly as close as possible to the supraorbital ridge and posteriorly along the convexity of the frontal bone

2.3.3 Dural Incision and Intradural Dissection

From this point the procedure is continued with the aid of the operating microscope. The dural incision is made symmetrically over each medial inferior frontal lobe just above the anterior edge of the bone opening. This incision has to be started at the maximum distance of 3–4 cm away from the midline; it is carried medially to reach the edge of the sagittal sinus.

In the vicinity of the superior sagittal sinus problems may be due to injury to the sinus bridging veins, or to its lacunar evaginations. When veins close to the sinus are exposed, whether to spare them should be considered with great care. Indeed, in such a manner damage to the bridging veins of the anterior frontal lobe can be avoided, so that these structures could be safely dissected aiming to prevent cerebral edema developing in the course of the operation. Nevertheless, if a bridging vein has to be sacrificed or is accidentally injured, bipolar coagulation is performed at a sufficient distance from the sinus (4–8 mm); the bleeding can also be managed with gentle compression from a hemostatic gauze, especially if it occurs directly at the sinus.

Generally, retraction on the mesial surface of the brain is needed for visualization of the falx cerebri below the sinus. This enable the passing of two sutures through the falx to the contralateral side under the sinus in order to tie them over it. Between these two ligatures, the sinus and the falx cerebri are cut down to its inferior border as anteriorly as possible to open up the operative field. As a rule, the inferior longitudinal sinus produces little or no bleeding, so that bipolar coagulation is sufficient. Complete transection of the falx provides the surgeon with an excellent and wide overview of the frontal base. Furthermore, for full utilization of the craniotomy, a relief incision with elevation sutures is placed in the corners.

Though, intradural maneuvers start with retraction of the frontal lobes in a lateral and slightly posterior direction with the aid of cottonoid sponges to protect the brain. At this point it is mandatory to proceed with sharp dissection of both olfactory tracts. The dissection should be performed in parallel alternating between the left and the right sides to reduce the risk of avulsion. During the approach to different lesions a certain degree of brain relaxation is needed and this is achieved by opening the sylvian fissure and the basal cisterns, and in the presence of high intracranial pressure, the lamina terminalis can be opened to release CSF from the third ventricle. After the release of CSF, the frontal lobe can be retracted more fully. The bifrontal craniotomy provides a good overview of the anterior skull base and gives access to the suprasellar and retrochiasmatic areas (Fig. 2.5). During the intradural procedure, the surgical field is filled with Ringer's solution at body temperature.

At the end of the procedure the dura mater and the skin are closed as in the unilateral subfrontal approach. The wide galea-periosteal flap obtained can be used for reconstruction of the anterior skull base to prevent CSF leakage. As a rule, bilateral subgaleal suction drains are positioned and left in place until third postoperative day.

2.4 Complications

The following complications may be encountered:
1. Epileptic seizures and neuropsychological deficit may occur if the cortex of the frontal lobes is damaged.
2. Anosmia may be caused by direct transection of the fila olfactoria during surgical manipulation or by ischemia if the feeding arteries from the ethmoidal arteries and supplying the olfactory nerves are damaged [8, 9].
3. Visual worsening due to surgical manipulation of the optic nerves.
4. Infections, CSF leakage, mucocele and pneumocephalus may occur if the dura mater and the frontal sinus are not properly closed [10].
5. Diabetes insipidus and hormone disturbance may occur if the pituitary stalk is damaged.
6. Hypothalamic dysfunction such as hyperphagia, hyperthermia, obesity and somnolence may occur if the vascular supply to the hypothalamus from small perforating arteries of the anterior communicating artery and from the superior hypophyseal arteries is damaged.
7. Periorbital swelling is commonly observed on postoperative days 2 to 3, but spontaneous resolution tends to occur over time.

2.5 Final Considerations

The classical unilateral or bilateral subfrontal approaches have their clear and definitive indications for the treatment of most of the lesions located in the anterior cranial fossa and in the supra- and parasellar area.

The extent and direction of tumor growth determines if the unilateral or the bilateral subfrontal approach should be used [11, 12].

In experienced hands this approach is a safe and reliable procedure giving excellent access to the main neurovascular structures of the anterior cranial base. Sometimes, particular anatomical conditions such as a prefixed chiasm or large tuberculum sellae can reduce the access to the sella turcica. Therefore the importance of an accurate preoperative neuroradiological assessment for optimum surgical planning is stressed.

The unilateral subfrontal approach can be used also for lesions with contralateral extension. The cutting of the falx above the crista galli and saving the superior sagittal sinus allows access to the contralateral side (Fig. 2.4).

Usually the approach is performed from the right side for the convenience of right-handed surgeons. The craniotomy should be very low and parallel to the orbital roof to avoid if possible opening of the frontal sinus, thus saving time in the reconstruction phase and reducing postoperative complications as infections, pneumocephalus, mucocele and CSF leakage. The dura mater should always be opened under microscopic magnification to better perform fine dissection so that the draining veins from the frontal lobe to the superior sagittal sinus are preserved, even if they must be stretched to achieve adequate exposure.

A self-retaining retractor, when used, should be gently placed on the frontal lobe surface in order to avoid olfactory filament avulsion from the cribriform plate [13]. To reduce the possibility of such an event, the olfactory cistern should be opened with sharp instruments in a proximal to distal direction in order to identify the bulb early. The surgeon should keep in mind that postoperative olfactory nerve dysfunction may not only be caused by disruption of the anatomical integrity of the nerves but also by direct compression with damage to the microvascular feeders coming from the ethmoidal arteries. Heavy and prolonged retraction should be avoided to reduce the risk of frontal lobe swelling. The degree of swelling is directly related to the force and duration of retraction.

We stress the importance of:
1. Head position: if the head is tilted back sufficiently, the brain tends to fall away from the roof of the orbit.
2. CSF drainage through a previously placed spinal lumbar needle and intraoperative early opening of the arachnoidal cisterns. Additional room can be provided by using osmotic diuretics and hyperventilation.

Once the ipsilateral optic nerve is visualized, the arachnoidal layer that bends the nerve to the frontal lobe is divided with sharp and blunt dissection to expose the contralateral optic nerve and backwards the chiasm. Often, exposure of the chiasm can be facilitated by opening the Sylvian fissure and the optocarotid cistern in order to separate the frontal and temporal lobes so that the frontal lobe can fall back farther.

At this point the tumor may be identified between the optic nerves, in either opticocarotid triangle, lateral to the carotid artery, and may extend around the pituitary stalk to the sella turcica and posteriorly in the third ventricle. The most frequent lesions in this area are meningiomas [14–17], suprasellar macroadenomas, craniopharyngiomas [18–20] and aneurysms [21].

In dealing with these lesions located in the anterior cranial fossa, the greatest risk to the patient comes from injury to the optic apparatus, the third nerve, the internal carotid arteries, the anterior communicating artery complex, the middle cerebral arteries, the basilar artery, the posterior communicating arteries and the choroidal arteries. These neurovascular structures could be embedded in or stretched by the tumor (Fig. 2.8). Optic nerves compressed or distorted by the mass should be never manipulated to avoid further visual loss. Moreover, the perforating arteries of the anterior circulation could be damaged because the surgeon fails to recognize them. None of the arteries should be coagulated until the surgeon is completely sure that they are arteries exclusively feeding the tumor.

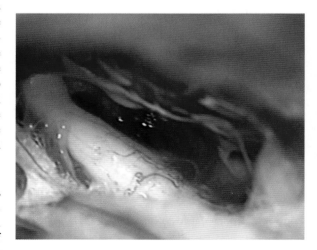

Fig. 2.8 Intraoperative microsurgical photograph showing both optic nerves diverging from the optic chiasm, with the left one stretched by a thin layer of arachnoid that still bends over it

Finally, both unilateral and bilateral subfrontal approaches, if from one side allow excellent visualization of the anterior cranial fossa with early control and management of the basal attachment of the lesion and of the proximal neurovascular structures, from the other side the surgeon has late visualization and control of the neurovascular structures dislocated at the posterior pole of the tumor.

References

1. McArthur LL (1912) An aseptic surgical access to the pituitary body and its neighborhood. JAMA 58:2009–2011
2. Frazier CH (1913) I. An approach to the hypophysis through the anterior cranial fossa. Ann Surg 57:145–150
3. Krause F (1914) Freilegung der Hypophyse. In: Krause F (ed) Chirurgie der Gehirnkrankheiten. Ferdinand Enke, Stuttgart, pp 465–470
4. Cushing H (1932) Intracranial tumors. Notes upon a series of two thousand verified cases with surgical-mortality percentages pertaining thereto. Charles C. Thomas, Springfield, MA
5. Wilson DH (1971) Limited exposure in cerebral surgery. Technical note. J Neurosurg 34:102–106
6. de Divitiis O, Angileri FF, d'Avella D et al (2002) Microsurgical anatomic features of the lamina terminalis. Neurosurgery 50:563–569; discussion 569–570
7. Yasargil MG (1996) Surgical approaches. In: Yasargil MG (ed) Microneurosurgery, vol IVB: microneurosurgery of CNS tumors. Georg Thieme, Stuttgart, pp 29–68
8. Bassiouni H, Asgari S, Stolke D (2007) Olfactory groove meningiomas: functional outcome in a series treated microsurgically. Acta Neurochir (Wien) 149:109–121; discussion 121
9. Sepehrnia A, Knopp U (1999) Preservation of the olfactory tract in bifrontal craniotomy for various lesions of the anterior cranial fossa. Neurosurgery 44:113–117
10. Nohra G, Jabbour P, Haddad A et al (2002) Subcranial subfrontal approach for the treatment of extensive cerebrospinal fluid leaks (in French). Neurochirurgie 48:87–91
11. Ardeshiri A, Wenger E, Holtmannspotter M, Winkler PA (2006) Surgery of the anterior part of the frontal lobe and of the central region: normative morphometric data based on magnetic resonance imaging. Neurosurg Rev 29:313–320; discussion 320–311
12. Erturk M, Kayalioglu G, Ozer MA (2003) Morphometry of the anterior third ventricle region as a guide for the subfrontal (translaminaterminalis) approach. Neurosurg Rev 26:249–252
13. Cardali S, Romano A, Angileri FF et al (2005) Microsurgical anatomic features of the olfactory nerve: relevance to olfaction preservation in the pterional approach. Neurosurgery 57:17–21; discussion 17–21
14. Chi JH, Parsa AT, Berger MS et al (2006) Extended bifrontal craniotomy for midline anterior fossa meningiomas: minimization of retraction-related edema and surgical outcomes. Neurosurgery 59:ONS426–433; discussion ONS433–424
15. Nakamura M, Roser F, Struck M et al (2006) Tuberculum sellae meningiomas: clinical outcome considering different surgical approaches. Neurosurgery 59:1019–1028; discussion 1028–1019
16. Nakamura M, Struck M, Roser F et al (2007) Olfactory groove meningiomas: clinical outcome and recurrence rates after tumor removal through the frontolateral and bifrontal approach. Neurosurgery 60:844–852; discussion 844–852
17. Spektor S, Valarezo J, Fliss DM et al (2005) Olfactory groove meningiomas from neurosurgical and ear, nose, and throat perspectives: approaches, techniques, and outcomes. Neurosurgery 57:268–280; discussion 268–280
18. Aryan HE, Ozgur BM, Jandial R, Levy ML (2005) Subfrontal transbasal approach and technique for resection of craniopharyngioma. Neurosurg Focus 18:E10
19. Maira G, Anile C, Colosimo C, Cabezas D (2000) Craniopharyngiomas of the third ventricle: trans-lamina terminalis approach. Neurosurgery 47:857–863; discussion 863–855
20. Shi XE, Wu B, Zhou ZQ et al (2006) Microsurgical treatment of craniopharyngiomas: report of 284 patients. Chin Med J (Engl) 119:1653–1663
21. Hernesniemi J, Ishii K, Niemela M et al (2005) Lateral supraorbital approach as an alternative to the classical pterional approach. Acta Neurochir Suppl 94:17–21

Supraorbital Eyebrow Approach

3

A Less Invasive Corridor To Lesions of the Anterior Cranial Fossa, Parasellar Region, and Ventral Brainstem

Andrew S. Little, Pankaj A. Gore, Aneela Darbar and Charles Teo

3.1 Introduction

The supraorbital eyebrow craniotomy is an anterolateral approach that allows the surgeon to address diverse pathology of the anterior cranial fossa, parasellar region, proximal sylvian fissure, ipsilateral circle of Willis, basal frontal lobe, and ventral brainstem. When supplemented with intracranial endoscopy, lesions of the lateral cavernous sinus, pituitary fossa, contralateral circle of Willis, and ipsilateral retroorbital space may be addressed. The goals of the approach are to treat neurosurgical lesions using a less-invasive technique, limit brain retraction and tissue trauma by exploiting anatomic corridors, offer comparable safety and efficacy relative to standard approaches, and yield a good cosmetic result.

Because of increased emphasis on smaller craniotomies tailored to specific pathology, the supraorbital craniotomy has evolved as a result of stepwise modifications to standard subfrontal and anterolateral approaches, which involve generous skin and bone flaps [1–10]. The supraorbital craniotomy is a "keyhole craniotomy" with important strengths and limitations [11]. This chapter reviews the surgical technique and provides case examples to illustrate how this approach may be correctly and incorrectly applied. The role of neuroendoscopy to expand operative indications is also discussed. The insights in this chapter represent practical advice from the senior author (C.T.), who has performed 170 procedures in children and adults.

3.2 Indications

Lesions appropriately approached by this keyhole craniotomy have been the subject of discussion in recent literature; the choice depends, in part, on surgeon preference and experience and, in part, on the anatomical constraints imposed by the exposure and the characteristics of the lesion (Table 3.1).

Aneurysms are the most commonly reported pathology [12–17]. In the largest aneurysm series to date, Reisch and Perneczky treated 229 (112 ruptured) lesions through this approach and reported a 2.2% rate of residua [12]. Their series included 21 patients with giant aneurysms and 50 patients with posterior circulation aneurysms. Intraoperative rupture occurred in four patients.

Brydon et al. recently reported their results in 50 patients with ruptured aneurysms. They applied the approach to anterior circulation lesions, with the exception of ophthalmic and middle cerebral artery lesions. They concluded that the approach offers the opportunity to repair ruptured aneurysms safely with minimal brain retraction [17]. Mitchell et al. described a series of 47 patients with unruptured anterior circulation aneurysms [14]. They did not treat patients with ruptured aneurysms or anterior projecting anterior communicating artery aneurysms.

Taken together, these reports indicate that clip ligation of selected anterior and posterior circulation aneurysms is feasible and achieves outcomes that are similar in experienced hands to the outcomes achieved using standard approaches; good occlusion rates are obtainable despite the smaller working area, and the surgeon is able to gain proximal and distal vessel control to secure intraoperative aneurysm rupture.

C. Teo (✉)
Centre for Minimally Invasive Neurosurgery, Prince of Wales Private Hospital, Randwick, New South Wales, Australia

Table 3.1 Selected case series utilizing the supraorbital approach.

Reference	Number of patients treated	Pathology addressed	Endoscope
[12]	450	Tumors (meningioma, craniopharyngioma, adenomas, brainstem), aneurysms	No
Teo et al., (unpublished)	170	Tumors (meningioma, craniopharyngioma, brainstem, third ventricle), trauma, aneurysms, orbital lesions	Yes
[13]	91	Anterior circulation aneurysms	No
[17]	50	Anterior circulation aneurysms	No
[14]	47	Anterior circulation aneurysms	No
[16]	37	Anterior circulation aneurysms	Yes
[19]	25	Tumors, trauma, tuberculoma, arteriovenous malformation	Yes
[20]	3	Frontal epidural abscess	No

Tumors of the parasellar region and anterior skull base can be safely addressed through the supraorbital approach. Our experience suggests that even large tumors intermingled with neurovascular structures can be removed. Furthermore, prominent vascularity is not a contraindication for the approach. The senior author has previously described his initial experience with neuroendoscopy and craniopharyngiomas, and has now treated 65 patients [18]. Total macroscopic excision was achieved in 60 (92%). These views are shared by Reisch and Perneczky who reported on 39 craniopharyngiomas and 23 pituitary adenomas [12]. They achieved gross total resection in 29 craniopharyngiomas (74%) and 19 adenomas (83%) with limited approach-related morbidity and excellent overall outcome. This corridor is also used for anterior skull-base meningiomas, including tumors of the orbital roof, tuberculum sella, and anterior clinoid process. Melamed et al. treated nine anterior skull-base meningiomas and noted satisfactory visualization, working space, and good resection rates with limited complications [19].

Other reported indications for the supraorbital approach include epidural abscess, orbital lesions, ventral midbrain tumors, and trauma. Noggle et al. reported three pediatric patients with frontal abscesses secondary to facial infections that were drained through this approach [20]. Caution should be used in treating dural or epidural lesions, such as abscesses, because the size of the craniotomy limits the area of dura that can be exposed. In these cases, the pathology was localized to beneath the flap and, therefore, appropriate. Orbital lesions that extend in proximity to the orbital roof may also be approached through the subfrontal corridor. The senior author has operated on 12 patients with intraorbital pathology such as meningiomas and hemangiomas. Neuroendoscopy and angled instruments are helpful to look over the orbital rim and achieve the caudally oriented operative trajectory.

In addition to orbital tumors, ventral midbrain lesions such as cavernomas and pilocytic astrocytomas are also accessible. This approach provides access to the cerebral peduncles by working through the window between basilar perforators. If resection of a brainstem lesion is planned, a contralateral trajectory often provides a better angle of attack [21]. The final class of pathology treated is anterior skull-base trauma. The supraorbital craniotomy has been used to repair skull-base fractures with associated spinal fluid leakage, address skull defects from penetrating injury, and remove bony fragments compressing the optic nerve [19].

3.3 Patient Selection

Appropriate patient selection is paramount when applying the supraorbital approach to intracranial pathology because it is a keyhole craniotomy with targeted access. In general, lesions of the anterior skull base, circle of Willis, parasellar region and cavernous sinus can be addressed, as is described above in the Introduction. However, there are several important caveats. Thoughtful planning, familiarity with alternative craniotomies, and careful evaluation of the benefits and disadvantages of the respective approaches will achieve the best result for the patient.

First, the size of the frontal sinus must be considered. When breached, the incidences of infection and CSF rhinorrhea are increased. Furthermore, a large frontal sinus displaces the craniotomy laterally altering the operative trajectory and limits the size of the bony opening. If the sinus is entered, Brydon et al. have shown that repair using bone putty may be successful [17].

The second limitation is a skull-base lesion that extends from the anterior cranial fossa to the middle fossa floor. Since the exposure provided by the supraorbital approach is primarily of the anterior fossa, the view of the middle fossa floor and lateral cavernous sinus tucked behind the lesser sphenoid wing is poor (Fig. 3.1). In our opinion, these lesions are better addressed through a standard pterional craniotomy or orbitozygomatic craniotomy, which provide greater exposure of the middle fossa floor and lateral cavernous sinus (Fig. 3.2). Reports of medial sphenoid wing meningiomas removed through this technique should be viewed cautiously [22].

The third limitation is represented by large olfactory groove meningiomas where gross total resection is desired. Because the ability to look cephalad through the supraorbital approach is limited by the orbital rim, these lesions may be better approached by other means, such as a bifrontal craniotomy or endonasal exposure. Furthermore, in order to address anterior midline structures, the surgeon must look over the orbital roof. Consider the orbital roofs as two mountains and the cribriform plate as the valley. The valley is deepest anteriorly, just behind the frontal sinus, and becomes shallower as it merges with the tuberculum sella posteriorly.

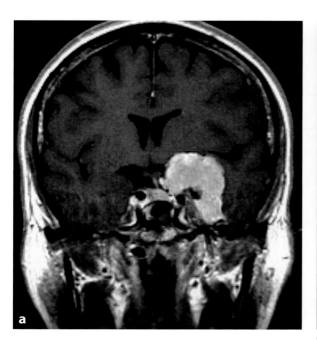

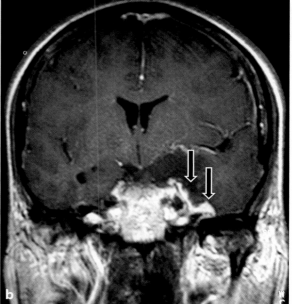

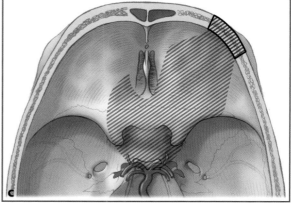

Fig. 3.1 Anatomical constraints of the supraorbital approach. **a**, **b** Coronal T1-weighted MR images with gadolinium contrast enhancement in a patient with a sphenoid wing meningioma: **a** preoperative; **b** postoperative (*arrows* residual tumor attached to the lateral cavernous sinus and floor of the middle fossa). This approach provides excellent access to the anterior cranial fossa and parasellar region, but visualization of the middle fossa is limited because of the sphenoid ridge. **c** Illustration of the skull base demonstrates appropriate targets (*hatched area*) for the supraorbital craniotomy. Other bony structures that limit exposure include the orbital roof, which impairs visualization of the medial anterior cranial fossa, and the posterior clinoid processes and tentorium, which limit infratentorial exposure

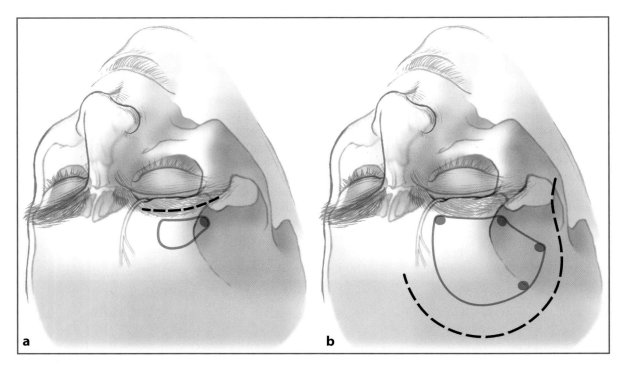

Fig. 3.2 Illustrations comparing the incision and bony exposure in a supraorbital craniotomy with those in a pterional craniotomy. **a** The supraorbital craniotomy utilizes the subfrontal corridor and involves a frontobasal burr hole and removal of a small window in the frontal bone. **b** The pterional craniotomy utilizes a frontotemporal incision and removal of the frontal and temporal bones and sphenoid wing. The pterional craniotomy primarily exploits the sylvian fissure

The deeper the valley or the more prominent the mountains, the more restricted the access.

The fourth limitation is superficial dural based tumors where the dural attachment or tail extends beyond the area visualized by the craniotomy. A standard frontotemporal incision and larger frontal craniotomy are needed in this instance in order to resect the dural tail. One important element of the keyhole concept is that the area of exposure is small at the craniotomy site, but it increases as one proceeds from the bone edge to deeper structures.

3.4 Anatomical Studies

Cadaveric studies have contributed to the refinement of the indications for supraorbital craniotomy and better delineated the relevant anatomy. When compared to the pterional and orbitozygomatic exposures using the circle of Willis as the surgical target, supraorbital craniotomy yields a similar working area [23]. As expected,

however, the maximum working angles are significantly less in the supraorbital craniotomy, suggesting that surgical freedom is constrained relative to standard approaches. These findings underscore the importance of a measured preoperative plan.

Kazkayasi et al. evaluated the anterior cranial landmarks to better define the safe zones for the craniotomy [24]. They studied the location of the supraorbital foramen/notch and its position relative to the frontal sinus in 30 adult skulls. In 33% of the skulls, the supraorbital foramen (the key medial landmark for planning the incision and craniotomy) was within the border of the frontal sinus. This work suggests that care must be taken to trace out the location of the frontal sinus as a routine step in preoperative planning rather than relying on anatomic surface landmarks.

Andersen et al. reviewed the courses of the supraorbital and supratrochlear nerves in ten cadavers [25]. They noted that both nerves have significant anatomical variability. Consequently, the nerves may be disrupted as part of the opening despite the use of anatomical landmarks for surgical planning. Therefore, patients should be counseled on the possibility of forehead numbness as a routine part of informed consent.

3.5 Application of Neuroendoscopy

Neuroendoscopy has been used by some practitioners to optimize the treatment of lesions managed through a supraorbital craniotomy. Neuroendoscopy helps address some of the limitations of the minimal access technique, namely, limited working angles and illumination in the depth of the operative field. The 0° endoscope provides a line-of-site view with high magnification and excellent illumination. We use the 30° endoscope and angled instruments to assess for tumor remnants around corners that are out of view of the microscope. The angled endoscope is also useful for evaluating the sella after pituitary adenoma removal, inspecting aneurysm ligation to ensure no perforators have been incorporated in the clip, and detecting aneurysm "dog ears" [13, 16]. Occasionally, we operate with the endoscope as the only source of light and visualization when the target lesion is deep-seated, such as third ventricular or midbrain pathology. Two examples of fully endoscopic technique have been provided by Kabil and Shahinian, who performed resections of two middle fossa arachnoid cysts and two sphenoid wing meningiomas [22, 26]. Menovsky et al. used an endoscopic technique for lesions of the interpeduncular fossa [27].

3.6 Surgical Technique

Several authors have published their technique for performing the supraorbital eyebrow craniotomy [8–10, 14, 15, 28]. Presented below are the steps that we follow supplemented with the modifications and suggestions of other groups (Figs. 3.2 and 3.3).

The patient is placed supine with 20° of reverse Trendelenberg position to facilitate venous drainage. The head is positioned with 20° of neck extension to allow the frontal lobe to auto-retract. The degree of head rotation towards the contralateral side is determined by the location of the pathology. Ipsilateral lesions require less head rotation (15–30°) than lesions of the olfactory groove and tuberculum sella (45–60°). After application of lubricant to the ipsilateral eye, a temporary tarsorrhaphy suture is placed to protect the cornea and sclera from the skin preparation agent. The hair is not shaved.

There are several options when making the initial skin incision. We prefer to make the incision within the eyebrow at its most superior margin. Others place the incision within a skin fold above the eyebrow arguing that it provides better access to the frontal floor [17]. The supraorbital notch can usually be palpated through the skin and serves as the medial limit of the skin incision. The incision is carried to the lateral margin of the eyebrow. If necessary, it can be extended up to 1 cm lateral to this point with a cosmetically pleasing result. Lateral exposure must be sufficient to place the frontobasal burr hole.

To maximize exposure, the skin edges are undermined. We prefer to incise the frontalis muscle in the line of the incision. Next, an inferiorly based U-shaped pericranial flap is incised and elevated. The margins of the skin incision are retracted with fish-hooks. The temporalis muscle is then elevated to expose the keyhole region and a small burr hole is placed to expose the frontal lobe dura. If a one-piece frontal craniotomy and orbital osteotomy is planned, the periorbita is also exposed with the burr hole. The supraorbital craniotomy is generally 2 to 3 cm wide and 1.5 to 2 cm high. The craniotomy must be large enough to accommodate fully opened bipolar forceps. When the supraorbital foramen/notch is lateral to the frontal sinus, it will serve as the inferomedial limit to the craniotomy. Otherwise, the craniotomy should be taken to the margin of frontal sinus without violating it. Frameless stereotactic guidance may be used to localize the frontal sinus. The base of the craniotomy should be taken as low as possible and parallel to the orbital roof. It is essential to drill flat the extradural bony ridges of the orbital roof prior to dural opening in order to maximize exposure.

The dura is opened in U-shaped fashion with its flap based inferiorly. No retractors are used. The proximal sylvian fissure and the interchiasmatic, opticocarotid, and carotid-oculomotor cisterns are opened for CSF release and brain relaxation. These latter three corridors are the primary working windows from the subfrontal approach. After the pathology of interest has been addressed, the dura is closed in watertight fashion. The bone is fixated with low-profile titanium plates. Demineralized bone matrix may be used to fill in the craniotomy line. Closure proceeds in layers. The skin is reapproximated by 3-0 nylon subcuticular closure without knots. The loose ends of this closure are tied over a nonadherent perforated plastic film dressing. The suture is removed on the fifth postoperative day.

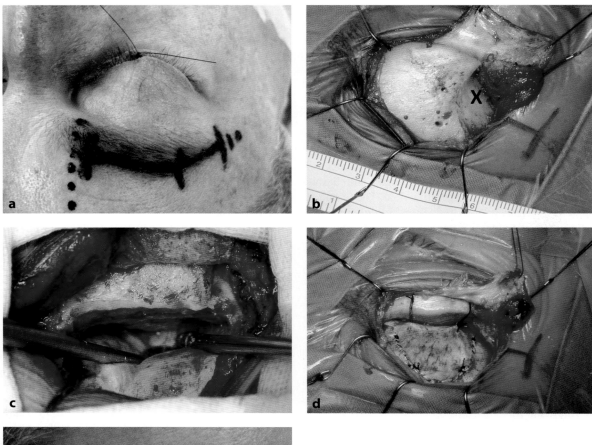

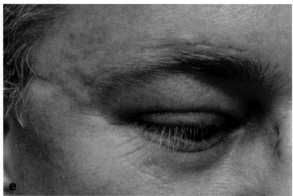

Fig. 3.3 Technique of the right supraorbital approach compiled from intraoperative photographs in several patients. **a** The incision is planned at the margin of the eyebrow (*solid line*) and can be extended laterally (*horizontal dashed line*) if needed with a good cosmetic result. The course of the supraorbital nerve is demonstrated (*vertical dashed line*). **b** A pericranial flap is reflected anteriorly and secured with sutures. The temporalis is elevated to expose the site for the frontobasal burr hole. A single burr hole is fashioned at position X. **c** The orbital roof is drilled flat to improve visualization. **d** At the conclusion, the C-shaped dural flap is closed water-tight and the bone is replaced with low-profile titanium plates. **e** Appearance of the incision at one year

The orbital rim can be removed to achieve a flatter operative trajectory and decrease brain retraction. Furthermore, it is possible to look in a more cephalad angle for tumors that extend up from the skull base. To incorporate the orbital rim with the craniotomy, the reciprocating saw is used to make a cut through the superior orbital rim at the medial limb of the craniotomy and through the lateral orbital rim just above the frontozy-gomatic suture. The orbital roof can be fractured through the burr hole. The disadvantages of removing the orbital roof include additional patient discomfort, and if there is a tear of the periorbita and dura during the bony work, the orbital fat can obscure visualization. Whether the surgeon chooses to remove the orbital rim or not, it is always advisable to drill down the ridges on the orbital roof to achieve the flattest possible trajectory.

3.7 Case Examples

3.7.1 Case 1

This healthy 72-year-old woman presented with left-sided hearing loss (Fig. 3.4). Imaging revealed a petro-clival meningioma with brainstem compression. Pre-operative MRI suggested that the basilar artery, left posterior cerebral artery, and deep veins were involved with tumor. We planned a two-stage approach to the lesion. In the first stage we utilized a supraorbital eyebrow craniotomy to resect the supratentorial compo-

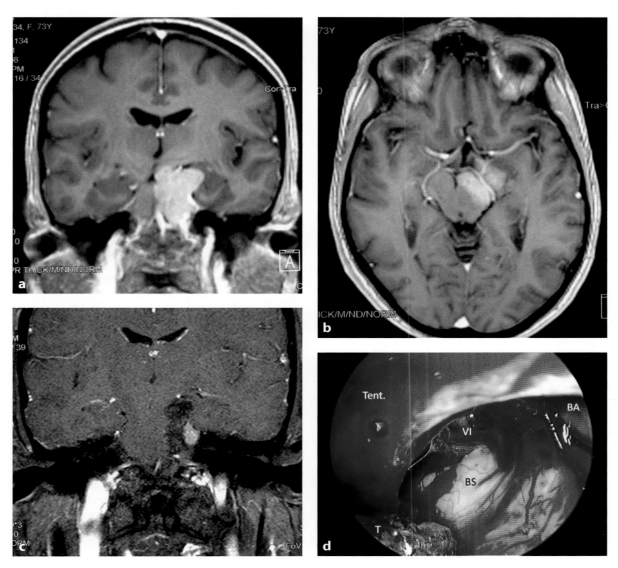

Fig. 3.4 Case example 1. **a – c** T1-weighted gadolinium enhanced MR images in a 72-year-old woman with a petroclival meningioma with brainstem compression (**a** preoperative coronal, **b** preoperative axial, **c** postoperative coronal). A supraorbital approach was planned as the first stage in a two-stage strategy with the modest goal of removing the supratentorial component of the tumor and separating it from the basilar perforators and proximal posterior cerebral artery before commencing with a retrosigmoid approach. **d** Intraoperative endoscopic view of the brainstem and abducens nerve. This case nicely illustrates the supratentorial access afforded by the approach, and highlights the limitations of exposure even when neuroendoscopy is used. Complete resection requires a second posterior fossa approach (*BA* basilar artery, *BS* brainstem, *T* tumor, *Tent.* tentorium, *VI* abducens nerve)

nent of the tumor and release the posterior cerebral artery and basilar artery. Because of the favorable tumor characteristics, we were able to resect the entire supratentorial component and most of the posterior fossa component using angled instrumentation supplemented with neuroendoscopy to look down the clivus. The abducens nerve and decompressed brainstem were observed at the conclusion of the procedure.

This case example highlights several important considerations. First, it demonstrates how angled instrumentation and neuroendoscopy can expand what is considered to be the traditional working area of an anterolateral approach. Second, it illustrates the limits of anatomic exposure caused by the tentorium and posterior clinoid processes; residual tumor is noted on the undersurface of the tentorium. The reader should note that the degree of resection achieved was greater than would be expected from a supratentorial approach because the tumor was soft and easily removed with suction.

3.7.2 Case 2

This 26-year-old man had a previous standard bicoronal incision and large frontal craniotomy for incomplete debulking of a left frontal, low-grade tumor (Fig. 3.5). The patient presented to our institution for a second opinion. Using the "two-point" rule that underscores the importance of picking a surgical trajectory that is in line with the long axis of the lesion, preoperative calculations showed that an anterior approach would be better than the superior approach adopted by the previous neurosurgeon. A complete macroscopic resection was accomplished using a supraorbital craniotomy.

This case example demonstrates how intraaxial tumors which present to the basal frontal lobe can be addressed through this approach.

3.7.3 Case 3

This 40-year-old man complained of retroorbital pain and diplopia, and was found to have a lesion within the right retroorbital space (Fig. 3.6). A complete removal was achieved through an eyebrow approach.

This case example demonstrates how lesions of the superior orbit and orbital apex may be addressed through this corridor. The craniotomy provides excel-

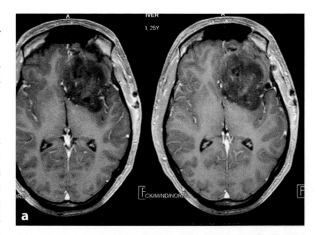

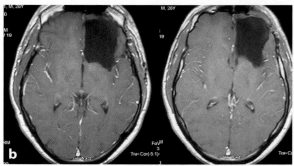

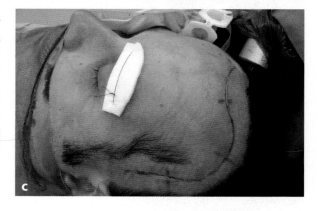

Fig. 3.5 Case example 2. **a**, **b** Axial T1-weighted gadolinium-enhanced MR images in a 26-year-old man with a frontal low-grade glioma resected through the supraorbital approach (**a** preoperative, **b** postoperative). **c** Immediate postoperative photograph contrasting the bifrontal incision used by another neurosurgeon and the eyebrow incision used to achieve a complete resection. In this case, the supraorbital approach afforded a more direct corridor to the tumor

lent access to the ipsilateral orbital roof, but angled instruments and neuroendoscopy are helpful for optimizing the caudally directed operative trajectory.

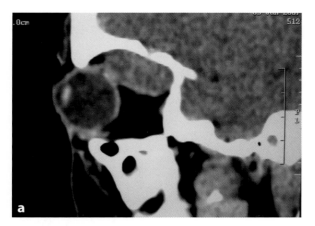

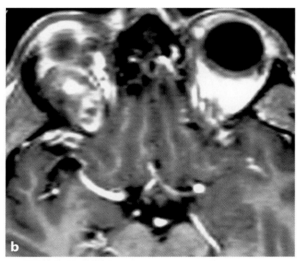

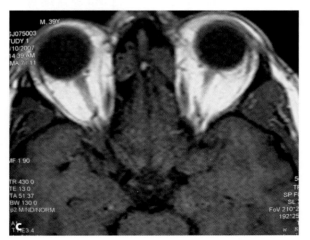

Fig. 3.6 Case example 3. **a**, **b** Preoperative sagittal CT image (**a**) and T1-weighted gadolinium-enhanced axial MR image (**b**) in a 40-year-old man with an intraorbital lesion adjacent to the orbital roof. **c** Complete resection was achieved through an eyebrow approach by removing the orbital roof and incising the periorbita

3.8 Complications and Complication Avoidance

3.8.1 Complications

The eyebrow supraorbital craniotomy has a unique set of approach-related complications. Unfortunately, most series lack a thorough assessment and do not distinguish between approach-related morbidity and overall morbidity, but some data are available from Reisch and Perneczky [12]. The most common approach-related complications are frontal numbness (7.5%) from injury to the supraorbital nerve and frontalis palsy (5.5%). Violation of the frontal sinus can cause CSF rhinorrhea (reported in 4% of patients). Rarely, patients will complain of painful mastication because of elevation of the temporalis muscle at the superior temporal line during the opening.

In addition to the complications described by Reisch and Perneczky, we have noted two others (Fig. 3.7). First, we have had two patients with burning of the eyebrow skin from the heat generated by the operating microscope light on 100% intensity. No such burns have been experienced since turning the illumination down to 70% and narrowing the cone of light. Second, we have had one patient with bone flap subsidence noted at the 3-year follow-up. This may be repaired with acrylic bone substitute if desired.

3.8.2 Complication Avoidance

To avoid supraorbital nerve injury, the skin incision should be limited medially by the supraorbital foramen/notch. It is nearly always possible to identify and preserve the supraorbital nerve during dissection as it emerges from its intraorbital course. Andersen et al. noted that the courses of the supraorbital and supratrochlear nerves are variable, so despite careful planning, surgeons should expect that a small percentage of patients will develop this minor adverse event despite meticulous dissection [25]. Occasionally, the supraorbital nerve is intentionally sacrificed because it can take a course over the planned craniotomy. Frontalis palsy is caused by inadvertent nerve section at the lateral aspect of the incision. Unlike the supraorbital nerve, the frontalis branch of the facial nerve is difficult to identify. Therefore, limiting the lateral extension of the incision can diminish the frequency of nerve palsy.

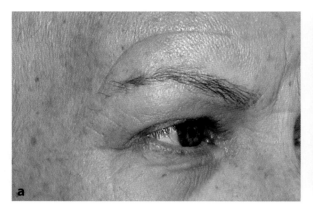

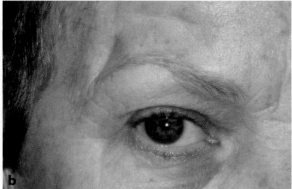

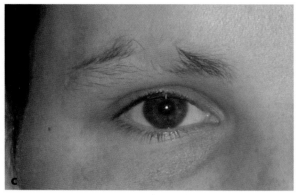

Fig. 3.7 Approach-related complications. **a, b** Photographs at 1 year (**a**) and 3 years (**b**) in a patient who had undergone resection of a parasellar lung metastasis demonstrating subsidence of the craniotomy. The incision was placed in a prominent skin crease in the patient's forehead. **c** Postoperative photograph in a male who sustained a burn from the microscope light

Of the reported complications, CSF rhinorrhea can be the most troublesome to manage. The incidence can be reduced by fashioning the craniotomy lateral to the frontal sinus. Neuronavigation can be used to mark the location of the sinus prior to the craniotomy. If the frontal sinus is violated, the mucosa can be stripped, the sinus packed with Betadine-soaked Gelfoam, muscle or fat, and covered with the vascularized pericranial flap harvested during the opening. If CSF leakage develops despite these maneuvers, lumbar drainage and re-exploration should be considered.

3.9 Criticisms of Supraorbital Eyebrow Craniotomy

As with other less-invasive techniques, understanding the limitations of the supraorbital approach is essential for good decision making. Knowledge of the criticisms will help the clinician refine patient selection and improve operative technique. The most common criticism is the decrease in surgical freedom offered by the eyebrow craniotomy compared to larger, standard approaches such as the pterional and orbitozygomatic craniotomies. The concern is that it will be more difficult for the surgeon to manage intraoperative complications. One frequently cited example is intraoperative rupture of an aneurysm. To obtain control, the surgeon may need to alter his surgical trajectory. As the literature has demonstrated, surgeons experienced with the approach are able expeditiously to manage intraoperative rupture. However, there is little space to accommodate a "third hand" for rapid suction if needed.

Another common criticism is that this approach is not suitable for complex skull-base lesions which are intimately involved with critical neurovascular structures. Some argue that different angles of view are required to fully visualize and protect them. Fortunately, the use of angled endoscopes may address this concern. The third criticism regards the incision; when it becomes infected the cosmetic result is suboptimal. An infected incision behind the hairline may ultimately yield a better result. Finally, and most importantly, it has not been demonstrated definitively that this approach offers improved morbidity when compared to standard approaches, though it is our impression that patients experience less postoperative pain and have a shorter hospital stay.

3.10 Practical Advice: Getting Started with Supraorbital Eyebrow Craniotomy

To gain expertise in the supraorbital craniotomy, we recommend starting with cadaveric dissections to develop a better understanding of the anatomical corridors and working angles. When applying the approach to patients, we recommend starting with standard approaches and paying close attention to the portion of the craniotomy actually used for access to various lesions. Gradually, the size of the craniotomy can be reduced and tailored to specific pathology as expertise develops. The first supraorbital craniotomies should be performed on patients with simpler pathology (i.e. cysts and small tumors) advancing to vascular lesions and large, deep tumors.

Since the angle of attack is different from standard frontolateral approaches, the surgeon must be prepared to alter his hand position for placing aneurysm clips, for example. Low-profile and bayoneted instruments are especially helpful in improving visualization at the tips. Concurrently, the surgeon should apply the endo-scope in all cases to learn how to exploit its superior illumination and ability to look around corners. We recommend using 0° and 30° endoscopes.

3.11 Summary

The supraorbital craniotomy is a keyhole approach to the anterior cranial fossa, parasellar region, circle of Willis, and ventral brainstem that has been successfully utilized to treat skull-base tumors, vascular lesions, traumatic lesions and arachnoid cysts. This approach exploits the normal subfrontal anatomic corridor and the basal cisterns to limit brain retraction and achieve wide exposure of the anterior cranial base with a satisfying cosmetic result. The technique is technically challenging, requiring stepwise training with progressively more limited craniotomies and lesions of increasing difficulty.

It is essential for the surgeon to understand the complications and limitations of the approach in order to select appropriate patients. Some practitioners have applied the endoscope to expand the indications for the approach because it improves visualization at the depths of the field and allows inspection of pathology hidden from the view of the operating microscope. Surgeons should familiarize themselves with the supraorbital craniotomy's unique approach-related morbidity in order to more effectively counsel patients.

References

1. Frazier CH (1913) I. An approach to the hypophysis through the anterior cranial fossa. Ann Surg 57:145–150
2. Krause F (1908) Chirurgie des Gehirns und ruckenmarks nach eigenen erfahrungen. Urban & Schwartzenberg, Berlin
3. Al-Mefty O (1987) Supraorbital-pterional approach to skull base lesions. Neurosurgery 21:474–477
4. Fujitsu K, Kuwabara T (1985) Zygomatic approach for lesions in the interpeduncular cistern. J Neurosurg 62:340–343
5. Maroon JC, Kennerdell JS (1984) Surgical approaches to the orbit: indications and techniques. J Neurosurg 60:1226–1235
6. Zabramski JM, Kiris T, Sankhla SK et al (1998) Orbitozygomatic craniotomy: Technical note. J Neurosurg 89:336–341
7. Yasargil MG, Fox JL, Ray MW (1975) The operative approach to aneurysms of the anterior communicating artery. In: Krayenbuhl H (ed) Advances and technical standards in neurosurgery. Springer, Vienna, pp 113–170
8. Reisch R, Perneczky A, Filippi R (2003) Surgical technique of the supraorbital key-hole craniotomy. Surg Neurol 59:223–227
9. Czirjak S, Nyary I, Futo J, Szeifert GT (2002) Bilateral supraorbital keyhole approach for multiple aneurysms via superciliary skin incisions. Surg Neurol 57:314–323
10. Jho HD (1997) Orbital roof craniotomy via an eyebrow incision: a simplified anterior skull base approach. Minim Invasive Neurosurg 40:91–97
11. Perneczky A, Muller-Forell W, van Lindert E, Fries G (1999) Keyhole concept in neurosurgery. Thieme, Stuttgart
12. Reisch R, Perneczky A (2005) Ten-year experience with the supraorbital subfrontal approach through an eyebrow skin incision. Neurosurgery 57 (4 Suppl):242–255
13. Lan Q, Gong Z, Kang D et al (2006) Microsurgical experience with keyhole operations on intracranial aneurysms. Surg Neurol 66 (Suppl 1):S2–S9
14. Mitchell P, Vindlacheruvu RR, Mahmood K et al (2005) Supraorbital eyebrow minicraniotomy for anterior circulation aneurysms. Surg Neurol 63:47–51
15. van Lindert E, Perneczky A, Fries G, Pierangeli E (1998) The supraorbital approach to supratentorial aneurysms: concept and technique. Surg Neurol 49:481–489
16. Paladino J, Pirker N, Stimac D, Stern-Padovan R (1998) Eyebrow approach in vascular neurosurgery. Minim Invasive Neurosurg 41:200–203

17. Brydon HL, Akil H, Ushewokunze S et al (2008) Supraorbital microcraniotomy for acute aneurysmal subarachnoid haemorrhage: results of first 50 cases. Br J Neurosurg 22:40–45

18. Teo C (2005) Application of neuroendoscopy to the surgical management of craniopharyngiomas. Childs Nerv Syst 21:696–700

19. Melamed I, Merkin V, Korn A, Nash M (2005) The supraorbital approach: an alternative to traditional exposure for the surgical management of anterior fossa and parasellar pathology. Minim Invasive Neurosurg 48:259–263

20. Noggle JC, Sciubba DM, Nelson C et al (2008) Supraciliary keyhole craniotomy for brain abscess debridement. Neurosurg Focus 24:E11

21. Little AS, Jittapiromsak P, Crawford NR et al (2008) Quantitative analysis of exposure of staged orbitozygomatic and retrosigmoid craniotomies for lesions of the clivus with supratentorial extension. Neurosurgery 62 (5 Suppl 2): ONS318–23

22. Kabil MS, Shahinian HK (2006) The endoscopic supraorbital approach to tumors of the middle cranial base. Surg Neurol 66:396–401

23. Figueiredo EG, Deshmukh V, Nakaji P et al (2006) An anatomical evaluation of the mini-supraorbital approach and comparisons with standard craniotomies. Neurosurgery 59 (4 Suppl 2):ONS212–20

24. Kazkayasi M, Batay F, Bademci G et al (2008) The morphometric and cephalometric study of anterior cranial landmarks for surgery. Minim Invasive Neurosurg 51:21–25

25. Andersen NB, Bovim G, Sjaastad O (2001) The frontotemporal peripheral nerves. Topographic variations of the supraorbital, supratrochlear and auriculotemporal nerves and their possible clinical significance. Surg Radiol Anat 23:97–104

26. Kabil M, Shahinian HK (2007) Fully endoscopic supraorbital resection of congenital middle cranial fossa arachnoid cysts: report of two cases. Pediatr Neurosurg 43:316–322

27. Menovsky T, Grotenhuis JA, de Vries J, Bartels RH (1999) Endoscope-assisted supraorbital craniotomy for lesions of the intrapeduncular fossa. Neurosurgery 44:106–110

28. Jallo GI, Bognar L (2006) Eyebrow surgery: the supraciliary craniotomy: technical note. Neurosurgery 50 (1 Suppl 1): ONSE157–158

Frontotemporal Approach

4

Giorgio Iaconetta, Enrique Ferrer, Alberto Prats Galino,
Joaquim Enseñat and Matteo de Notaris

4.1 Introduction

The frontotemporal approach, popularized by Yasargil
for the treatment of intracranial aneurysms [1], is still
one of the most versatile and widely used approaches
in contemporary neurosurgery. It has also been employed for a large number of other applications, such
as lesions of the sellar region, the cavernous sinus, and
the anterior and middle cranial fossa, and as a basic
module for more complex approaches to the skull base.
The widely recognized advantage of the frontotemporal
craniotomy is the enhanced exposure of deep neurovascular structures, which offer a shorter and wider view
of the surgical target. The immediate release of cerebrospinal fluid from the basal cisterns and the early visualization of the neurovascular structures result in a
significant reduction in brain retraction and preservation of the normal vascular anatomy. Furthermore, it allows the early identification of the ipsilateral internal
carotid artery, thus providing an early proximal vascular control.

Although Krause [2] and Dandy [3] were among the
first to describe and publish the frontotemporal craniotomy, the real father of this approach was George J.
Heuer [4], a pioneer in neurosurgery at the John Hopkins Hospital. He was the first full-time assistant in the
Hunterian Laboratory directed by Harvey Cushing,
who trained him in neurosurgery [5]. He developed this
craniotomy to resect chiasmatic lesions, which included
hypophyseal, optic nerve and suprasellar tumors. How-

ever, one century has elapsed since this early formula-
tion; the indications provided by George J. Heuer still
remain adequate.

Modern neurosurgical techniques have been compared for years to balance the need to minimize brain
retraction and maximize surgical exposure [1, 6, 7]. The
development of the neurosurgical operative environment is actually driven principally by parallel evolution
in science and technology. Important tools including
neuroendoscopic techniques as well as neuronavigation
and advanced intraoperative imaging, reflect the effort
to reduce morbidity and brain trauma, and to optimize
the position, reduce the size and tailor the shape of the
craniotomy.

4.2 Positioning

The hair should be cut before the patient enters the operating room. Shaving the whole head might be unnecessary; we prefer only to shave the area of the skin incision a couple of centimeters behind and in front. The
patient is placed in the supine position on the operating
table with the legs propped up on pillows. The head is
rotated to the side contralateral to the approach by approximately 30° and fixed to the Mayfield-Kees pin
headrest. The two-pin arm is placed on the contralateral
side. The anterior pin is placed over the frontal bone
inside the hairline, close to the pupillary line, and the
posterior pin is placed within the parietal bone, above
the superior temporal line, taking care to avoid penetration of the temporal muscle which would increase
instability of the head and postoperative discomfort.
The single pin is fixed behind the ear, superior to the

G. Iaconetta (✉)
Dept of Neurological Science, Division of Neurosurgery
Università degli Studi di Napoli Federico II, Naples, Italy

P. Cappabianca et al. (eds.), *Cranial, Craniofacial and Skull Base Surgery.*

mastoid process, within the parietal bone. The vertex of the head is then tilted down 10–15° such that the malar eminence is almost the highest point of the operative field (Fig. 4.1). Once the patient is well fixed to the operating table to ensure the position while the table is tilted, the torso is then flexed downward so that the head is slightly above the level of the heart to favor venous flow.

During these maneuvers the surgeon should take care not to overstretch the arteries and veins of the neck, to avoid possible impairment of venous drainage, as well as of the esophagus and trachea. The cervical segment of the spine should not be rotated to the extreme in any direction. Once the head is definitively positioned and secured to the Mayfield-Kees head-holder, no more adjustments should be made as they may be dangerous for the cervical spine. Correct positioning ensures an optimal viewing angle to the central cranial base thus minimizing retraction of the frontal and temporal lobes, which naturally fall away respectively from the orbital roof and from the sphenoid ridge.

Neurophysiological monitoring may play an important role when surgery has to be performed around or within the cavernous sinus and superior orbital fissure, to avoid damage to the cranial nerves. Positioning of electrodes on the extraocular muscles is useful for monitoring the abducens, trochlear and oculomotor nerves. The surgeon must entertain the possibility of temporal occlusion of the internal carotid artery, in which case somatosensory evoked potentials and electroencephalography are extremely helpful for intraoperative monitoring and a permissible temporary occlusion time. Cerebral blood flow monitoring is also useful to control the supply of the cortical areas during occlusion of the vessel.

Meticulous scrubbing of the skin and draping concludes this step of the approach.

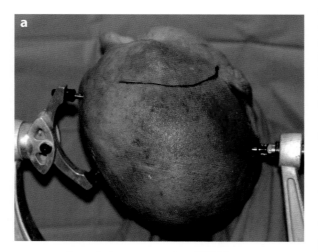

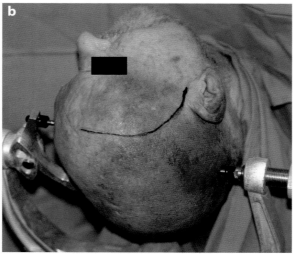

Fig. 4.1 Patient positioning and skin incision. The head is rotated to the side contralateral to the approach by approximately 30° and fixed to the Mayfield-Kees pin headrest

4.3 Skin Incision

The skin incision for the standard frontotemporal approach starts approximately 0.5–1 cm anterior to the tragus advancing in a curvilinear shape as far as the midpupillary line at the hairline–forehead interface (Fig. 4.1). If a more extended posterior exposure of the middle fossa is needed, a question mark skin incision reaching the midline is preferable.

A relaxing skin incision should be made in order to avoid inadvertent penetration of the pericranium and of the temporal fascia over the frontal and the temporal regions, respectively. We prefer to dissect the area close to the ear, always subgaleal, by means of blunt or finger dissection to avoid damaging the superficial temporal artery and the frontotemporal branch of the facial nerve. The incision is made in short segments (2–3 cm), while an assistant pushes the borders of the incision to prevent bleeding, Raney clips are applied to the rim of the scalp. This maneuver allows bleeding to be controlled while performing the skin incision. Once the galeocutaneous layer has been dissected, three different methods of temporal muscle dissection can be performed: interfascial, subfascial, or submuscular.

4.4 Anatomical Basis for Preservation of the Superficial Temporal Artery and the Frontal Branch of the Facial Nerve

The soft tissues covering the frontal area comprise skin, subcutaneous tissue, galea aponeurotica (also called epicranial aponeurosis), loose connective tissue and pericranium. The temporal region is an extremely complex anatomical area and the terminology used to describe it is often confusing. Therefore we believe that some anatomical remarks are mandatory. The skin of the temporal area is variable in thickness consisting of five layers covered by an outermost horny layer. These layers are on top of the dermis, which consists of collagenous and elastic fibers with hair follicles, sebaceous glands and rare sweat glands. Just below is located the subcutaneous fatty tissue which is thicker over the zygomatic arch. The thickness of the scalp varies from 4 to 9 mm. Under the subcutaneous tissue the galea pericranii is identifiable. In this area this tissue is called the temporoparietal fascia which is considered to be part of the superficial muscle–aponeurotic system. Within it runs the superficial temporal artery and the frontotemporal branch of the facial nerve. The temporalis fascia is attached in an arched fashion to the superior temporal line, to the lateral surface of the frontozygomatic process and to the medial surface of the zygoma.

Directly beneath this there is loose areolar tissue (also called subgaleal fascia or subgaleal space) which is connective tissue that becomes thin and fatty in correspondence with the zygoma and is in continuity with the subcutaneous fat below the zygomatic arch. The pericranium in the temporal region, at the level of the superior temporal line, splits into two layers, one deeper, beneath the temporal muscle in contact with the temporal squama (frequently confused in the surgical literature with the deep temporal fascia), and the other more superficial, covering the muscle, called the temporal fascia (called by many authors the superficial temporal fascia). This layer, in turn, splits into two separate superficial and deeper laminae, which enclose the superficial temporal fat pat (corresponding to the so-called intrafascial fat pad reported in the literature). There are two well recognized fat pads over the temporalis muscle. The first, already described above, is located within the duplication of the temporal fascia. The second is sited more deeply between the fascia and the temporalis muscle. It is in continuity with the fat tissue of the infratemporal fossa, the cheek and the orbit. It continues medially to the temporalis muscle forming a sort of thin pillow between the temporal squama and the medial surface of the muscle and contains the deep temporal vessels and nerves. These fat pads can vary in thickness, from very thick to extremely thin.

4.5 Anatomy of the Facial Nerve and Superficial Temporal Artery within the Temporal Region

The division of the facial nerve into the temporal and zygomatic branches takes place within the parotid gland. The temporal branch suddenly pierces the parotid-masseteric fascia below the zygomatic arch dividing into its three terminal rami: anterior which innervates the corrugator supercilii and orbicularis oculi muscles; middle, known also as the frontal branch, which innervates the frontalis muscle; and posterior which innervates the anterior and superior auricular and the tragus muscles (this branch has no clinical relevance in humans).

The point where the temporal branch of the facial nerve gives rise to the anterior and middle rami is located 2–2.5 cm anterior to the tragus, while the frontal ramus pierces the galea to reach the frontal muscle 1–3 cm posterior to the lateral canthus. The temporal branch is located within the temporoparietal fascia, cranially, and, in proximity to the zygoma in the loose areolar tissue, over the superficial lamina of the temporal fascia. Knowledge of this anatomy is essential to avoid postoperative cosmetic deficits.

Bernstein and Nelson in a very detailed anatomical study on the temporal branch of the facial nerve stated that: "the temporal branch of the facial nerve lies within an area bounded by a line from the earlobe to the lateral edge of the eyebrow inferiorly and a second line from the tragus to the lateral coronal suture just above and behind the highest forehead crease." It is very important to remark that the frontal ramus of the temporal branch of the facial nerve crosses the zygomatic arch approximately 2 cm anterior to the tragus and runs 1 cm caudal and parallel to the frontal branch of the superficial temporal artery. This vessel, therefore, could be a useful landmark indicating the position of the frontal nerve (Fig. 4.2).

The superficial temporal artery also shows a high degree of variability in its course. It is a terminal branch

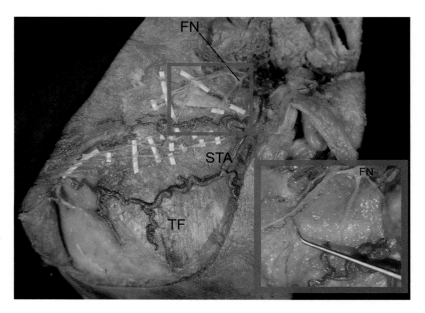

Fig. 4.2 Right frontotemporal craniotomy. Dissection of the entire course of the facial nerve. Inside the blue box the frontal branch of the facial nerve is exposed. *FN* facial nerve, *STA* superficial temporal artery, *TF* temporal fascia

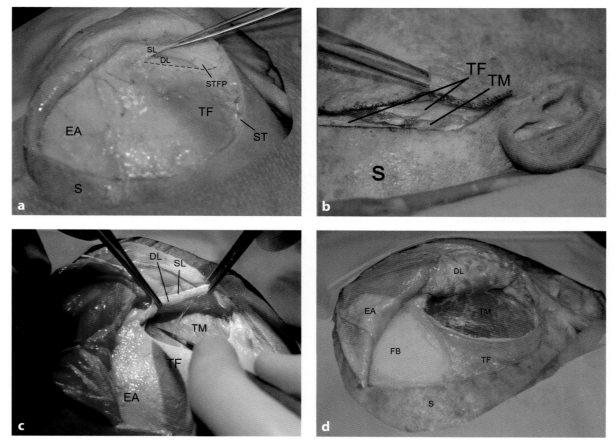

Fig. 4.3 Right frontotemporal craniotomy. Different techniques of dissection of the temporal muscle: **a** interfascial; **b** submuscular; **c, d** subfascial. *DL* deep layer of the temporal fascia, *EA* epicranial aponeurosis, *FB* frontal bone, *S* skin, *SL* superficial layer of the temporal fascia, *ST* subcutaneous tissue, *STFP* superficial temporal fat pad, *TF* temporal fascia, *TM* temporal muscle

of the external carotid artery, running close to the tragus within the subcutaneous tissue and bifurcating in the temporal region 2 cm above the zygomatic arch. The frontal branch gives rise to many twigs in the frontal area and finally anastomoses with the supraorbital artery of the ophthalmic artery. The parietal branch supplies the parietal, temporal and occipital areas, anastomosing with the contralateral parietal branch and with the posterior auricular and occipital arteries. Collateral branches of the superficial temporal artery are the transverse artery of the face, the temporal artery, and the zygomatic-orbital artery.

Preserving vessel integrity is mandatory to obtain a well-vascularized galeopericranial flap and to perform, if necessary, an extracranial–intracranial bypass grafting procedure.

4.6 Temporal Muscle Dissection Methods

4.6.1 Interfascial

This technique was extensively described by Yasargil at the beginning of the 1980s. The scalp is dissected from the pericranium and then reflected anteroinferiorly toward the orbit and fixed to fish-hooks until the orbit rim is exposed. Care must be taken to avoid damage to the supraorbital nerve, which runs in the supraorbital notch just below the junction of the medial third and lateral two-thirds of the upper orbital rim. The pericranium covering the frontal region is incised in a triangular shape, pedicled anteriorly and reflected toward the orbit.

The superficial lamina of the temporalis fascia is incised from the most anterior part of the inferior temporal line as far as the root of the zygoma and then reflected anteriorly with the scalp, exposing the superficial fat pad between the two laminae (Fig. 4.3a). This maneuver is necessary to ensure the preservation of the frontotemporal branch of the facial nerve passing just above the superficial lamina inside the loose areolar tissue. The anterior quarter of the temporal muscle is still covered by the deeper lamina of the temporal fascia, which is incised and dissected from the frontozygomatic process and zygoma. When the muscle has been stripped away from the temporal fossa, it is reflected backwards and inferiorly to expose the pterion, the temporal squama, the sphenoid wing, and part of the parietal, frontal and zygomatic bones.

4.6.2 Submuscular

The initial step of the approach is the same as described above. After skin incision, dissection is performed in the subgaleal plane to expose the temporal fascia. When the superficial layer of the temporal fascia comes into view, the temporal muscle is incised (Fig. 4.3b) and dissected free from the temporal bone, leaving the temporal fascia with its fat pads in situ covering the muscle. Using periosteal elevators and following the submuscular plane, the dissection should be performed following the direction of the fibers to avoid tearing the muscle from the deeper part of the temporal fossa, close to the zygoma, in the direction of the superior temporal line. During this maneuver, we never use monopolar coagulation to avoid temporal muscle atrophy caused by injury to its vascular supply. Once fish-hooks are fixed to the muscle, the bony temporal surface is widely exposed (Fig. 4.4b). Moreover, the risk of injury to the frontotemporal branch of the facial nerve is lower with the submuscular approach.

4.6.3 Subfascial

This technique allows wide exposure of the zygoma and is particularly useful if a *combined orbitozygomatic* craniotomy is planned. It allows the muscle to be mobilized fully so as not to hinder exposure. The incision over the temporal fascia is performed close to the temporal line and parallel to the skin incision in a semilunar fashion and includes both superficial and deep laminae (Fig. 4.4c). The fascial layers, with the superficial fat pad inside, are elevated together and reflected forward (Fig. 4.4d). Therefore, the dissection of the temporal fascia must proceed to reach the superior border of the zygoma and the frontozygomatic suture. At this point, the deep layer is incised along the medial aspect of the zygoma. If necessary, the zygomatic bone can be removed to enhance the exposure of the middle fossa. We always perform preplating to avoid repositioning problems of the zygoma. The temporal muscle is then stripped from the infratemporal fossa using the same retrograde technique as described above. The temporalis muscle may later be incised, leaving a cuff of fascia at the superior temporal line, for reapproximation or totally mobilizing the muscle free from the bone (Fig. 4.4). This technique avoids any injury to the frontal branches of the facial nerve, and provides a low and wide basal extension of the craniotomy.

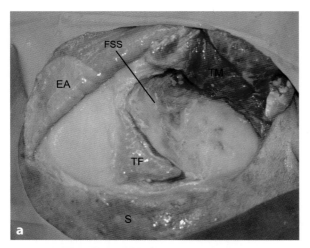

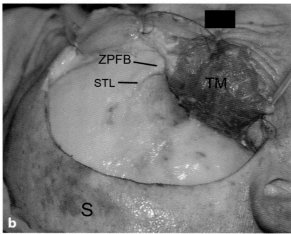

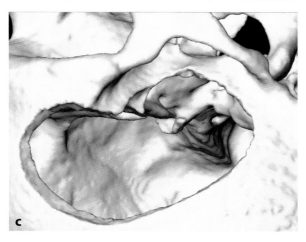

Fig. 4.4 Temporal muscle transposition (**a**, **b**) and CT scan 3-D reconstruction of the frontotemporal craniotomy (**c**). *EA* epicranial aponeurosis, *FSS* frontosphenoidal suture, *S* skin, *STL* superior temporal line, *TF* temporal fascia, *TM* temporal muscle, *ZPFB* zygomatic process of the frontal bone

4.7 Craniotomy

Using a high-speed electric drill (Midas Rex, Fort Worth, Texas), we first perform the standard keyhole described by Dandy [3] as we prefer, for a standard pterional craniotomy, to leave the orbital roof intact. The burr hole is placed just above the frontosphenoidal suture, below the superior temporal line and posterior to the frontozygomatic suture (Fig. 4.5a,d). Care should be taken to distinguish between the frontozygomatic and frontosphenoidal sutures. This burr hole is usually located 8 to 10 mm above the MacCarty's keyhole, which is situated over the frontosphenoidal suture, approximately 1 cm behind the frontozygomatic junction (Fig. 4.5b) [8]. When placed appropriately, this burr hole allows exposure of both the frontal dura and the periorbita (Fig. 4.5c), and it is particularly suitable when performing a frontotemporoorbitozygomatic craniotomy.

We usually place a single burr hole taking care to keep the dura mater intact. A craniotome is then inserted into the burr hole and the first cut is made from the frontal keyhole, and carried toward the supraorbital notch to approximately 2 cm above the orbital rim. Staying lateral to the supraorbital notch decreases the risk of frontal sinus penetration; however, penetration may be unavoidable in the presence of a well-pneumatized frontal sinus. The cut is continued downward in a curvilinear fashion, over the parietal bone finishing over the sphenotemporal suture. At this point, we usually prefer to complete the craniotomy using a high-speed drill to groove the last part of the bone over the zygomaticsphenoidal suture and then spanning the greater wing of the sphenoid near the line of the zygoma. This groove ensures a precise and safe fracture line across the sphenoid when raising the bone flap (Fig. 4.4c).

The bone flap is elevated gently and the dura is detached from the inner surface with a blunt dissector. When the flap has been removed the lesser wing of the sphenoid is drilled down to optimize the most basal trajectory to the skull base (Fig. 4.6a, b; Fig. 4.7). In order to perform this maneuver, it is often necessary to release cerebrospinal fluid by cutting the dura on the frontal and temporal surfaces for 0.5–1 cm. Under surgical microscope magnification, using a diamond burr, we flatten the orbital roof with great caution to avoid unplanned entry into the orbit. The greater sphenoid wing is also flattened on its posterior ridge, as shown in Fig. 4.7, a three-dimensional reconstruction of the approach.

Possible complications related to these maneuvers included bleeding from the orbitomeningeal artery

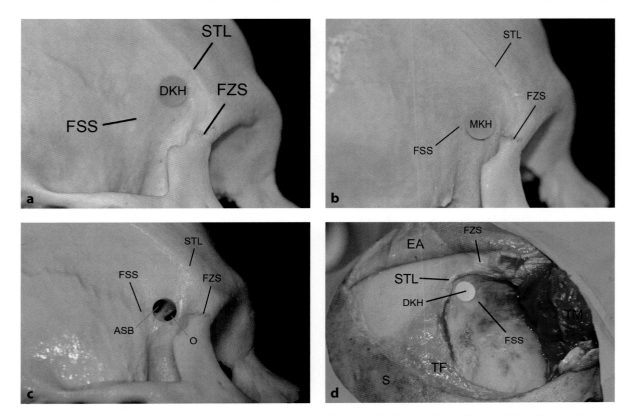

Fig. 4.5 Positioning of the keyhole. **a, d** The Dandy point is placed just above the frontosphenoidal suture, below the superior temporal line and posterior to the frontozygomatic suture. **b, c** The MacCarty point is situated over the frontosphenoidal suture, approximately 1 cm behind the frontozygomatic junction. *ASB* anterior skull base, *DKH* Dandy keyhole, *EA* epicranial aponeurosis, *FSS* frontosphenoidal suture, *FZS* frontozygomatic suture, *MKH* MacCarty's keyhole, *O* orbit, *S* skin, *STL* superior temporal line, *TF* temporal fascia, *TM* temporal muscle

branches, an anastomotic vessel of the ophthalmic artery reaching the middle meningeal artery, and the inadvertent penetration of the orbit and the frontal sinus. The orbitomeningeal artery can be coagulated or packed with bone wax; the high-speed drill with diamond burr is also useful in reducing bleeding. The opening of the orbit is generally not a problem and can be managed quite easily simply by placing a small piece of muscle to close the hole. If the frontal sinus is entered, the mucoperiosteal layer has to be completely removed and the cavity has to be filled with muscle or fat and sealed with fibrin glue to avoid the formation of a frontal mucocele. These maneuvers allow retraction of the frontal lobe away from the orbital roof and maximize the exposure of the skull base. Once this step has been completed, dural take-up sutures can be placed circumferentially to minimize the bleeding from the epidural space (Fig. 4.6a).

4.8 Dural Opening

The dural incision is made in the usual semicircular fashion. The dural flap is then reflected toward the orbit and sphenoid ridge and retracted using fish-hooks (Fig. 4.6c). A slight retraction of the frontal lobe allows exposure of the carotid, and the chiasmatic and lamina terminalis cisterns (Fig. 4.8a). Early release of cerebrospinal fluid from these cisterns allows optimal brain relaxation. The dissection of the sylvian fissure is typically undertaken in a proximal-to-distal fashion. Usually the arachnoid covering the sylvian fissure is very thin, but sometimes may be thicker in which case the neurovascular structures are not perfectly identifiable. Dissection is generally recommended at the frontal side because the superficial middle cerebral veins course on its temporal aspect. Retracting the frontal lobe, these

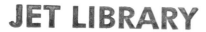

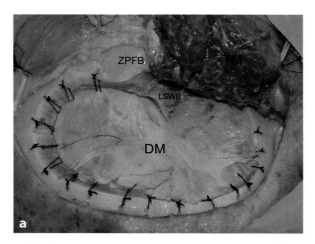

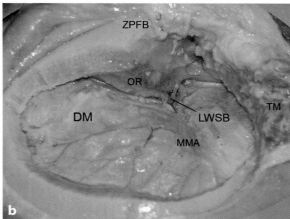

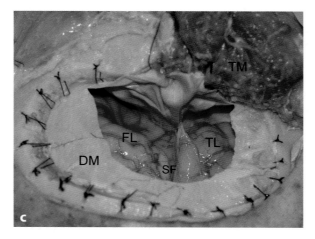

Fig. 4.6 a Craniotomy. **b** When the flap has been removed the lesser wing of the sphenoid is drilled down to optimize the most basal trajectory to the skull base. **c** Dural opening. *DM* dura mater, *FL* frontal lobe, *MMA* middle meningeal artery, *LWSB* lesser wing of the sphenoid bone, *SF* sylvian fissure, *TL* temporal lobe, *TM* temporal muscle, *ZPFB* zygomatic process of the frontal bone

veins are left intact (inadvertent injury can result in brain swelling). It is essential to preserve the superficial middle cerebral venous system. While retracting the frontal lobe, the surgeon should take care to avoid excessive displacement and stretching of the olfactory nerve which can be seriously damaged. The superficial middle cerebral veins receive the deep middle cerebral vein and frontal veins and drain into the sphenoparietal sinus, into the cavernous sinus or also into the basal vein of Rosenthal, and rarely into the vein of Labbé or into the transverse sinus.

Dissection of the sylvian fissure begins at the level of the opercular part of the inferior frontal gyrus, as described by Yasargil. Once the fissure has been entered, the dissection continues in the direction of the middle cerebral artery. Deep within the sylvian fissure, the frontal lobe often protrudes laterally, indenting the temporal lobe; in such a case, to avoid parenchymal damage, the fissure has to be opened following the distal branches of the middle cerebral artery. Once the sylvian fissure is completely opened, the entire circle of Willis, and the anterior cerebral artery and its branches come into view (Fig. 4.8b). If the approach has been performed correctly, a wide exposure of the sellar, parasellar, suprasellar and retrosellar areas is achieved (Fig. 4.9). Both carotid arteries, the middle and anterior cerebral artery and their branches, the anterior communicating artery, Heubner's recurrent arteries, the anterior choroidal artery, the posterior communicating artery, the basilar artery, the posterior cerebral artery (P1 and P2 segments), the superior cerebellar artery, the olfactory nerve, both optic nerves and chiasm, the third nerve, the pituitary stalk, and the anterior and posterior clinoids are exposed (Fig. 4.10). Once the Liliequist's membrane has been opened, the interpeduncular cistern is entered and the basilar artery and its branches come into view and also the third nerve is exposed (Fig. 4.11).

4.9 Endoscope-Assisted Technique

Endoscope-assisted microsurgery has gained wide acceptance for the management of cerebral aneurysms with favorable results in terms of reduction of both morbidity and mortality rates. This minimally invasive technique has enhanced the visualization of blind corners around the aneurysm, and of perforating arteries and small vascular variations, and helps in precise positioning of the clip during microsurgical procedures. There are several

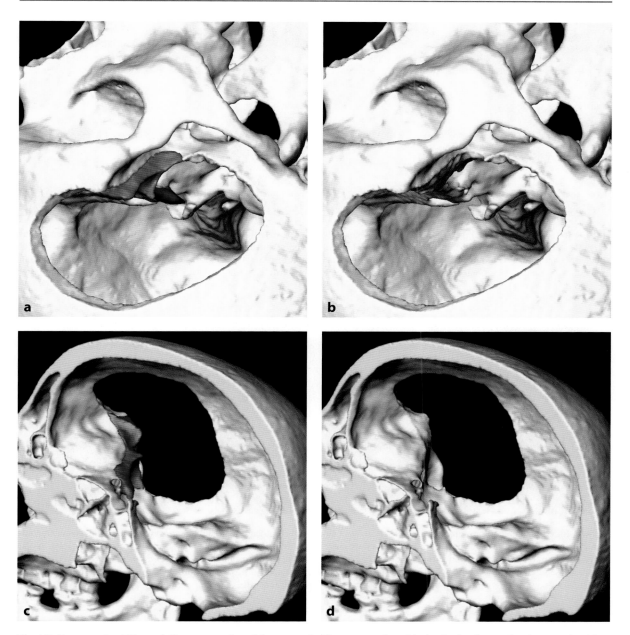

Fig. 4.7 Postoperative CT scan 3-D reconstruction of the approach. The greater sphenoid wing is also flattened on its posterior ridge.

advantages of this technique: it provides excellent illumination in deep planes, it visualizes the blind corner enabling observation of perforators of the other side, it confirms the precise position of the clip, it provides a favorable view of posterior circulation aneurysms (especially those of the basilar tip), and it results in a small craniotomy with minimal brain retraction.

For visualization of posterior circulation aneurysms, we usually introduce a 45° endoscope in a corridor between the carotid artery and the oculomotor nerve (Fig. 4.12a). Through this route access to the basilar bifurcation is feasible.

In patients with a basilar tip aneurysm, the endoscope enables the surgeon to visualize both the pos-

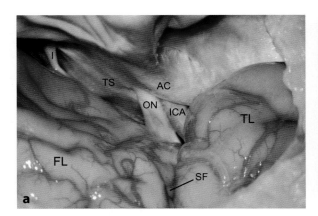
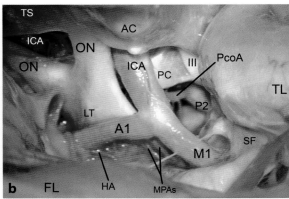

Fig. 4.8 Intradural exposure; right approach. Before (**a**) and after (**b**) opening of the Sylvian fissure. *A1* first segment of the anterior cerebral artery, *AC* anterior clinoid, *FL* frontal lobe, *HA* Heubner's artery, *I* olfactory tract, *III* oculomotor nerve, *ICA* internal carotid artery, *LT* lamina terminalis, *M1* first segment of the middle cerebral artery, *MPAs* perforating arteries, *ON* optic nerve, *P2* second segment of the posterior cerebral artery, *PC* posterior clinoid, *PcoA* posterior communicating artery, *SF* sylvian fissure, *TL* temporal lobe, *TS* tuberculum sellae

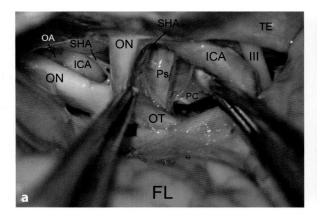
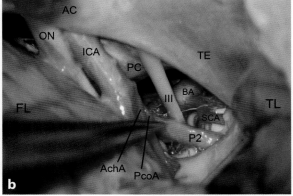

Fig. 4.9 Intradural exposure; right approach. **a** Instruments enlarging the optocarotid area. **b** Displacing medially the posterior communicating artery, exposing the contents of the interpeduncular cistern. *AC* anterior clinoid, *AchA* anterior choroidal artery, *BA* basilar artery, *FL* frontal lobe, *ICA* internal carotid artery, *III* oculomotor nerve, *OA* left ophthalmic artery, *ON* optic nerve, *OT* optic tract, *P2* second segment of the posterior cerebral artery, *PC* posterior clinoid, *PcoA* posterior communicating artery, *Ps* pituitary stalk, *SCA* superior cerebellar artery, *SHA* superior hypophyseal artery, *TE* tentorial edge, *TL* temporal lobe

Fig. 4.10 Intradural exposure; right approach; enlarged view. *A1* first segment of the anterior cerebral artery, *A2* second segment of the anterior cerebral artery, *AC* anterior clinoid, *AcoA* anterior communicating artery, *BA* basilar artery, *FL* frontal lobe, *HA* Heubner's artery, *ICA* internal carotid artery, *III* oculomotor nerve, *LT* lamina terminalis, *M1* first segment of the middle cerebral artery, *OA* left ophthalmic artery, *ON* optic nerve, *P2* second segment of the posterior cerebral artery, *PC* posterior clinoid, *PcoA* posterior communicating artery, *SCA* superior cerebellar artery, *SHA* superior hypophyseal artery, *TE* tentorial edge, *TL* temporal lobe, *TS* tuberculum sellae

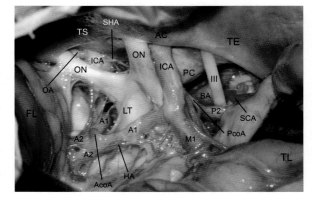

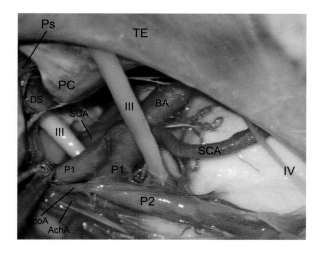

Fig. 4.11 Intradural exposure; right approach; close-up view of the interpeduncular fossa. *AchA* anterior choroidal artery, *BA* basilar artery, *DS* dorsum sellae, *III* oculomotor nerve, *IV* trochlear nerve, *P1* first segment of the posterior cerebral artery, *P2* second segment of the posterior cerebral artery, *PC* posterior clinoid, *PcoA* posterior communicating artery, *Ps* pituitary stalk, *SCA* superior cerebellar artery, *TE* tentorial edge

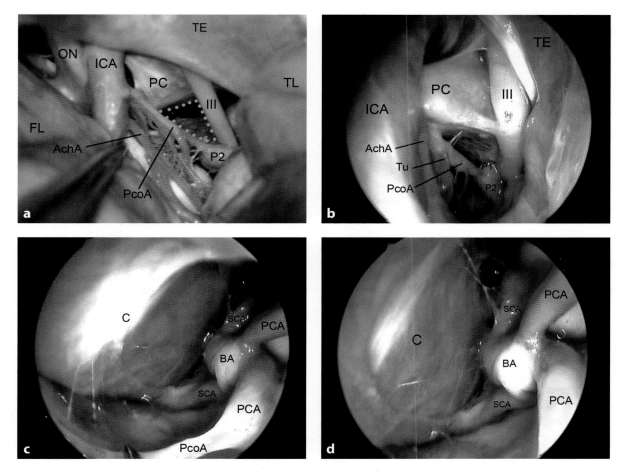

Fig. 4.12 Intradural exposure; right approach; microsurgical (**a**) and endoscopic (**b–d**) views. *AchA* anterior choroidal artery, *BA* basilar artery, *C* clivus, *FL* frontal lobe, *ICA* internal carotid artery, *III* oculomotor nerve, *ON* optic nerve, *P1* first segment of the posterior cerebral artery, *P2* second segment of the posterior cerebral artery, *PC* posterior clinoid, *PCA* posterior cerebral artery, *PcoA* posterior communicating artery, *SCA* superior cerebellar artery, *TE* tentorial edge, *TL* temporal lobe, *Tu* thalamoperforating artery; green dotted triangle area for entry of the endoscope into the interpeduncular fossa

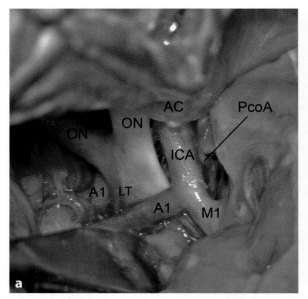

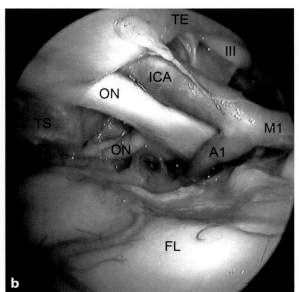

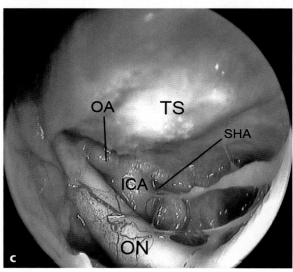

Fig. 4.13 Intradural exposure; right approach; microsurgical (**a**) and endoscopic omolateral (**b**) and contralateral (**c**) views. *A1* first segment of the anterior cerebral artery, *AC* anterior clinoid, *ICA* internal carotid artery, *FL* frontal lobe, *III* oculomotor nerve, *LT* lamina terminalis, *M1* first segment of the middle cerebral artery, *OA* left ophthalmic artery, *ON* optic nerve, *PcoA* posterior communicating artery, *SHA* superior hypophyseal artery, *TE* tentorial edge, *TS* tuberculum sellae

terior cerebral and the superior cerebellar arteries of the contralateral side as well as the ipsilateral posterior communicating artery and its perforators (Fig. 4.12b–d).

Another important role of the endoscope-assisted technique is the direct surgical clipping of superior hypophyseal and ophthalmic aneurysms without drilling of the anterior clinoid process (Fig. 4.13b,c). The microscopic view of these aneurysms may be obstructed by the ipsilateral internal carotid artery and the optic nerve (Fig. 4.13a).

4.10 Dura, Bone and Wound Closure

The dura mater can be sutured with a 4-0 silk suture using a single, interrupted or continuous suture. In this case intermittent knots are required every 3–4 cm for a perfect watertight closure, which is absolutely imperative. When the surgeon is convinced that there is no bleeding from the epidural space, also because of the transosseous tunnel which secures the dura elevated against the bony margin (Fig. 4.14a), the bone flap can be repositioned and fixed with single 0 silk sutures in the usual manner, with holes in both the free flap and the bone margin (Fig. 4.14b, c), or otherwise using miniplates and screws, or the different devices available on the market. The space created by the bone drilling can be filled with synthetic bone substitute.

Reapproximation of the temporal muscle requires caution and care to avoid atrophy and asymmetry. If a narrow myofascial cuff is attached to the bone at the level of the superior temporal line, after gentle repositioning of the muscle on the temporal fossa, it is sutured using single stitches to approximate and fix the muscle and then the fascia, taking care to preserve the

vascular supply and to achieve a good anatomical approximation (Fig. 4.14b). If the muscle has been disinserted completely from the temporal line, and there is no myofascial cuff, we place eight to ten holes corresponding to the temporal line using a high-speed drill (Fig. 4.14c); some authors place holes passing through the free bone flap, in which case the muscle has to be fixed before stabilizing the bone flap, or a silk suture with two needles at the extremities has to be used in order to pass through the muscle, since the flap has already been positioned. We prefer to place a couple of holes above and below the temporal line in order to

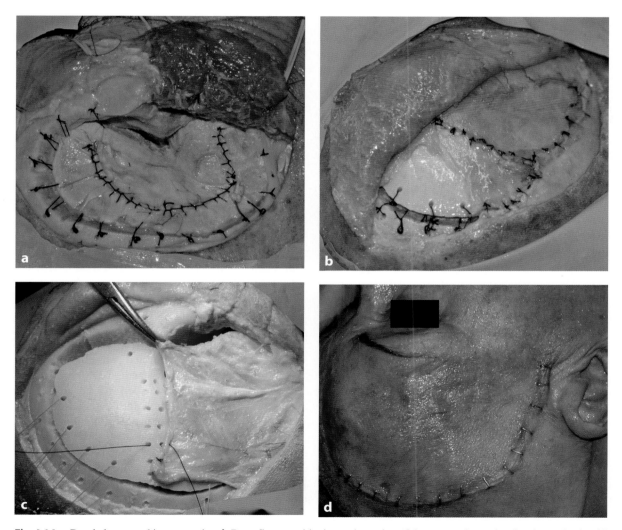

Fig. 4.14 **a** Dural closure and its suspension. **b** Bone flap repositioning and suturing of the temporal muscle when its tendon is still in sight. **c** Technique for temporal muscle closure when its tendon has been disinserted from the bone. **d** Skin closure with staples

obtain two tunnels in a diagonal direction, inclined more than 90°, then we pass a 3-0 vicryl stitch and fix the border of the muscle in correspondence with the superior temporal line. The suture of the temporal fascia concludes this step.

After reflection of the scalp and removal of the fish hooks, the subcutaneous tissue is sutured using 3-0 suture single stitches, then the cutaneous margins are reapproximated and sutured using a stapler or 2-0 silk suture or metal clips (Fig. 4.14d). A 24-hour subgaleal low suction drainage can be useful.

In conclusion, we can say that the main dangers and complications of the frontotemporal approach include: injury to the facial nerve and superficial temporal artery during the step of the skin incision, blood loss from the skin flap due to inadequate hemostasis, injury to the dura due to the craniotome while preparing the bone flap, injury to the vessels and nerves due to clumsy maneuvers, damage to the frontal and temporal lobes due to excessive retraction of the spatulas, intraparenchymal and/or subdural hematoma due to inadequate hemostasis, epidural hematoma due to a slack elevation suture of the dura, and hematoma of the soft tissues.

4.11 Extradural Anterior Clinoidectomy

Removal of the anterior clinoid process can be very useful for eradication of tumors or clipping of aneurysms located in the supra- and parasellar region by providing a wider surgical corridor to the optic nerve and carotid artery, reducing the need for brain retraction. The anterior clinoid is located at the medial end of the lesser sphenoid wing. It represents the lateral wall of the optic canal and covers the superior wall of the cavernous sinus.

Before starting the clinoidectomy it is extremely important to study a high-resolution CT scan to determine if there is a ring of bone formed by the junction of the anterior and middle clinoid processes, which surrounds the carotid artery before it becomes intradural. Removal of the clinoid in such a case carries a high risk of injury to the carotid artery. Another reason is to determine if the clinoid is pneumatized. Medial to the anterior clinoid is the optic nerve and laterally there is the superior orbital fissure.

After standard craniotomy and flattening of the sphenoid ridge and orbit, as described before, we usually first outline the superior orbital fissure, then we dissect the dura from the clinoid medially to expose the ridge of the optic canal and the falciform ligament. We drill the optic canal in order to expose 2–3 mm of the intraorbital segment of the nerve using a diamond. Obviously these maneuvers have to be performed under microscope magnification. We drill the bone of the optic canal coursing parallel to the nerve and never transversally from the medial to lateral limits of the nerve, because we have found that this involves less risk to the nerve, and we never push but just peel away the bone which is very thin, to avoid penetrating or drilling the nerve. Irrigation is extremely important to avoid burning it. It is not necessary, in our opinion, to drill more medially, since it may be possible to enter the ethmoid sinus, and for this reason the nerve is unroofed more on its superior and lateral surfaces (Fig. 4.15).

At this point we start drilling from the lateral border of the nerve, making a right angle to the course of the optic canal, in the direction of the superior orbital fissure. The drilling needs a lot of irrigation to preserve the anatomical structures which are in proximity to the anterior clinoid (optic nerve, carotid artery, oculomotor nerve). During drilling with the tip of the diamond burr, if the drill is temporarily stopped, we can feel if the process is still tightly adherent or if it has started to move. When it has moved, using a microdissector, we create a plane between the dura sited under the clinoid and the clinoid itself in order to remove it completely en bloc using a small rongeur.

Often we can observe bleeding coming from the cavernous sinus which can be stopped by packing with Gelfoam. A small piece of optic strut usually remains sited lateroinferiorly to the optic nerve; in this case and even if the en bloc removal is not possible, the remaining bone has to be drilled out very cautiously step by step.

Once the clinoid is completely removed, associated with flattening of the orbit, superiorly and laterally, the surgical corridor to the sellar and parasellar regions is markedly widened. After the standard dural opening for a pterional approach has been performed as described above, we cut the dura following the direction of the sylvian fissure toward the optic nerve, splitting the dura in two sheets, the frontal and the temporal, in order to have simultaneous intra- and extradural control of the optic nerve and carotid artery, and opening of the optic sheath and distal dural ring allows further mobilization of the two anatomical structures.

Complications related to the extradural anterior clinoidectomy include: opening of the ethmoid sinus or extensive drilling of the optic strut which lead into the

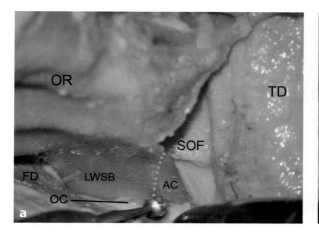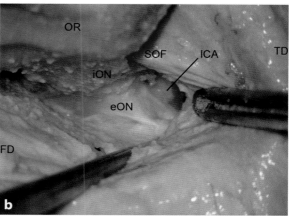

Fig. 4.15 Microsurgical view; extradural anterior clinoidectomy. **a** Exposure and drilling of the anterior clinoid process and optic canal under microscope magnification. **b** Widened space after complete removal of the AC. *AC* anterior clinoid, *eON* extracranial intracanalar optic nerve, *FD* frontal dura, *ICA* internal carotid artery, *iON* intraorbital optic nerve, *LWSB* lesser wing of sphenoid bone, *OC* optic canal, *OR* orbit roof, *SOF* superior orbital fissure, *TD* temporal dura

sphenoid sinus with consequent rhinorrhea (which is repaired using muscle strips and fibrin glue); oculomotor paresis due to manipulation of the third nerve which is in contact with the inferolateral surface of the clinoid; visual disturbance and quadrantanopsia as a consequence of manipulation of the ophthalmic artery; damage to the optic nerve due to the heat of drilling or to manipulation; injury to the carotid artery and/or ophthalmic artery; pneumocephalus; and rupture of aneurysms. Among 50 procedures we have experienced four cases of temporary oculomotor paresis, one case of severe visual deficit related to the drilling procedure, two cases of injury to the optic nerve due to its manipulation, and three cases of rhinorrhea due to paranasal sinus opening.

In our opinion, anterior clinoidectomy requires a certain level of experience which has to be obtained by cadaveric dissection.

4.12 Intradural Anterior Clinoidectomy

The main indication for intradural clinoidectomy is for aneurysm clipping. If the aneurysm is located at the basilar tip, on the carotid-ophthalmic artery, intracavernously, or on the internal carotid artery-posterior communicating artery, sometimes there is not enough space to apply the aneurysm clip or even a temporary

clip. For this reason it is absolutely necessary to remove as much bone as possible in order to enlarge the surgical corridor, and the anterior clinoid represents an obstacle. Its removal allows 4–6 mm more of the carotid artery to be exposed before entering the cavernous sinus. Usually after a standard frontotemporal approach and opening of the cisterns, we cut the dura covering the base of the clinoid in proximity to the optic canal running from the optic nerve in the direction of the superior orbital fissure.

Once this procedure is completed, we transect the dura in the middle of the clinoid process from the base toward the clinoid apex drawing a sort of T shape (Fig. 4.16a). In this way we dissect and split the dura over the clinoid into two sheets, medial and lateral, which we reflect, respectively, medially on the optic nerve, and laterally on the carotid artery to protect these structures.

Once the clinoid process has been exposed, cottonoid sponges are placed around the area to be drilled and on top of them we put a piece of surgeon's glove for more protection, then we can drill it totally or partially which is enough to provide more room. We always drill parallel to the optic nerve and to the carotid artery (Fig. 4.16b,c). This is the advantage of this procedure: to drill what we need under direct visual control of the anatomical structures. We have also used this procedure in meningiomas of the sphenoid ridge with huge reactive hyperostosis and bone infiltration.

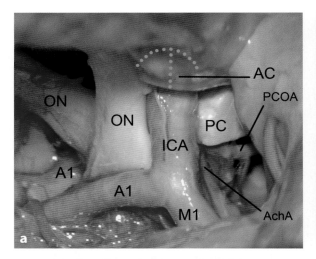

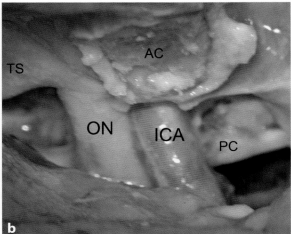

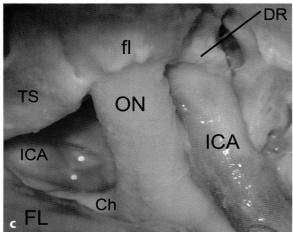

Fig. 4.16 Microsurgical view; intradural anterior clinoidectomy. **a, b** After the dura above the anterior clinoid process has been transected in a "T" shape (**a**), we usually drill always parallel to the optic nerve and to the carotid artery (**b**). **c** The distal ring is finally exposed. *A1* precommunicating anterior cerebral artery, *AC* anterior clinoid, *AchA* anterior choroid artery, *Ch* optic chiasm, *DR* distal ring, *fl* falciform ligament, *FL* frontal lobe, *ICA* internal carotid artery, *M1* first tract of the middle cerebral artery, *ON* optic nerve, *PC* posterior clinoid, *PCOA* posterior communicating artery, *TS* tuberculum sellae

In such cases it is extremely difficult to perform the extradural approach, because of bleeding and difficulty in orientation since the bony landmarks are lost. In these cases we prefer intradural drilling which we consider safer than extradural, but the latter has, in our opinion, some advantages: the dura protects the intradural structures which with intradural drilling are exposed to the risk of direct damage, the procedure is faster than intradural drilling because no delicate structures that can be damaged are in direct contact with the drilling burr, and because of the anatomy we find that the extent of bone removal is greater after the extradural procedure.

The same complications observed with the extradural procedure can also occur during and after the intradural approach.

4.13 Posterior Clinoidectomy

Removal of the posterior clinoid may be necessary in patients with a low basilar tip aneurysm or in those with sphenopetroclival tumors. Sometimes the bony prominence of this process which may be redundant, reduces the surgical corridor to the interpeduncular space, so there is inadequate room to place clips or to remove segments of tumor located posteriorly to the clivus. When we consider this maneuver necessary, we incise the dura covering the clinoid process at its base, then, as we do in intradural anterior clinoid drilling, we make a perpendicular incision from the base in the direction of the apex of the clinoid, creating a sort of T shape (Fig. 4.17a).

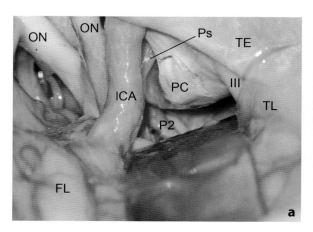
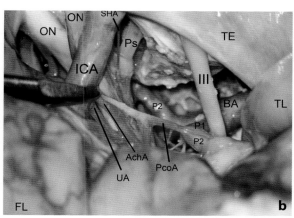

Fig. 4.17 Microsurgical view; posterior clinoidectomy. **a** Transection of the posterior clinoid process tip dura. **b** Anatomic exposure after posterior clinoidectomy. *AchA* anterior choroidal artery, *BA* basilar artery, *FL* frontal lobe, *ICA* internal carotid artery, *III* oculomotor nerve, *ON* optic nerve, *P1* precommunicating tract of the posterior cerebral artery, *P2* postcommunicating tract of the posterior cerebral artery, *PC* posterior clinoid, *PcoA* posterior communicating artery, *Ps* pituitary stalk, *SHA* superior hypophyseal artery, *TE* tentorium, *TL* temporal lobe, *UA* uncal artery

After dissecting the two sheets, medial and lateral, and reflecting them, we place cottonoid sponges around the clinoid with a piece of surgeon's glove on top of them, and with a small diamond burr start drilling from the tip of the clinoid process in the direction of the base, removing the bone we consider necessary to create sufficient space (Fig. 4.17b). Adequate irrigation is necessary. Great care has to be taken to avoid direct damage to the third nerve or to the vessels in close proximity to the clinoid. Bleeding can be controlled by bipolar coagulation or by using hemostatic tools in the event of penetration into the sphenopetroclival venous gulf [9].

4.14 General Considerations

The frontotemporal approach can be used to treat a large number of pathologies. It is beyond the scope of the present chapter to give a detailed discussion for every type of these lesions. Therefore, we present a discussion of general principles and recent applications for the most common pathologies approached through this route.

4.14.1 Vascular Lesions

The frontotemporal craniotomy can be considered the most significant and versatile approach in vascular surgery. In fact, 95% of aneurysms occur within the circle of Willis, usually in relation to the anterior and posterior communicating arteries and the bifurcations of the internal carotid, middle cerebral, and basilar arteries [10].

In our experience, a subfascial method of temporal muscle dissection and a tailored craniotomy provide adequate access to the anterior circle of Willis [11], excellent for aneurysms of the supra- and infraclinoidal internal carotid artery, the anterior communicating artery, and the middle cerebral artery. In selected cases basilar bifurcation aneurysms can be approached via this route.

The critical step to gain adequate exposure of the lesion is to disclose the floor of the anterior cranial fossa, this, in turn, requires accurate planning for keyhole placement, a wide craniotomy and extensive removal of the lateral sphenoid ridge and clinoid processes. When the cisterns are widely opened and the cerebrospinal fluid is drained, the surgeon has to define the anatomy of the aneurysm in order to choose the right corridor for the clip to be used. Sometimes ventricular drainage can be useful for minimizing the need for brain retraction.

For vascular pathology we always advocate a wide opening of the sylvian fissure that can be achieved using different techniques: a medial to lateral transsylvian approach following the middle cerebral artery from the proximal to the distal part, and opening the sylvian fissure from lateral to medial by following the distal branches of the middle cerebral artery. We favor dissecting the sylvian fissure through a small incision in the superior temporal gyrus with subpial dissection and identification of the distal branches of the middle cerebral artery, which can be followed proximally to the aneurysm. Otherwise, the surgeon can begin the dissection using one of the techniques mentioned above and change the approach if technical difficulties occur during the operation. It is important to proceed to one of the techniques depending on the location, direction and morphology of the aneurysm as well as the concomitant presence of subarachnoid hemorrhage or intraparenchymal hematoma.

Recent advances in instrumentation and neuroimaging have led to the use of microscope-integrated intraoperative near-infrared indocyanine green videoangiography during aneurysm surgery (Figs. 18 and 19). Furthermore, in many cases, this method is very useful to ensure vessel patency or complete occlusion of the aneurysm or malformation.

4.14.2 Meningiomas

These tumors account for about 20% of all primary brain tumors originating in the central nervous system, making them the most common. Meningiomas of the sphenoid wing, of the tuberculum sellae and planum sphenoidale, of the olfactory groove, of the orbital roof, and intracavernous, frontosphenoidal or temporosphenoidal tumors can be approached using frontotemporal craniotomy (Fig. 4.20).

Removal of these lesions follows the general principles of extraaxial brain tumor surgery, that is to devascularize the mass from its dural attachment, to dissect the meningioma from the brain following the arachnoidal plane, and to disconnect the leptomeningeal feeding vessels. In our opinion it is safer to debulk the tumor far from vital structures at the beginning of surgery, particularly if they are not in direct and close-up view. We advocate the use of bipolar for

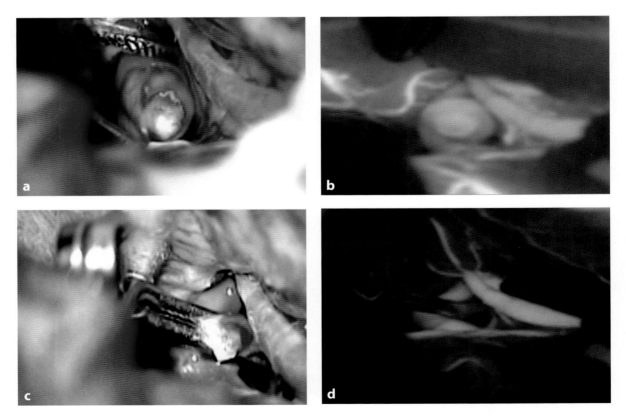

Fig. 4.18 Microsurgical view; middle cerebral artery aneurysm before (**a**) and after (**c**) clipping. Microscope-integrated intraoperative near-infrared indocyanine green videoangiography of the same case before (**b**) and after (**d**) clipping

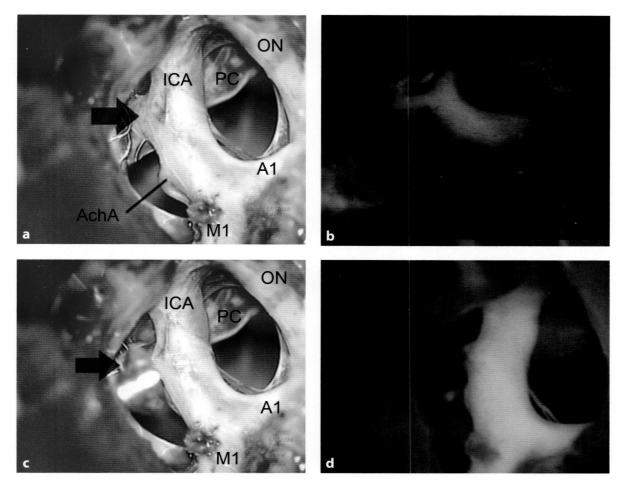

Fig. 4.19 Microsurgical view; posterior communicating artery aneurysm after clipping (**a**, **c**). Microscope-integrated intraoperative near-infrared indocyanine green videoangiography of the same case (**b**, **d**). *A1* first segment of the anterior cerebral artery, *AchA* anterior choroidal artery, *ICA* internal carotid artery, *M1* first segment of the middle cerebral artery, *ON* optic nerve, *PC* posterior clinoid

shrinking and coagulating, and ultrasonic aspirator for debulking. The dura infiltrated by the tumor has to be resected when the mass has been removed. The high-speed drill can be employed in the presence of hyperostotic or infiltrated bone. A diamond burr and generous irrigation are recommended.

4.14.3 Craniopharyngiomas

Craniopharyngiomas are histologically benign neuroepithelial tumors of the CNS and comprise approximately 3% of all intracranial tumors in adults, but 69%

in children. These lesions arise from squamous cell embryological rests found along the path of the primitive adenohypophysis and craniopharyngeal duct. Although histologically benign, these tumors frequently recur after surgical treatment. In addition, due to their specific location near critical intracranial structures (usually in strict relationship with the optic nerves, pituitary stalk and hypothalamus), both the tumor and the related medical and surgical complications can cause significant morbidity.

In our experience, the best treatment for these lesions is radical surgical excision. We usually approach the craniopharyngiomas via a standard frontotemporal approach because of proximal blood control of the in-

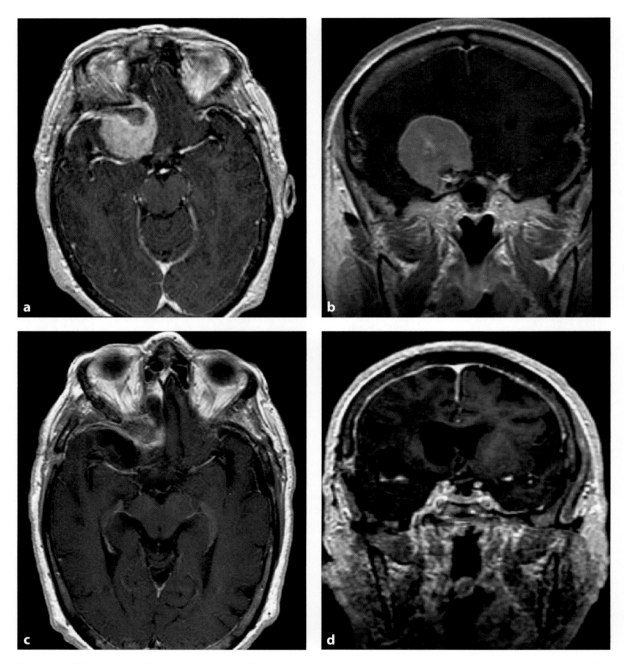

Fig. 4.20 MR images of a clinoidal meningioma. Preoperative (**a**, **b**) and postoperative (**c**, **d**) images show complete removal of the lesion

ternal carotid artery and optic nerves is advisable to safely dissect the tumor (Fig. 4.21). Sometimes it is necessary to combine this craniotomy with other approaches such as transsphenoidal, subfrontal interhemispheric or transcallosal.

4.15 Special Considerations

The frontolateral approach is generally utilized in the anterior circulation, for basilar tip aneurysms, and for lesions involving the sellar, parasellar, suprasellar and pre-

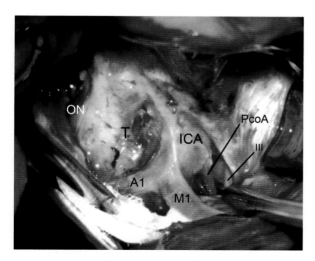

Fig. 4.21 Microsurgical view. Intraoperative exposure of an intra- and suprasellar craniopharyngioma. *A1* precommunicating tract of the anterior cerebral artery, *ICA* internal carotid artery, *III* oculomotor nerve, *M1* first tract of the middle cerebral artery, *ON* optic nerve, *PcoA* posterior communicating artery, *T* tumor

pontine regions. Furthermore, extrinsic tumors arising or invading the sphenoid ridge, the tuberculum sellae, the olfactory groove, the cavernous sinus, and the superior orbital fissure are approached through this route. This approach can also be used for intrinsic lesions of the anterior frontal, frontoorbital and superior temporal gyri. Advances in surgical technique, anesthesia, neuroimaging, and more recently endovascular techniques, may increase the success of treating lesions of these areas.

The extent and safety of the surgical procedure depend upon accurate preoperative planning and a rigor-

ous, methodical, step-by-step approach to the target, which should be secured with minimal manipulation to the surrounding structures. The main complications of this surgery are diplopia due to damage to the third, fourth and sixth cranial nerves, visual deficits due to direct or thermal injury from drilling of the optic nerve, damage to the carotid artery and its branches, lesions of the brain due to excessive brain retraction, and cerebrospinal fluid rhinorrhea.

The surgeon must obtain a complete and detailed history from the patient and/or parents. The history, in concert with a well-performed physical examination, is the basis for a diagnosis and treatment plan. Preoperative laboratory studies should include endocrine evaluation of lesions involving the sellar and parasellar areas consisting of baseline serum hormonal values.

General imaging studies include a thin-slice CT scan with 3-D reconstructions that can reveal abnormalities of the bone (erosion, hyperostosis) and tumor calcification. A gadolinium-enhanced brain MRI scan of intracranial lesions is fundamental to reaching the correct diagnosis, and coronal 3-D and sagittal or coronal 2-D phase-contrast imaging may also be used to show the relationship to adjacent arterial (displacement, occlusion) and venous (infiltration, occlusion) structures.

Cerebral angiography is effective if the lesion encroaches on the carotid or other major intracranial arteries or a major venous sinus. It is used to better assess whether arteries and venous sinuses are patent. In the case of meningioma and other vascular tumors and malformations, angiographic embolization of appropriate feeding vessels can decrease blood loss during operative resection and may contribute to complete lesion removal.

References

1. Yasargil MG (1984) Microneurosurgery, vol 1. Thieme, Stuttgart
2. Krause F (1908) Chirurgie des Gehirns und Rückenmarks: Nach eigenen Erfahrungen, vol I. Urban and Schwarzenberg, Berlin
3. Dandy WE (1918) A new hypophysis operation. Devised by Dr. G. J. Heuer. Bull John Hopkins Hosp 29:154–155
4. Heuer GJ (1920) Surgical experience with an intracranial approach to chiasmal lesions. Arch Surg 1:368–381
5. Borden WB, Tamargo RJ (2002) George J Heuer: forgotten pioneer neurosurgeon at the Johns Hopkins Hospital. J Neurosurg 96:1139–1146
6. Figueiredo EG, Deshmukh P, Zabramski JM et al (2005) Quantitative anatomic study of three surgical approaches to the anterior communicating artery complex. Neurosurgery 56:397–405; discussion 397–405
7. Gonzalez LF, Crawford NR, Horgan MA et al (2002) Working area and angle of attack in three cranial base approaches: pterional, orbitozygomatic, and maxillary extension of the orbitozygomatic approach. Neurosurgery 50:550–555; discussion 555–557
8. MacCarty CS (1961) The surgical treatment of intracranial meningiomas. Charles C. Thomas, Springfield
9. Iaconetta G, Fusco M, Samii M (2003) The sphenopetroclival venous gulf: a microanatomical study. J Neurosurg 99:366–375
10. Rhoton AL Jr (1980) Anatomy of saccular aneurysms. Surg Neurol 14:59–66
11. Yasargil MG, Fox JL (1975) The microsurgical approach to intracranial aneurysms. Surg Neurol 3:7–14

Orbitozygomatic Approach

5

Renato J. Galzio, Manfred Tschabitscher and Alessandro Ricci

5.1 Introduction

The orbitozygomatic (OZ) approach is an extension of the basic frontotemporal (FT) approach, which is associated with an OZ osteotomy and eventually with zygomatic arch resection. We emphasize that the basic FT approach, for us as for other authors, always includes resection of the sphenoid bridge (frontotemporopterional craniotomy).

Several different names have been used in the literature to identify the OZ craniotomy, including supraorbital, orbitocranial, orbitopterional (OPt), cranioorbital, cranioorbitozygomatic, frontoorbitozygomatic, frontotemporoorbitozygomatic (FTOZ), and others. The difference in the described flaps and techniques is subtle and the main purpose is to provide increased exposure beneath the frontal and temporal lobes.

The OZ approach is a combined anterolateral approach, which perfectly adheres to the conceptual principle of skull-base surgery of removing bone in order to minimize iatrogenic trauma. As any other approach to the cranial base, it provides a wide working room, a short working distance, a straight access and the possibility of handling the lesion from different angles of view with minimal manipulation and retraction of critical perilesional neurovascular structures.

Removal of the supraorbital rim to access the pituitary through a frontal craniotomy was described by McArthur in 1912 [1] and Frazier in 1913 [2]. Yasargil in 1969 introduced the pterional approach [3] and in

1975 combined this approach with a lateral orbital osteotomy to access anterior communicating artery (ACoA) aneurysms [4]. Jane et al. in 1982 extended the indications for supraorbital craniotomy to tumoral and vascular lesions located in the anterior cranial fossa and in the sellar, parasellar and orbital regions [5]. Pellerin et al. in 1984 [6], Hakuba et al. in 1986 [7] and Al-Mefty in 1987 [8] reported their experience with the use of OZ craniotomy, extending its indications to the treatment of lesions located not only in the anterior and middle cranial fossae, but also to those in the upper clival and nearby posterior cranial fossa regions. Since then, the approach has been widely adopted and a number of variations and modifications have been reported. The OZ craniotomy can either be performed in one single piece [6-12] or in two separate pieces [4, 5, 13, 14].

Some investigators have suggested osteoplastic craniotomies to avoid temporalis muscle atrophy, especially in the pediatric population [15-17]; however, most authors suggest nonpedunculated osteotomies because this is the simplest way to perform the flap and because careful dissection of soft tissues generally does not produce worse cosmetic results.

The addition of zygomatic arch resection has been proposed to achieve a wider access to the infratemporal fossa, for lesions deeply located in the central skull base or for high-positioned or very complex basilar artery aneurysms. The zygomatic arch can be resected together with the OZ flap or as a separate piece, attached to the masseter muscle insertion or completely detached [13, 14, 18-22].

In 2004, we reported that forced mouth opening associated with the OZ approach may provide a wider exposure of the infratemporal fossa and of the lateral splanchnocranial spaces, allowing the removal of ex-

R.J. Galzio (✉)
Dept of Health Sciences, University of L'Aquila, and
Dept of Neurosurgery, San Salvatore Hospital, L'Aquila, Italy

P. Cappabianca et al. (eds.), *Cranial, Craniofacial and Skull Base Surgery.*
© Springer-Verlag Italia 2010

tensive benign tumors expanding into multiple intracranial and extracranial compartments, without adding destructive procedures affecting the mandibular bone and avoiding associated transfacial approaches [23].

There are a number of quantitative anatomical studies and reports of computed 3D virtual reconstructions that objectively demonstrate the increased operative exposure and the widening of the angles of attack resulting from orbital rim removal, OZ osteotomy and/or zygomatic arch dislocation [24-26].

The OZ approach is indicated in the treatment of challenging vascular and neoplastic lesions. Potential complications may be related both to the complexity of the treated pathology and to the operative procedure. Careful technique, based on precise performance of the surgical steps, is mandatory to achieve satisfactory results. The OZ craniotomy may be tailored and adapted according to site, extension and size of the lesion to be treated.

The OZ approach is the most widely used and studied cranial base approach and a number of modifications have been described. It is useful for each surgical team to standardize their technique. We consider cadaveric dissections extremely important to achieve adequate surgical skills in skull-base surgery. We have evolved and better focused our technique in the Institute of Anatomy and Cell Biology of the Medical University of Vienna.

In our institution we essentially use two different variants of the approach: the complete OZ (FTOZ) approach, performed in two pieces, and a more limited single-piece craniotomy (OPt). These approaches are described in detail, focusing on the surgical steps and also considering the indications, advantages, possible complications and their prevention. Knowledge of the anatomical structures, layers and regions, and of the origin and course of arteries and nerves, makes possible the best preparation for these approaches and allows adequate reconstruction, preserving function and esthetics and avoiding complications. Finally, an anatomical note of the anterolateral cranial region is introduced.

5.2 Anatomy of the Anterolateral Cranial Region and Related Structures

Frontal, parietal, temporal, zygomatic and sphenoid bones, connected through their respective sutures, form the anterolateral aspect of the skull. The pterion is the most important cephalometric landmark of this region; it indicates the point where the frontal, parietal, temporal, and sphenoid bones meet (Fig. 5.1). The periosteum covering the skull is termed the pericranium. At the level of the temporal bone, the periosteum strictly adheres to the inner surface of the temporalis muscle [27]. The floor of the anterior cranial fossa is mainly formed by the orbital process of the frontal bone, which is somewhat convex with a number of (orbital) crests, that may be more or less developed. The frontal crest is located anteriorly in the midline. This bony ridge separates the two sides and gives attachment to the falx cerebri, which contains the origin of the superior and inferior sagittal sinuses. The central portion of the anterior fossa is much deeper and is formed by the ethmoid bone, with the medial area being the cribriform plate and the lateral area being the fovea ethmoidalis, which represents the roof of the ethmoid sinus. The crista galli is centrally located to separate the two cribriform plates that show multiple perforations transmitting the olfactory nerve filaments. The foramen cecum is located between the frontal crest and the crista galli. Usually fibrous dural attachments plug this blindly ending foramen, although rarely it may contain a persistent anterior nasal emissary vein (normally existing in young children).

Lateral to the cribriform plate, the cribroethmoid foramina give passage to the anterior, middle and posterior ethmoidal arteries. The posterior portion of the anterior fossa is formed by the upper part of the body and lesser wings of the sphenoid bone. Centrally lies the planum or jugum sphenoidale, which constitutes the roof of the sphenoid sinus, bordered posteriorly by the anterior chiasmatic sulcus. Laterally, the lesser wing of the sphenoid roofs the optic canal, which transmits the optic nerve with its dural sheath to the orbit, and forms a sharp posterior bony border, in which the sphenoparietal sinus is hosted. The anterior clinoid process, the medial end of the lesser sphenoid wing, covers the anteromedial portion of the cavernous sinus containing the internal carotid artery (ICA), where this artery forms its final loop before entering the dura. The anterior clinoid process gives attachment to the tentorium cerebelli. The butterfly-shaped middle cranial fossa extends from the lesser wing of the sphenoid to the petrous ridge of the temporal bone, formed by the body and greater wings of the sphenoid bone and by the squamous and petrous portions of the temporal bone. It is bounded in front by the anterior chiasmatic sulcus, the anterior clinoid processes and the posterior margins of the lesser wings of the sphenoid,

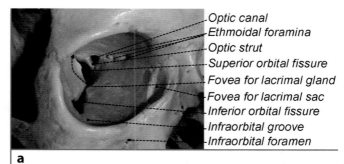

Optic canal
Ethmoidal foramina
Optic strut
Superior orbital fissure
Fovea for lacrimal gland
Fovea for lacrimal sac
Inferior orbital fissure
Infraorbital groove
Infraorbital foramen

a

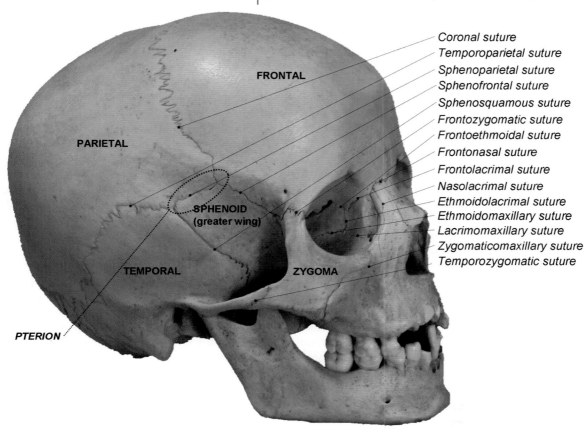

FRONTAL

PARIETAL

SPHENOID
(greater wing)

TEMPORAL

ZYGOMA

PTERION

Coronal suture
Temporoparietal suture
Sphenoparietal suture
Sphenofrontal suture
Sphenosquamous suture
Frontozygomatic suture
Frontoethmoidal suture
Frontonasal suture
Frontolacrimal suture
Nasolacrimal suture
Ethmoidolacrimal suture
Ethmoidomaxillary suture
Lacrimomaxillary suture
Zygomaticomaxillary suture
Temporozygomatic suture

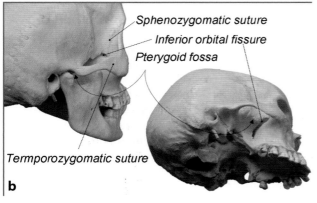

Sphenozygomatic suture
Inferior orbital fissure
Pterygoid fossa

Termporozygomatic suture

b

Fig. 5.1 Anterolateral aspect of the skull and relative sutures with the particulars of the internal surface of the orbit (**a**) and of the inferior orbital fissure (**b**)

behind by the dorsum sellae and the posterior border of the petrous bone, and laterally by the sphenoparietal and temporoparietal sutures. It is traversed by the squamosal, sphenoparietal, sphenosquamosal, and sphenopetrosal sutures.

The central part of the middle fossa shows in front the prechiasmatic sulcus (chiasmatic groove) and the tuberculum sellae. The prechiasmatic sulcus ends on either side at the optic foramen, which transmits the optic nerve and ophthalmic artery to the orbital cavity. The tuberculum sellae is a transverse ridge that separates the chiasmatic groove anteriorly from the sella turcica posteriorly. The sella turcica is a deep rounded depression that cradles the pituitary gland. On either side of the sella turcica, the carotid groove contains the sigmoid curve of the ICA as it courses from the petrous apex through the cavernous sinus. The sella turcica is bounded posteriorly by a quadrilateral plate of bone, the dorsum sellae, the upper angles of which are the posterior clinoid processes, that afford further attachment to the tentorium cerebelli. The posterior biclinoidal line is a line passing between the apex of the two posterior clinoidal processes. It is an important landmark that can be visualized in preoperative neuroimaging studies. Below each posterior clinoid process, a notch for the abducens nerve is found. Occasionally a middle clinoid process exists that can be bridged to the anterior clinoid, so forming a caroticoclinoid foramen, through which passes the ICA.

The lateral parts of the middle fossa are the wider portion of the middle skull base and are marked by depressions and crests and traversed by furrows for the anterior and posterior branches of the middle meningeal vessels. These furrows begin near the foramen spinosum, where the middle meningeal artery enters the cranium, and the anterior runs forward and upward to the sphenoidal angle of the parietal bone, while the posterior runs laterally and backward across the squama temporalis and the parietal bone. There are several depressions and elevations in the floor of the middle cranial fossa. The trigeminal impression, containing the stem of the trigeminal nerve, is located anterolateral to the foramen lacerum at the apex of the petrous ridge. Posterior to this, the eminentia arcuata overlies the superior semicircular canal. The tegmen tympani, a thin bone plate roofing the middle ear, is situated anterolateral to the eminentia arcuata, with the hiatus and the groove of the greater superficial petrosal nerve (GSPn) located in between. The groove of the GSPn courses obliquely from posterior to anterior and from lateral to medial, directed towards the foramen lacerum, and represents an impor-

tant landmark because it courses parallel and immediately superior and lateral to the canal containing the ICA in its horizontal intrapetrous portion.

A number of important foramina are found in the mesial floor of the middle cranial fossa. Anteriorly is the superior orbital fissure (SOF), which leads to the orbital cavity. Inferior and lateral to the SOF, the foramen rotundum transmits the maxillary division (V2) of the trigeminal nerve; this is in effect a canal of about 4 mm length. Posterolateral to the foramen rotundum, the foramen ovale transmits the mandibular division (V3) and the motor branch (V3m) of the trigeminal nerve together with the lesser superficial petrosal nerve. The foramen spinosum lies posterior and lateral to the foramen ovale. Upmost medially, where the petrous apex articulates with the sphenoid bone, an irregularly rounded opening to the carotid canal is formed, which represents the cranial outlet of the foramen lacerum (Fig. 5.2) [27-30].

In the mesial surface of the middle cranial fossa is lodged the cavernous sinus. An accurate description of this complex structure is beyond the scope of this chapter. Briefly, it is a hexagonal lacunar venous (it is a matter of discussion whether it is plexiform or sinusoidal) structure with proper dural walls. The anterior wall is hidden under the anterior clinoid process, the superior and lateral walls are continuous, with the tentorial edge in between, The superior wall is entered by the third cranial nerve and, more posterior and lateral, by the fourth cranial nerve, and the lateral wall is formed by two different dural layers: an external one, represented by the dura of the temporal lobe, and a thinner connective internal layer strictly adherent to the periosteum of the sphenoidal bone. The ICA and the first division of the trigeminal nerve penetrate the cavernous sinus through this wall. The medial wall corresponds to the dura propria covering the sella turcica. The inferior wall is formed by the periosteum of the sphenoid bone in the angle between the body and great wing. The posterior wall lies between the middle and posterior fossa, represented by the petroclinoid fold, through which the sixth cranial nerve penetrates inside. The cavernous sinus contains the intracavernous ICA and the sixth cranial nerve, located medially to the internal layer of the lateral wall, while the third and fourth cranial nerves and the first division of the trigeminal nerve cross inside it, located between the two layers of the lateral wall.

The ICA originates from the common carotid artery at the level of the third/fourth cervical vertebrae and enters the carotid canal of the petrous bone. It ascends vertically for about 5 mm and then turns anteromedially

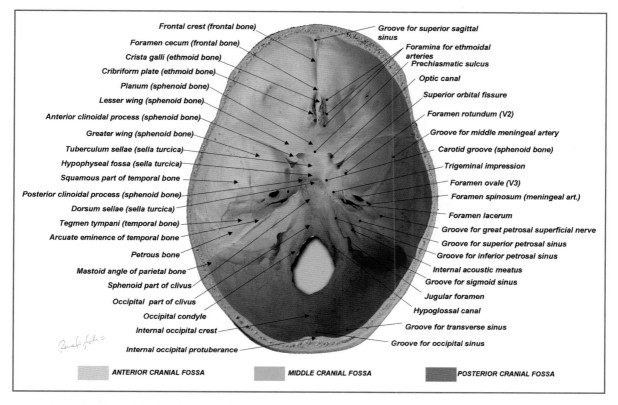

Fig 5.2 Internal surface of the skull base with the three cranial fossae and the main bone landmarks

(posterior loop) into the horizontal portion, medial to the eustachian tube and slightly inferior and anterolateral to the cochlea. The horizontal portion of the intrapetrous ICA runs obliquely from posterior to anterior and from lateral to medial in a bony canal, which may be dehiscent in its superior wall, under Meckel's cave to enter the cavernous sinus laterally and from below. In the cavernous sinus the ICA is embedded in the venous plexus and forms three loops: lateral, medial and anterior. The ICA penetrates the basal frontal dura lateroinferiorly to the optic nerve entrance in its canal. The superior wall of the cavernous sinus forms a fibrous ring (internal ring) around the ICA, while the dura mater forms a second superior ring (external ring), less firmly attached. The cervical ICA gives no branches, but its intrapetrous portion gives off caroticotympanic and pterygoid branches. The intracavernous ICA provides a number of branches mainly supplying the cranial nerves contained in the cavernous sinus, the pituitary, and the tentorial and clival dura (Fig. 5.3) [28, 29, 31].

The orbit is the cavity containing the eye and related structures. It is limited by four walls: superior, inferior, medial and lateral. The superior wall, or orbital roof, is formed by the orbital process of the frontal bone. The superior bony margin of the orbit is defined by the (supra)orbital rim. In its medial portion is located the supraorbital notch or foramen, from which the supraorbital nerve emerges. The lateral wall is formed by the zygomatic and sphenoidal bones, the inferior wall corresponds to the orbital portion of the maxillar and palatine bones, while the medial wall is formed by the ethmoidal and lacrimal bones. In the orbital cavity there are two fissures and one canal. The SOF, located in the posterior part of the orbital wall, between the greater and the lesser wings of the sphenoid, transmits from the cranial cavity the ophthalmic, oculomotor, trochlear and abducens nerves, as well as the superior ophthalmic vein. The inferior orbital fissure (IOF) is a cleft between the greater wing of the sphenoid and the orbital surface of the maxilla for passage of the zygomatic and infraorbital nerve and vessels. The maxillary division

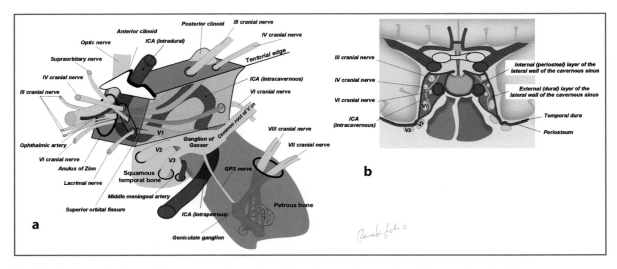

Fig 5.3 Schematic drawings of the cavernous sinus viewed from the lateral aspect (**a**) and in coronal section (**b**)

(V2) of the trigeminal nerve, in effect, enters the pterygopalatine fossa through the foramen rotundum, which is separated from the SOF by a bony bridge called the maxillary strut. After a short course in the pterygopalatine fossa, the maxillary nerve enters the IOF in its middle portion to become the infraorbital nerve, which runs together with the infraorbital artery in the infraorbital groove (sulcus infraorbitalis). The groove anteriorly acquires a bony roof and becomes the infraorbital canal, which leads to the infraorbital foramen.

The optic canal contains the optic nerve with its dural sheath and the ophthalmic artery. The optic strut is a thin lamina of bone located in the inferomedial wall of the optic canal, which separates it from the infraclinoid ICA at level of the anterior loop. The lacrimal gland lies in the fovea located in the superolateral angle. The lacrimal sulcus, the groove-like beginning of the nasolacrimal canal, and the fossa of lacrimal sac are located in the superomedial portion of the orbit, between the anterior and posterior lacrimal crests, near the anterior ethmoidal foramen, which gives passage to the anterior ethmoidal nerve and vessels. The periostium of the orbital cavity is termed the periorbita and is solidly adherent to the bone at the inlet and outlet of the orbit. It contains the oculomotor muscles and nerves, the first branch of the trigeminal nerve and the optic nerve and eyeball, which is contained in a gliding connective tissue membrane (Tenon's capsule). The terminal branch of the ophthalmic nerve exits the periorbita and passes to the frontal region through the supra-

orbital notch, that sometimes forms a true foramen (Fig. 5.1, parts A and B) [27, 30].

Over the outer anterolateral aspect of the skull, two different muscular layers are found. The deep craniofacial muscular layer is represented by the masticatory muscles, all innervated by the motor branch of the third division of the trigeminal nerve (V3), that comes out from the foramen ovale, and mainly vascularized by branches from the maxillary artery. The temporalis muscle, the most important of the masticatory muscles providing for more than 50% of the mandibular action, has its inferior attachment in the coronoid process of the mandible while its distal fibers are attached at the level of the superior and the inferior temporal lines; the muscle lies directly on the periosteum; it is covered by a fascia muscularis propria, which represents the inner layer of the superficial temporal fascia, attached superiorly to the superior temporal line and inferiorly to the inner margin of the zygomatic arch. Proper arteries (deep temporal arteries, branches of the internal maxillary artery) and nerves (deep temporal nerves) of the temporal muscle course in its deep surface, immediately over the subperiosteal plane.

The masseter muscle is attached superiorly to the zygomatic arch (mainly formed by the zygomatic process of the temporal bone) and inferiorly to the mandibular angle. This muscle is also provided with a proper muscular fascia and receives innervation and vascularization from its deeper surface. The other masticatory muscles, lateral and medial pterygoid muscles, lie in the subtemporal pterygoid space. The superficial musculoaponeurotic layer (epicranius muscle) lies over the deep muscular layer. It is formed by the mimic muscles, innervated by the frontal branch of the facial nerve and vascularized mainly by the superficial temporal artery (STA). The galea aponeurotica is the common tendon of all these muscles. Over the temporalis muscle the galea constitutes the external layer of the superficial temporal fascia (fascia temporalis superficialis): it is attached inferiorly to the outer margin of the zygomatic arch and superiorly shows reinforced adhesions to the proper muscular fascia at level of its insertion in the superficial temporal line.

The superficial aponeurotic layer represents the continuation of the fascia cervicofacialis superficialis, which contains all the facial mimic muscles, including the orbicularis oculi. The facial nerve (cranial nerve VII) in its intraparotid portion gives rise to the frontotemporal branch, which innervates the frontal muscles and partly the orbicularis oculi (also innervated by the zygomatic branch). The frontotemporal branch crosses over the zygomatic arch approximately 2 cm anterior to the tragus, within 1 cm from the anterior division of the STA and runs in the fat pad contained between the galea and the fascia temporalis propria. The derma and skin are innervated anterolaterally by the supraorbital nerve (the thickest distal branch of V1, which conveys sensation from the forehead, conjunc-

tiva, upper eyelid and frontal sinus) and posterolaterally by the auriculotemporal nerve (distal branch of V3, coming from the foramen ovale, crossing over the posterior root of the zygomatic arch and running posterior to the STA and anterior to the tragus in the supragaleal plane) [32-34]. Figure 5.4 depicts the relationships of the arteries and nerves of the superficial planes of the anterolateral cranial region with the temporal muscle and its fascial layers.

5.3 Operative Technique

5.3.1 Frontotemporoorbitozygomatic Approach

We prefer to perform the FTOZ approach as a two-piece nonosteoplastic craniotomy not only because it results simpler, but also because it may be more easily adapted and tailored, based on the specific pathology to be treated. Moreover the two-piece OZ craniotomy allows more extensive orbital roof removal and better visualization of the basal frontal lobe, so that the risks of enophthalmus and poor cosmetic results are reduced [26].

We rarely use lumbar drainage, which in any case is contraindicated in the presence of a large supratentorial

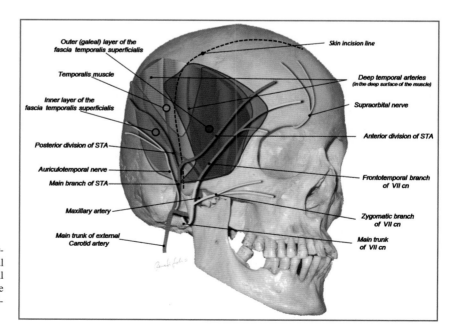

Fig 5.4 Relationships of the arteries and nerves of the superficial planes of the anterolateral cranial region with the temporal muscle and its fascial layers (*STA* superficial temporal artery).

mass, obstructive hydrocephalus and a ruptured aneurysm operated on in the immediate posthemorrhagic period. Controlled cerebrospinal fluid (CSF) removal, on the other hand, relaxes the brain and minimizes the use of retraction in the treatment of unruptured (or not recently bleeding) complex aneurysms and in parasellar and juxta-clival lesions.

Orotracheal intubation is used, with the tube coming out from the contralateral angle of the mouth and securely fixed by plasters to the skin to avoid its migration.

The patient is placed supine with a soft gelatin roll under the ipsilateral shoulder to reduce neck torsion and to improve venous drainage. The arms, secured at the patient's side, are padded to avoid pressure on nerves and arteries. Both legs are slightly flexed at the knee to avoid hyperextension injury, and are wrapped with sequential compression devices to reduce venous stasis and to prevent thromboembolic complications. The operating table is adjusted so that the trunk and head are elevated about 20° for additional improvement of cerebral venous outflow. Once secured to a Mayfield three-point headrest, taking care that the pins are kept far away from the planned incision site, the head is extended backward over the neck about 10-15° so that the malar eminence remains the highest point in the operative field; this maneuver allows the frontal and temporal lobes to fall by gravity away from the bony basal structures for better surgical access with minimal need for retraction. Finally the head is rotated 15-60° to the contralateral side. The degree of rotation is dictated by the location and extension of the targeted lesion: 30° rotation brings the perpendicular axis of vision directly to the anterior clinoidal process, at the point where the optic nerve enters its canal and the ICA becomes intradural; rotation is increased for lesions involving the middle anterior fossa and the lateral fossa, decreased for lesions involving the orbital, juxtasellar and clival regions. During the operation, with the head-holder rigidly fixed to the table, the head position may be altered to optimize the surgical view by turning and/or tilting the table itself; the angle of the microscope can also be manipulated to obtain multidirectional viewing. Figure 5.5 shows the position of the patient on the operating table.

The soft tissues of the superficial planes are prepared in the interfascial mode [32]. The skin incision is started below the posterior root of the zygomatic arch, 1 cm anterior to the tragus, continued superiorly along the line of the posterior third of the temporal muscle, and then frontally curved toward the opposite superior temporal line, in a bicoronal fashion, remaining whenever possible at least 1 cm behind the hairline. The position of this incision preserves the main trunk of the STA, that courses behind it together with the auriculotemporal nerve over the galea, and the frontotemporal branch of the facial nerve, which is located in the areolar fat between the outer (galea) and inner (fascia muscularis propria) layers of the superficial temporal fascia, crossing over the zygomatic arch about 2 cm anterior to the tragus.

The skin flap is sharply dissected from the galea and reflected anteroinferiorly. Acute folding of the flap may interfere with the blood supply and subsequently cause bad scarring of the skin incision. The scalp posterior to the incision is undermined and a flap formed by galea and pericranium is incised from below and along both superior temporal lines, carefully dissected subperiosteally preserving the periosteal blood supply, and turned downward. This galeal-pericranial flap will be available during the reconstructive phase for paranasal sinus repair and prevention of CSF leakage. The inferior limits of the lateral incisions of the flap are at least 2.5 cm distal to the orbitozygomatic suture to preserve the frontotemporal branch of cranial nerve VII, which remains below. At this level, the outer (galea) and inner (fascia temporalis propria) layers of the fascia temporalis superficialis are then incised together in an oblique direction toward the posterior root of the zygomatic arch. The inferior portion of the incised superficial temporalis fascia (with the frontotemporal branch of the facial nerve inside its two layers) is reflected inferiorly together with the galeal-pericranial flap. Sharp subperiosteal dissection further exposes the orbital rim to the zygoma. The supraorbital nerve, which may be in a notch or in a true foramen, is reflected with the flap. Small osteotomes or a high-speed drill are used to free the nerve and its accompanying vessels, if it is contained in a foramen.

A second incision is performed posteriorly in the fascia temporalis superficialis, comprising both its external and internal layers, from the superior temporal line to the posterior zygomatic root, along the posterior third of the temporal muscle. The fascial incisions join at the posterior root of the zygomatic arch and the temporalis fascia (with all its layers) remains adherent to the superior temporal line attachment, forming a triangle with two free sides joining at the inferior vertex. The superior portion of the fascia temporalis superficialis is dissected free from the outer surface of the temporal muscle and elevated superiorly while remaining attached to the superior temporal line to form a large fascial cuff that will be used later for reconstruction.

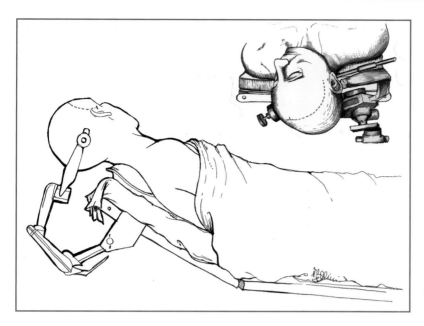

Fig 5.5 Positioning of the patient on the operating table

The inferior portion of the same fascia is reflected down with the galeal-pericranial flap to completely expose the lateral part of the orbital rim, the temporal process of the zygomatic bone and the zygomatic arch, which is dissected subperiosteally preserving its attachment to the masseter muscle. Subsequently, the zygomatic arch may be sectioned at its extremities using an oscillating saw, a Gigli saw or a thin high-speed drill, and turned down attached to the masseter muscle; the zygomatic cuts should be oblique for secure reattachment of the arch; preplating the bone at the level of the cutting lines makes its reconstruction easier.

The temporal muscle is then sectioned posteriorly along the direction of its fibers. A second superior incision is performed in the muscle at the level of its attachment to the inferior temporal line to leave a narrow muscular cuff for subsequent reconstruction. The muscle is mobilized from the calvaria using a subperiosteal elevator. This subperiosteal dissection is better performed in a retrograde fashion, from inferior to superior and from posterior to anterior in order to better preserve the deep arterial feeders and nerves that course in the medial surface of the temporalis muscle just superficially to the periosteum; to minimize muscle atrophy, monopolar cauterization has absolutely to be avoided [14, 32-34]. The temporalis muscle is then turned downward. The lateral wall of the orbit becomes evident and can be freed from the last attachments of the

temporal muscle until the anterolateral portion of the IOF is exposed at the level of the suture between the greater wing of the sphenoid and the zygomatic bone. If the zygomatic arch has been sectioned, the muscle is passed between its residual extremities and further retracted. Resection of the zygomatic arch is not always performed; it is only indicated when a wide exposure of the lower middle fossa is programmed.

The periorbita is then freed from the supralateral orbital margin to a depth of 2.5 to 3 cm; the periorbita is continuous with the frontal periosteum and preserving the base of the pericranial flap during its former preparation is helpful in defining the periorbital plane and in keeping it intact during its separation from the roof and lateral wall of the orbit. The periorbita is most adherent at the level of the frontozygomatic suture, and once freed at this point a plane is defined for further dissection. The periorbital dissection is thereafter best started laterally, taking care not to endanger the lacrimal gland, which is located just medial to the suture. Medially, the trochlear swing sling insertion must be preserved. Dissection of the periorbita is brought laterally to expose the lateral borders of the superior and inferior orbital fissures. Disruption of the periorbita allows the yellowish orbital fat to come out. Bipolar coagulation may be used to reduce bulging cumbersome fat if the disruption is small, but large breaks in the periorbita have to be repaired with absorbable sutures. Violation of the periorbita leads to increased postoperative periorbital swelling and bruising and may increase the risk of late enophthalmus. After the periorbita is freed, the galeal-pericranial and temporalis muscle flaps are retracted, together with the underlying scalp flap, with downward directed hooks to fully expose the anterolateral bony surface of the skull.

The FTOZ craniotomy is then performed. A frontotemporal flap is prepared first, with drilling of the sphenoid ridge as routinely performed for a standard pterional approach. The osteotomy can be extended anteriorly and medially toward the frontal midline or inferoposteriorly toward the temporalis fossa, as needed to expose the targeted lesional area. Because the FTOZ approach is used to treat particularly complex and extensive lesions, normally the osteotomy is extended medially to the supraorbital notch in the frontal region and is pushed low and posterior in the temporal area. Usually three burr holes are made using a cranial perforator or a round-tipped high-speed drill. The first hole is placed in the frontal bone immediately behind the frontozygomatic suture. The second burr hole is placed in the lowermost exposed squamous temporal bone, just posterior to the sphenosquamosal suture, about 2 cm anterior to the posterior root of the zygomatic arch. The third burr hole is placed at the level of the temporoparietal suture, anterior to the temporal line. Some bone dust may be retained when the holes are made, to be placed along the reapposed bony edges of the frontotemporal craniotomy during reconstruction. The dura mater underlying the holes is then dissected free with a subperiosteal elevator; if it is strongly adherent to the bone of the inner cranial surface, a further fourth hole is placed just lateral to the midline in the frontal bone above the nasion; this hole has to expose the frontal dura immediately lateral to the superior sagittal sinus, eventually perforating both the anterior and posterior walls of the frontal air sinus.

Using the drill and small osteotomes to remove the bony bridge formed by the greater wing of the sphenoid, a basal craniectomy joining the first two holes is performed. With a high-speed powered craniotome, the second and third holes are connected. The osteotomy is initially directed horizontally and posteriorly in the squama of the temporal bone for 2 to 3 cm and is then curved superiorly toward the temporoparietal hole. An osteotomy is then cut from the third hole to the superior orbital rim, in a curved fashion directed from posterior to superior, passing behind the musculofascial cuff, and then anteroinferiorly toward the frontal basis medial to the supraorbital notch; the roof of the orbit will stop the

craniotome. When a fourth hole has been placed, the osteotomy ends at its level. In most cases the lower part of this osteotomy will enter the frontal sinus, severing its external and internal walls.

Finally, an osteotomy is made starting at the burr hole located in the frontal bone near the OZ suture and directed, just above and parallel to the orbital rim, toward the frontal ending of the previous bony cut (or toward the fourth hole). Periosteal elevators are used to further dissect the dura from the inner bony surface and to remove the frontotemporal flap. After mobilization of the flap, the frontal sinus is exposed. Its posterior wall is then removed, the mucosa is exenterated and the ostium of the frontal sinus is plugged with muscle or fat held in place with fibrin glue. These maneuvers constitute the so-called "cranialization" of the sinus and all instruments used to perform it, and thereafter exposed to the nonsterile environment of the air sinus, are kept separate and resterilized while surgical team redresses.

Usually, the dura is secured to the bone with multiple sutures passed through tiny holes drilled all along the frontoparietal edge of the craniotomy. The basally exposed dura is then dissected with small subperiosteal elevators from the frontal floor (until the anterior clinoid process and the distal entrance of the optic canal are fully exposed), from the sphenoid ridge (until the lateral portion of the SOF is exposed), and from the anterolateral and inferior borders of the temporal fossa (until the foramen rotundum, ovale and spinosum and also the petrous portion of the temporal bone, if necessary, are exposed). Brain detension, obtained by administration of osmotics and diuretics and rarely by CSF subtraction, is helpful in this phase. The residual medial portion of the sphenoid bridge is drilled away until the SOF is reached. A small artery (recurrent meningeal branch of the ophthalmic artery or orbitomeningeal artery) is invariably seen passing from the temporal dura to the orbit at the lateral edge of the SOF and represents a valuable landmark for dural dissection. The lateral and superior borders of the SOF are enlarged using punches and small osteotomes to be successively connected with the bony cuts for the OZ osteotomy. In particular, the most deep and medial portion of the orbital roof overlying the orbital entrance of the optic nerve is rongeured away. The bony crests in the orbital process of the frontal bone are also drilled away if they are exuberant. The bone of the temporal fossa is then drilled or rongeured away until the medially located foramina are seen and eventually freed. Normally we prefer to drill these bony structures under microscopic magnification, particularly while proceeding to the depth.

The OZ osteotomy can then be performed. The first cut is made with a thin-pointed drill at the level of the inferior aspect of the lateral orbital rim, just over the zygomatic root of the arch (which has been previously sectioned), directed toward the anterolateral border of the IOF. The IOF may be difficult to expose when the angle between the external surface of the lateral wall of the orbit and the outer anteroinferior border of the temporal fossa, just overlying the pterygoid space, is particularly tight. In this infrequent case, a notch may be drilled in the temporal floor, inferior and lateral to the foramen rotundum, to better control the anterolateral portion of the IOF. A second osteotomy is then performed from the IOF to the lateral edge of the SOF; this cut, sectioning the inferomedial part of the greater sphenoid wing, is more easily performed if the SOF has been previously enlarged, exposing the periorbita at the level where it is continuous with the temporal dura. A third osteotomy is then cut in the medial aspect of the orbital roof, under direct visualization, from the superior orbital rim to the superior edge of the SOF, which also has been previously enlarged medially to expose the periorbita at the point where it becomes continuous with the dura propria of the optic nerve; this cut is started just medial to the supraorbital notch and passes lateral to the frontoethmoidal suture, taking care to avoid injury to the trochlear insertion of the superior oblique muscle. All cuts are performed with a thin-tipped drill or alternatively a reciprocating saw.

While performing the osteotomies, a malleable spatula is placed between the bone and the dissected periorbita to prevent its laceration, avoiding any pressure on the orbital contents. Also the frontal and temporal dura, detached from the bone, is elevated during the osteotomies and eventually protected with malleable retractors applied with minimal pressure. The use of cottonoids placed over the dura or periorbita has to be avoided during this operative time, because they could become entangled in the drill point and violently rotated endangering the exposed structures. After completion of the osteotomies, the OZ flap is freed from any residual dural and periorbital deep adhesion and mobilized outward. Figure 5.6 shows the preparation of a total OZ craniotomy in a cadaveric specimen.

At this point the basal frontal and medial temporal dura is completely exposed, separated from the periorbita by a bony bridge formed superiorly by the roof of the optic canal and the anterior clinoid process and laterally by the most posterior residual of the lateral orbital wall. From this point any surgical maneuver is conducted under magnification. The optic canal is opened extradurally using small rongeurs to skeletonize the dura propria of the optic nerve. The anterior clinoid process is drilled, together with the optic strut, using small diamond-tipped burrs to expose the subclinoid portion of the ICA. These maneuvers are performed in most cases because they allow better mobilization of the ICA and optic nerve after the dural opening, which facilitates the surgical treatment of lesions extensively involving the anterior and middle cranial base or expanding into the parasellar region and/or the interpeduncular cistern. We prefer not to use the drill to unroof the optic canal in order to avoid damage to the sheath of the optic nerve. The anterior clinoid process is drilled from its superior wall and from its inner portion, leaving a thin bony sheet around its borders that is successively broken and removed with small dissectors.

After complete removal of the clinoid process, troublesome bleeding from the cavernous sinus can be controlled by plugging the cavity with small pieces of microfibrillar collagen (Avitene; MedChem Products, Woburn, MA) avoiding compression of the ICA. The anterior clinoid process may be pneumatized, communicating with the sphenoid sinus. The ethmoid and sphenoid sinuses may also be entered when the planum sphenoidale is further drilled medial to the optic canal. Each communication with the paranasal sinuses will be closed during the reconstructive phase. If needed, the dura covering the temporal floor may be elevated, exposing the foramina spinosum, ovale and rotundum. The middle meningeal artery, coming out from the foramen spinosum, may be sectioned. Dissection of the dura posterior to the foramen ovale exposes the GSPn as it exits the geniculate ganglion from the facial hiatus; endangering or sectioning this nerve may cause ipsilateral ocular anhydrosis. The GSPn is sectioned only in the rare cases in which the horizontal intrapetrous portion of the ICA has to be exposed (for example, when a short high-flow by-pass is prevented in the treatment of an extensive intracavernous neoplasm).

The intradural or the extradural route may be then used, eventually in combination, to treat the targeted pathology. The extradural route is particularly indicated in the treatment of neurinomas involving the temporal fossa and of meningiomas expanding in the sphenocavernous region. In these cases, when a wide exposure of the temporal fossa and eventually of the infratemporal spaces is needed, mobilization of the zygomatic arch is mandatory (Fig. 5.7). The intradural route is more frequently used. The dura mater is widely opened in a standard fashion (C-shaped incision based anteriorly) and used to retract inferiorly the periorbita with the in-

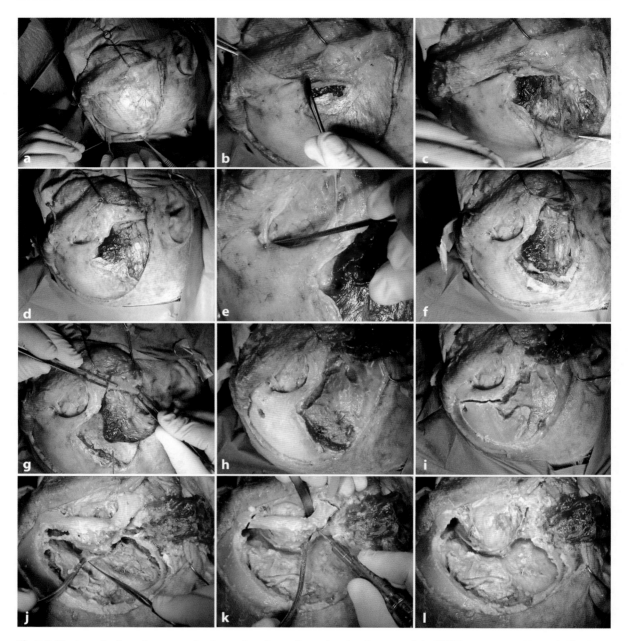

Fig 5.6 Photographs from the preparation in a cadaveric specimen showing the steps of the FTOZ approach. **a** The scalp flap is retracted and the galeal and pericranial flap is being incised. **b** The galeal-pericranial flap has been reflected and both the outer and the inner layers of the fascia temporalis superficialis are incised. **c** The posterior border of the fascia temporalis superficialis has been incised and turned upward to form a triangle based along the superior temporal line. **d** The inferior part of the fascia temporalis superficialis has been subperiosteally dissected and turned inferiorly, completely exposing the orbital rim, zygoma and zygomatic arch. **e** The supraorbital nerve is exposed in its canal. **f** The supraorbital nerve has been mobilized and retracted inferiorly with the pericranial flap; the temporal muscle is dissected along the direction of its fibers and incised at the level of the inferior temporal line leaving a small muscular cuff. **g** The temporal muscle has been dissected in a retrograde fashion and the zygomatic arch resected. **h** The temporal muscle has been reflected trough the resected extremities of the zygomatic arch; the burr holes have been placed and the sphenoid bridge has been resected joining the first and second holes. **i** The frontotemporal craniotomy has been prepared joining the holes using a craniotome. **j** The frontotemporal flap has been removed, exposing the opened frontal sinus; the dura is dissected from the orbital roof, sphenoid bridge and temporal floor. **k** The orbitozygomatic craniotomy is prepared. **l** The orbitozygomatic flap has been removed, exposing the periorbita, and frontal and temporal dura

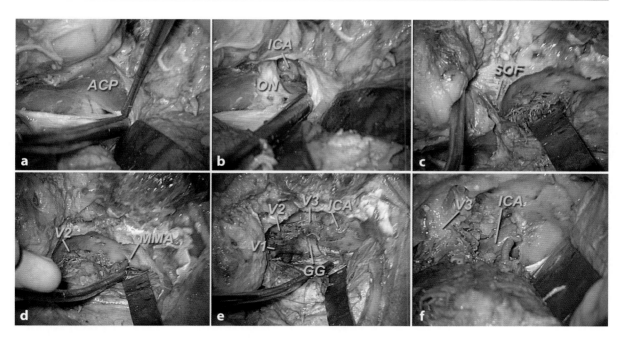

Fig 5.7 Photographs from the preparation in a cadaveric specimen showing the extradural intracranial preparation of the FTOZ approach. **a** The dura is dissected from the small bony bridge separating the periorbita from the frontal dura at the level of the orbit apex formed by the roof of the optic canal and the anterior clinoid process (*ACP*). **b** The optic canal has been unroofed exposing the optic nerve (*ON*); an anterior clinoidectomy has been performed exposing the subclinoidal portion of the internal carotid artery (*ICA*). **c** The superior orbital fissure (*SOF*) has been completely opened revealing the temporal dura in continuity with the periorbita at the level of the orbitomeningeal artery. **d** The dura is dissected from the temporal floor exposing the second division of the trigeminal nerve (*V2*) entering the foramen rotundum and the middle meningeal artery (*MMA*) entering the cranium from the foramen spinosum. **e** The middle meningeal artery has been sectioned and the temporal dura has been elevated to show the three divisions (*V1, V2, V3*) of the trigeminal nerve, the gasserian ganglion (*GG*) and the distal portion of the primary root of the trigeminus. **f** The horizontal portion of the ICA is exposed under V3 before its entrance into the cavernous sinus by drilling its canal

traorbital contents, to gain further basal working room. The sylvian fissure is widely opened as a rule and further space may be gained by opening the dura propria of the optic nerve and incising the dural ring encircling the ICA at its intradural entrance. Intradural mobilization of the optic nerve and ICA allows the surgical corridor located between these structures (interoptico-carotid cistern) and the corridor between the ICA siphon and the third cranial nerve (laterocarotid cistern) to be enlarged.

The third cranial nerve may be further mobilized by sectioning the insertion of the dura at the tentorial notch lateral to the nerve. This maneuver may enlarge the working space lateral to the ICA (moving laterally the third cranial nerve) and also may create a surgical corridor lateral to the nerve (if it is retracted medially). The posterior clinoid process can be resected to gain access toward the upper clival region and/or the interpedun-

cular cistern. This maneuver is particularly useful to expose complex and low-lying distal basilar aneurysms. It has to be emphasized that the posterior clinoid process is located inside the cavernous sinus. It can only be resected, using a diamond-tipped drill and small punches, after the overlying dura has been incised and rebated. Troublesome bleeding from the cavernous sinus is stopped by plugging with pieces of microfibrillar collagen. The cavernous sinus may be opened either extradurally or intradurally (Fig. 5.8).

On completion of the surgical procedure, a watertight dural closure is performed. Dural defects can be repaired with free pericranial grafts harvested from posterior to the undermined skin flap. If the ethmoid or sphenoid sinuses have been opened during the approach or removed because of pathological involvement, these sinuses are also cranialized and packed with autologous fat grafts and fibrin glue, as previously

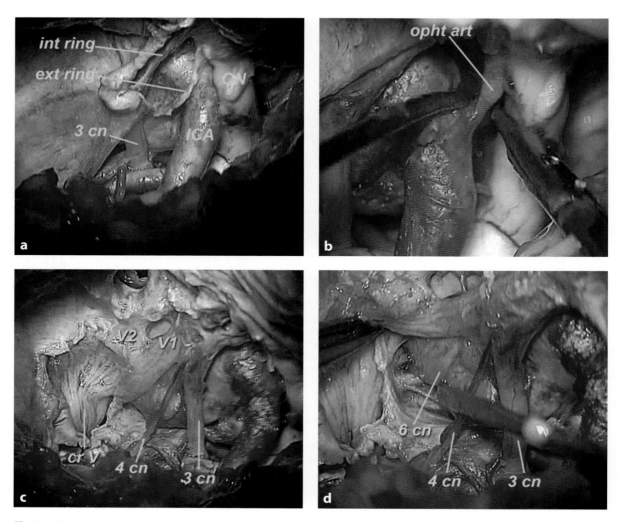

Fig 5.8 Photographs from the preparation in a cadaveric specimen showing the intradural preparation of the cavernous sinus. **a** Opening the dura medially to the third cranial nerve (*3 cn*) clearly reveals the external dural ring (*ext ring*) and the internal dural ring (*int ring*) encircling the internal carotid artery (ICA; *ON* optic nerve). **b** after incision of the dural rings the ICA may be mobilized exposing the ophthalmic artery (*opht art*) under the optic nerve. **c** The cavernous sinus is completely exposed and the third cranial nerve (*3 cn*), the fourth cranial nerve (*4 cn*) and the first branch of the trigeminal nerve (*V1*) are clearly evident on the lateral aspect of the ICA; removing the temporal dura over the sellar floor also reveals the common root of the trigeminal nerve (*cr V*) and the second branch of the same nerve (*V2*). **d** The sixth cranial nerve (*6 cn*) is clearly visible with the dural portion (external wall) of the cavernous sinus, in which are contained V1, 4 cn and 3 cn, moved medially

performed with the opened frontal sinus. The OZ flap is reapposed and fixed with titanium miniplates and screws. The pedicled anterior galeal-pericranial flap is then turned, extended to cover the cranialized frontal sinus and any other defect in the anterior cranial fossa, and sutured to the basal frontal dura. The dura is suspended with stay sutures also to the superior edge of the OZ bone and to the undersurface of the temporal muscle; one or two central dural tack-ups are also placed. The frontotemporal flap is then reattached using miniplates and screws or other rigid fixation devices (Craniofix; B. Braun Aesculap, Tuttlingen, Germany). Eventual bony defects in the frontal region, as when a hole has been placed at this level, are hidden with shaped titanium plates. Bone dust may be placed to fill gaps along the edges of the craniotomy for cosmetic reasons and to favor osteogenesis. The temporalis muscle is returned to its anatomic position and sutured to the muscular cuff and to its posterior sectioned portion. The zygomatic arch, if sectioned and displaced, is repositioned using the previously implanted miniplates. The fascia is reconstructed suturing its sectioned edges. A drain is placed over the reconstructed fascia and the scalp incision is closed in two layers.

5.3.2 Orbitopterional Approach

This method combines the frontotemporal craniotomy with the superolateral orbitotomy into one single bone flap. Patient positioning and preparation are the same as described for the FTOZ approach. The head is usually rotated 30-40°. The scalp incision is similar to the one used for the complete OZ approach, but extended less toward the contralateral side, starting at the level of the posterior root of the zygomatic arch and normally ending at the midline. We also use the interfascial preparation to perform this more limited OZ approach, although subfascial preparation is recommended by some authors. We use the submuscular, and sometimes the subfascial, preparation for the standard pterional approach [8, 11, 14, 33]. However, we prefer the interfascial preparation for any OZ approach because this preparation better exposes, in our opinion, the superolateral aspect of the orbit and its contents.

The scalp flap is dissected, with sharp and blunt dissection, from the galea and from the outer layer of the fascia temporalis superficialis. A full-thickness incision of the galea and the pericranium is then performed anterior to the superior temporal line, starting about 3 cm above the superolateral edge of the orbit and stopping 1 or 2 cm below the skin incision. A second incision is made from the inferior limit of the first one, perpendicular to it, directed to the midline. The superficial and deep layers of the fascia temporalis superficialis are then incised from the same level to the posterior root of the zygomatic arch. The three incisions form an inverted T. The superiorly incised pericranium is then dissected from the frontal bone and everted superiorly and medially. A subfascial dissection of the inferior portion of the temporal muscle is performed and the fascia temporalis superficialis is turned downward together with the inferior frontal pericranium, which has been incised with the galea and subperiosteally dissected from the orbital rim.

The superolateral border of the orbit is then exposed from the ascending frontal process of the zygoma to the supraorbital notch (or foramen). The frontotemporal branch of the facial nerve is left intact, mobilized inferiorly between the two layers of the fascia temporalis superficialis. This fascia is then detached from the superficial temporal line, dissected from the outer surface of the temporalis muscle and everted posteriorly and laterally. The incised fascial flap, including both its superficial and deep layers, forms a posteriorly based triangle with two free sides joining at its anteroinferior limit on the superior temporal line, above the frontozygomatic suture. This preparation of the fascia temporalis allows a better final reconstruction of the fascial plane. It is somewhat different from the one used for the FTOZ approach, where the fascial cuff forms a triangle based at the superior temporal line with the two free edges joining posteroinferiorly at the level of the posterior root of the zygomatic arch.

We use this last preparation routinely whenever opening of the frontal sinus is prevented and a pericranial flap is needed to cover the defect. Preoperative knowledge of frontal sinus extension from neuroimaging is essential and navigation may help in the decision. In any case the exposed temporalis muscle is posteriorly incised. Dissection of the muscle along the course of the fibers in its inferior portion limits the section to its superolateral portion. The muscle is then incised along its attachment to the inferior temporal line, leaving a small muscular cuff for final reconstruction. The muscle is then dissected free in a retrograde fashion and mobilized posteroinferiorly away from the skin flap. The periorbita, continuous with the anteroinferiorly everted pericranium, is dissected from the bone of the orbital rim and roof from lateral to medial to a depth of about 2.5-3 cm from the ascending zygomatic process to the supraorbital notch. It is rarely necessary to mobilize the supraorbital nerve when it passes through a foramen; this is done only if the prevented craniotomy is to be extended medial to the nerve exit.

The craniotomy is then performed. A keyhole burr hole is placed over the frontosphenoidal suture 1 cm behind the frontozygomatic suture. This hole is made with a ball-pointed high-speed drill so that its upper half exposes the periorbita and its inferior half exposes the frontal dura, with the bony orbital roof in between. This hole (MacCarty's keyhole) is located about 1 cm behind the point where the frontal keyhole for a standard craniotomy is usually placed to allow a deeper dissection of the periorbita [9, 35]. Two accessory holes are made: one in the lowest exposed squamous temporal bone just superior to the posterior root of the zygomatic arch, and the other at the level of the temporoparietal suture inferior to the temporal line. All the holes will be hidden under the temporalis muscle after reconstruction. A thin craniectomy is then performed using the drill and small punches from the inferior edge of the cranial half of the pilot keyhole along the sphenoid bridge.

After the dura has been dissected using curved periosteal elevators from the inner surface of the skull bone, an osteotomy is performed using a craniotome from the second to the third holes and continued toward the superior orbital rim, usually lateral to the supraorbital notch. The craniotome is stopped by the

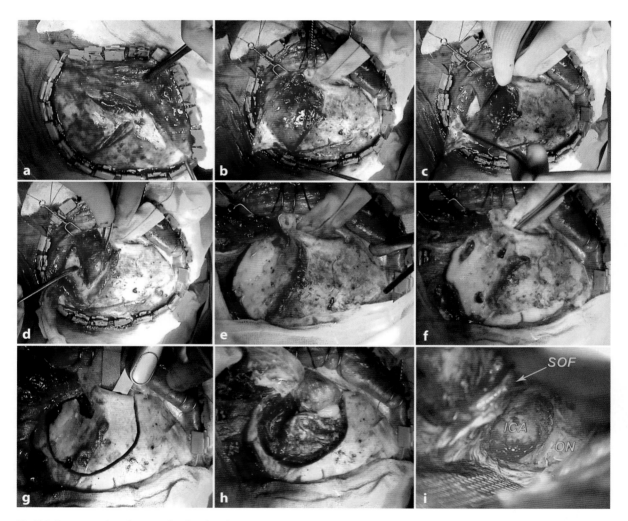

Fig 5.9 Intraoperative photographs showing the preparation for the orbitopterional approach (*left side*). **a** The scalp flap has been turned and the galea and pericranium are incised along the superior temporal line and from about 2.5 cm above the supraorbital rim to the midline, while both layers of the fascia temporalis superficialis are incised toward the posterior zygomatic root, forming an inverted T. **b** The superior border of the pericranial flap has been turned upward and the fascia temporalis superficialis has been reflected downward forming a posteriorly based triangle. **c** The temporal muscle is incised. **d** The temporal muscle is dissected in a retrograde fashion. **e** The temporal muscle is reflected inferiorly to expose the lateral wall of the orbit. **f** The burr holes have been placed; the MacCarty burr hole reveals inferiorly the periorbita and superiorly the frontal dura. **g** Osteotomies have been performed and the final cut in the orbital roof is made with a reciprocating saw. **h** The bone flap is removed showing the periorbita, and the frontal and temporal dura. **i** Opening of the superior orbital fissure (*SOF*), optic canal unroofing and anterior clinoidectomy are performed showing the medial loop of the internal carotid artery (*ICA*) lateral to the optic nerve (*ON*)

orbital roof. A second cut is made using the craniotome from the inferoposterior temporal hole to the inferior edge of the craniectomy performed over the sphenoid ridge, along the floor of the middle fossa. The frontal basal dura is then dissected with a small subperiosteal elevator, penetrated from the cranial part of the Mac-Carty's hole from the inner bony surface. With a thin-tipped drill a cut is then made in the lateral orbital rim, inferior to the frontozygomatic suture flush with the malar eminence, directed superiorly to the burr hole. The anterosuperior orbital rim is also sectioned medial to the supraorbital notch where the craniotome stopped. Finally, the thin bone of the orbital roof is sectioned using a drill or an oscillating saw and protecting the periorbita with a malleable spatula to join the limits of the previously placed cuts in the orbital rim. We strongly advise against the practice sometimes suggested of forcibly fracturing the orbital roof, because the uncontrolled line of fracture may involve the SOF and/or the optic canal endangering the critical structures contained inside; moreover, orbital roof section performed under direct vision allows a larger orbital osteotomy [8, 12, 16].

After the residual dural and periorbital adhesions have been dissected from the bone, the craniotomy flap can be removed. The flap must be elevated proceeding medial to lateral to avoid the mobilized orbital roof being driven into the inferior frontal lobe. If needed, additional bone may be removed piecemeal or by drilling to reach the superolateral edge of the SOF. The larger the residual defect in the orbital roof after reconstruction, the higher is the risk of postoperative enophthalmus or pulsatile exophthalmus. We recommend performing the cut in the orbital roof as deep as possible proximal to the SOF.

If the dura is difficult to dissect from the inner cranial bone and at risk of laceration during the cranial osteotomies, the procedure may be converted to a two-piece OPt craniotomy: a fourth burr hole is placed in the frontal bone over the supraorbital notch and joined with the craniotome to the pilot hole in a cut passing behind the orbital rim. The anterolateral orbital rim and roof are then mobilized performing osteotomies as described above, but under direct vision from the subfrontal aspect. OPt craniotomy is also better performed as a two-piece method in patients in whom thick orbital crests and walls are evident on preoperative neuroimaging studies.

After the OPt craniotomy has been mobilized, the optic canal may be opened and the anterior clinoid process drilled, as described above for the FTOZ approach. Obviously, the OPt approach provides a less-

extensive operative field. The middle fossa is well exposed only in its anterior portion, but all maneuvers already described after dural opening (i.e. mobilization of the optic nerve and ICA, section of the tentorial dural notch lateral to the entrance of the third cranial nerve, transcavernous posterior clinoidal process resection, wide sylvian fissure opening, etc.) may be performed.

After the operative procedure has been completed, careful reconstruction has to be achieved. The dura mater is sutured or grafted in a watertight fashion and definitively suspended. The OPt bony flap is reapposed and rigidly affixed to the edges of the craniotomy, taking special care to place the orbital rim at an adequate height and to avoid sinking. Bony edges are reapproximated nearer at the level of the anterolateral cut in the frontal region. The temporalis muscle and fascia are cautiously sutured along the incised edges and the scalp incision is closed in multiple layers. Figure 5.9 shows the operative preparation of a single-piece OPt craniotomy.

5.4 Indications

The fundamental principle of cranial base approaches is that improved operative exposure and reduced brain retraction can be achieved through increased bone resection. However the increased exposure is gained at the expense of a greater risk of cosmetic deformity, functional incompetence and other complications. Exactly tailoring the extent of bone resection to the particular requirements of the pathology to be treated reduces risks and complications while maintaining the advantages of the skull-base approach. This is the reason we use, and describe, different modifications of the OZ approach.

The OPt variant is the most limited of these approaches. It exposes the superolateral orbit cavity, the entire anterior cranial fossa and the anterior part of the middle cranial fossa, the sellar and parasellar region and, if the posterior clinoidal process is resected, the upper clival region. Exposure of these extradural compartments gives access to a number of intradural structures: the olfactory and optochiasmatic pathways, the pituitary, the ICA siphon and the arterial branches of the anterior circulation with the anastomosing circle of Willis and the upper basilar artery, the inferior portion of the frontal lobe and the anteromedial portion of the temporal lobe; the cavernous sinus in its anterosuperior part is also exposed.

The OPt approach is indicated in the treatment of lesions involving the orbital apex and the superior orbital

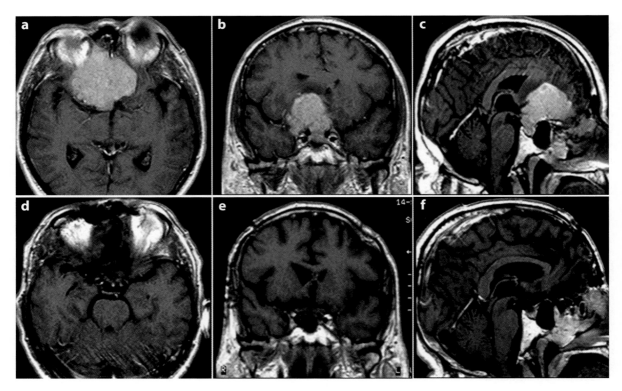

Fig 5.10 Preoperative (**a**, **b**, **c**) and postoperative (**d**, **e**, **f**) MRI scans of a meningioma occupying the medial bilateral orbital floor, jugum and tuberculum sellae in a 36-year-old patient with pituitary dysfunction and visual loss. This tumor was completely removed via an orbitopterional approach

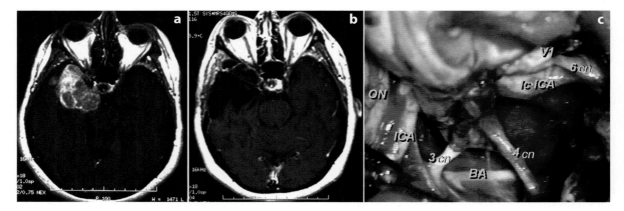

Fig 5.11 Preoperative (**a**) and postoperative (**b**) MRI scans of a right sphenocavernous meningioma removed via the orbitopterional approach. Intraoperative image (**c**) shows the right cavernous sinus opened from its superior wall and the intracavernous portion of the tumor (unusually soft in consistency) completely removed, with preservation of the third (*3 cn*), fourth (*4 cn*) and sixth (*6 cn*) cranial nerves and of the first branch of the trigeminal nerve (*V1*) in their intracavernous course. The intracavernous portion of the internal carotid artery (*Ic ICA*) also appears intact. the optic nerve (*ON*), internal carotid artery (*ICA*) and basilar artery (*BA*) in their intradural course are also completely free from tumor residuals. This 37-year-old patient complained preoperatively of atypical trigeminal neuralgia, which disappeared after the operation; no adjunctive definitive neurological deficit was observed at follow-up

cavity, both intra- and extraconal, of small to medium-sized extraaxial expansive lesions involving the inner and middle greater sphenoidal wing and the sellar fossa, of aneurysmal lesions, and of lesions intraaxially located at depth in the frontal and temporal lobes. Removal of the orbital roof enlarges the subfrontal angle of vision and lowers the skull-base trajectory making the working space shallower and wider as compared with the standard pterional craniotomy. The OPt approach is well suited to the treatment of meningiomas involving the jugum sphenoidale, the tuberculum sellae, the clinoidal process and the anteromedial sphenoid

wing (Fig. 5.10). Meningiomas involving the cavernous sinus (sphenocavernous meningiomas) can be also treated, in the case of soft parenchymal lesions, opening its superior wall lateral to the entrance of the third cranial nerve (Fig. 5.11).

Pituitary tumors with prevalent suprasellar and laterosellar expansion and craniopharyngiomas at the same location not suitable for the transphenoidal route are also best treated through the orbital modification of the OZ approach. This approach can be used to treat limited and well-circumscribed extra- or intraaxial tumors (i.e. cavernous angiomas, gangliogliomas, amarthomas) located

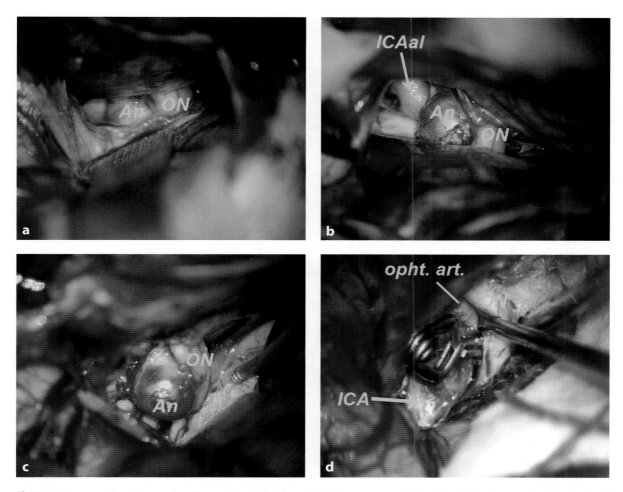

Fig 5.12 Intraoperative photographs of a very large left infraophthalmic aneurysm. A left orbitopterional approach with extradural optic canal unroofing and anterior clinoidectomy was performed. **a** After dural opening, the aneurysm (*An*) is exposed lateral to the optic nerve (*ON*). **b** The dura mater overlying the removed anterior clinoidal process is incised, revealing the anterior loop of the internal carotid artery (*ICAal*) in the Dolenc's triangle. **c** The aneurysm is better exposed after mobilization of the optic nerve. **d** A clip is apposed at the base of the aneurysm with preservation of the ophthalmic artery (*opht. art.*). This 19-year-old patient presented with visual deficit in the right eye, and showed a good postoperative recovery

deep in the inferior portion of the frontal lobe or in the mesial portion of the temporal lobe. The wide subfrontal exposure provided by the OPt approach allows full visualization of the ACoA complex without brain retraction. Difficult ACoA aneurysms can then be treated with minimal opening of the sylvian fissure and reduced resection of the gyrus rectus, and also if upwardly directed and deeply embedded in the frontal lobe. Complex carotid bifurcation aneurysms can also be exposed with minimal retraction. Optic canal unroofing and anterior clinoidal process resection allow intradural mobilization of the optic nerve and ICA and make this approach ideal for the treatment of subchiasmatic carotidoophthalmic aneurysms and of large and giant proximal carotid siphon aneurysms (Fig. 5.12). We prefer to perform anterior clinoidectomy via the extradural route, but not for bleeding lesions in the acute stage or for very large aneurysms directly lying on the planum sphenoidale [36].

The FTOZ approach may be performed with or without zygomatic arch mobilization. This approach maximizes exposure of the middle fossa and allows better exposure of the lateral portion of the posterior fossa. It is mainly indicated for the treatment of large lesions located in the temporal floor, also involving the anterior fossa and/or the orbit walls and cavity. The total OZ approach is also indicated for the treatment of lesions expanding medially from the anterior and middle fossa towards the tentorial edge, whatever their

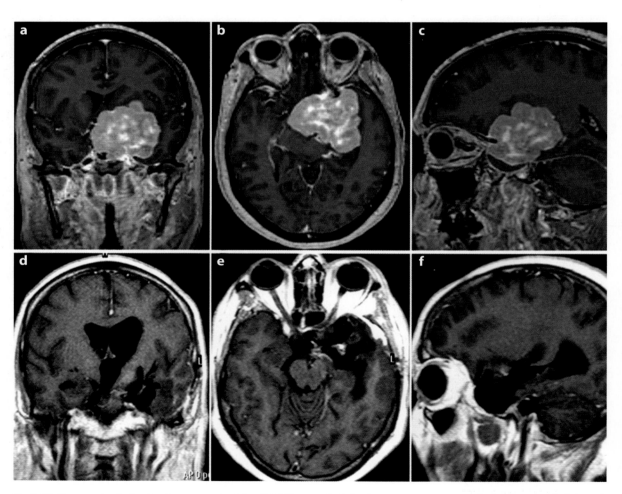

Fig 5.13 Preoperative (**a**, **b**, **c**) and postoperative (**d**, **e**, **f**) MRI scans of a left sphenopetrocavernous meningioma approached through a FTOZ craniotomy without zygomatic arch resection. This 58-year-old patient presented with a mild right-sided hemiparesis, and no adjunctive deficit was noted after the apparently total removal

size. Sphenopetrous and sphenopetroclival meningiomas with prevalent expansion in the middle fossa, as well as other extradural and intradural extraaxial tumors at the same location (e.g. chordomas, chondromas, dermoids), are typical lesions that can be resected using this approach (Fig. 5.13). Eventual extension of these lesions into the posterior fossa can be reached via a transcavernous posterior clinoidectomy and/or by drilling the petrous bone medial to the carotid canal in Kawase's triangle [38]. For very large tumors the way for a complete resection is progressively created by the exeresis itself.

Pituitary tumors and craniopharyngiomas with retrosellar extension are also indications for this approach. Tumors of the optochiasmatic pathways sometimes show wide exophytic expansions into the lateral and retrosellar cisterns and are well suited to the FTOZ approach. Very large fifth cranial nerve schwannomas completely occupying the middle cranial fossa, including its more anterior portion, are also best treated with this approach, which allows the exeresis of these lesions through a completely extradural or a combined extra- and intradural route (Fig. 5.14). Smaller trigeminal neurinomas in the middle fossa are best treated

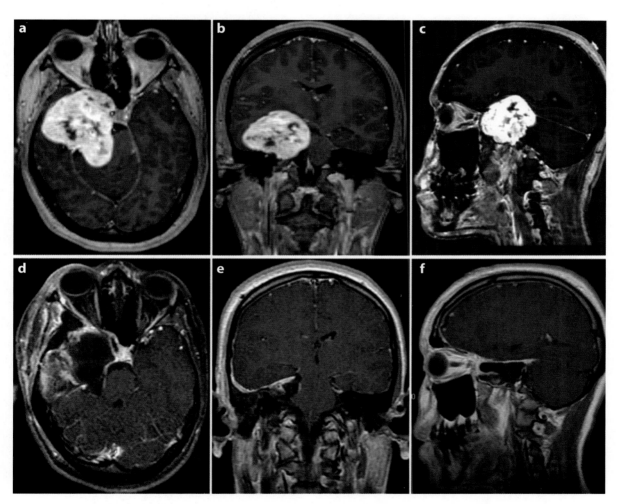

Fig 5.14 Preoperative (**a**, **b**, **c**) and postoperative (**d**, **e**, **f**) MRI scans of a large right trigeminal neurinoma expanding into the middle and posterior fossa and bordering the deepest portion of the anterior fossa. The lesion was completely resected via a totally extradural route using a FTOZ approach with zygomatic arch resection. This 17-year-old girl presented with visual disturbance progressively worsening over one year until vision loss; only after the appearance of facial dysesthesias was the patient referred for neuroradiological investigation

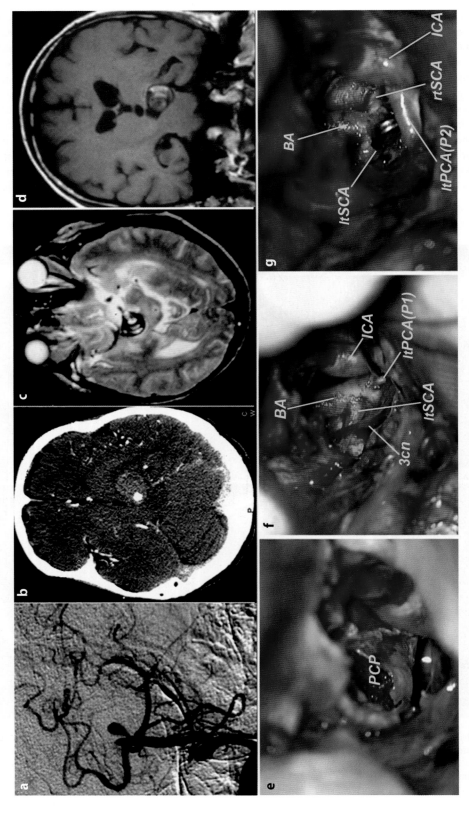

Fig 5.15 Preoperative angiogram (**a**), contrast-enhanced CT scan (**b**) and MRI scans (**c, d**) of a very large partially thrombosed aneurysm arising from the distal basilar artery. The lesion was approached via a left FTO craniotomy completed with optic canal unroofing and anterior extradural clinoidectomy. Intraoperative images (**e–g**): **e** after opening the dura, the posterior clinoid process (*PCP*) inhibits a clear view of the basilar artery (*BA*) is revealed in the surgical corridor between the internal carotid artery (*ICA*) and of the parental artery; **f** after removal of the PCP the basilar artery (*BA*) is revealed in the surgical corridor between the internal carotid artery (*ICA*) and third cranial nerve (*3cn*), with the aneurysm originating at the level of the junction between the left superior cerebellar artery (*ltSCA*) and the precommunicating tract of the left posterior cerebral artery [*ltPCA(P1)*]; **g** the aneurysm is clipped at the level of the implant base working below the postcommunicating tract of the left posterior cerebral artery [*ltPCA(P2)*], also preserving flow in the contralateral superior cerebellar artery (*rtSCA*) and in the right posterior cerebral artery (not visible in the image). This 43-year-old women presented with progressive right hemiparesis and third cranial nerve paresis; she progressively recovered after the operation

with a simple tranzygomatic approach. Basilar aneurysms can also be treated with a FTOZ approach, which allows control of these lesions from the subtemporal and the anterior surgical corridors. Transcavernous posterior clinoidectomy provides further access to the interpeduncular fossa. This maneuver is essential to visualize basilar aneurysms lying below the posterior biclinoidal line, but it also may be performed to visualize the upper portion of the basilar artery, where a temporary clip can be applied [39] (Fig. 5.15).

The FTOZ approach with zygomatic arch resection allows multidirectional viewing and surgical dissection

of deeply located lesions via the three fundamental anterolateral routes: transsylvian, subfrontal and subtemporal. The addition of zygomatic arch mobilization to the FTOZ approach is required when tumoral lesions extend into the deepest portion of the tentorial edge and toward the lateral part of the posterior fossa. Lesions with infratemporal expansion are also best treated with zygomatic arch resection. Removal of the zygomatic arch lowers the angle of vision in the treatment of basilar artery aneurysms highly projecting over the posterior biclinoidal line, allowing complete control of the aneurysm with minimal brain retraction. The combina-

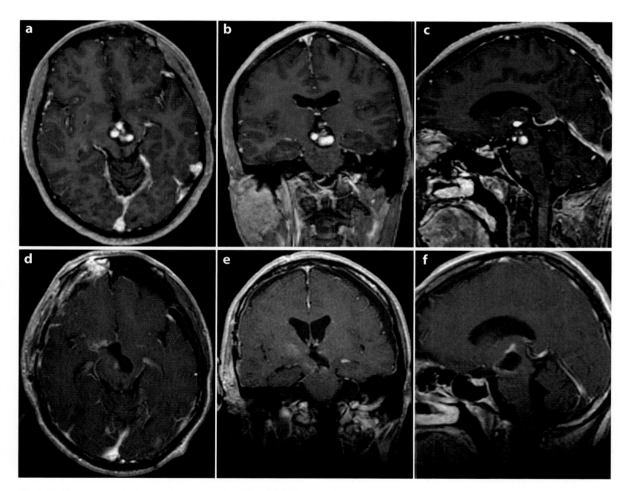

Fig 5.16 Preoperative (**a, b, c**) and postoperative (**d, e, f**) MRI scans of a cavernous angioma ventrally located in the rostral midbrain. The lesion was approached via a FTOZ craniotomy with zygomatic arch resection which allowed entry to the midbrain from the safe zone located in the superomedial portion of the mesencephalic tegmentum in the most anterior portion of the right cerebral peduncle. This 31-year-old man had several episodes of right-sided hemiparesis with subsequent partial recovery. After the last, more serious, hemiparetic onset the patient also showed left-sided third cranial nerve paresis. Progressive recovery of both the hemiparesis and the third cranial nerve paresis was noted after the operation

tion of the surgical perspectives permitted by this approach allows access to lesions located in the ventral midbrain through safe surgical corridors (Fig. 5.16).

We have described a further modification of the total OZ approach, consisting of forced opening of patient's mouth to expose the infratemporal pterygoid region and the posterolateral wall of the maxillary sinus. This modification can be useful in the treatment of benign tumors encompassing both the neurocranial and splachnocranial compartments [23].

5.5 Complications and Complication Avoidance

Complications are related to improper surgical maneuvers during the true operative phase or to the procedural preparation of the OZ craniotomy.

Accurate preoperative planning is essential to reduce morbidity. Preoperative neuroimaging provides precise information about the origin, location, extension and possible nature of the lesion, as well as about lesional relationships with neighboring neurovascular structures and osteodural landmarks. MRI and CT scans are complementary studies, and both have to be performed when dealing with the complex pathologies requiring a skull-base approach; bone windows on the CT scan also have to be performed. Magnetic resonance angiography, angio-CT and/or digital subtraction angiography are used to determine the functional status of the lesional and perilesional vasculature, both arterial and venous. Proper tumor vascularization, encasement of arteries and perforators and venous outflow have to be confirmed before any procedure is performed. For aneurysms, standard angiography is better supplemented with an angio-CT scan with 3-D reconstruction to achieve complete spatial orientation. In tumors and vascular lesions in which collateral circulation has to be assessed, a balloon occlusion test is performed with clinical neurological evaluation associated with EEG and SPECT or xenon CT scanning. We rarely use preoperative embolization, which remains indicated for lesions highly vascularized from branches of the external carotid artery (middle meningeal, internal maxillary and/or ascending pharyngeal arteries), as is the case in juvenile angiofibromas and rarely in meningiomas, or from the tentorial branches of the petrocavernous ICA. Embolization of the STA is inadvisable because it may cause problems in the blood supply to the skin flap [8, 12]. Saving the deep temporal branches of the internal maxillary artery during embolization procedures prevents secondary hypotrophy of the temporal muscle.

Virtual tridimensional computed reconstruction of the special anatomy of each single patient is helpful. Navigation is useful both for accurate preoperative planning and to achieve precise orientation during surgical maneuvers. The use of adjunctive intraoperative methodologies (i.e. intraoperative Doppler sonography, videofluoroangiography, endoscopic assistance) and neurophysiological monitoring further reduce complications.

Mortality and morbidity rates depend on many variables, including the patient's preoperative clinical condition and lesional features. Preoperative evaluation includes clinical, endocrinological and metabolic assessment. Neurological examination with documentation of visual acuity, ocular motility, olfactory function, facial sensation and situation of facial and masticatory muscles is necessary to determine any preoperative deficit in the cranial nerves that can be injured during the operative procedure. The nature, location, extension, vascularity and consistency of the pathology influence the operative results. The larger the tumor and the harder its consistency, the worse the surgical conditions. Retrochiasmatic and deep locations, arterial and nerve encasement and invasion of the cavernous sinus usually carry a higher risk of complications and a lower probability of total removal. Intra- or postoperative brain swelling can occur not only as a consequence of arterial injury, but also secondary to obstruction of the venous outflow. Elevation of the temporal lobe may endanger the infratemporal veins and especially the vein of LabbÈ, which should be preserved; a cautious subpial dissection of this vein along its inferior portion in the temporal lobe as far its entrance into the sigmoid sinus may eventually be performed. Postoperative epidural hematomas are prevented by accurate dural suspension and avoiding excessive cerebral detension during the procedure. Both excessive and too-limited exposure of the lesion are to be avoided.

Complications directly related to the preparation of the OZ craniotomy are mainly esthetic and functional. Application of strong hemostatic clips, aggressive coagulation of superficial vessels, occlusion of the posterior trunk of the STA and acute folding of the scalp flap can all endanger the blood supply and cause bad scarring of the skin incision. Interfascial preparation and accurate subperiosteal elevation of the myofascial planes from the orbital rim and zygomatic arch prevent injury to the frontotemporal and zygomatic divisions of the facial nerve. If a galeal-pericranial flap is prepared, incision of its inferior border has to be stopped at least 2.5 cm above the frontozygomatic suture to avoid section of aberrant branches of the frontotemporal division of cranial nerve VII.

Postoperative hypotrophy of the temporalis muscle may be a consequence of direct injury to muscle fibers by improper dissection or excessive retraction, ischemia from interruption of the primary arterial supply, denervation and inappropriate muscle tension. Careful subperiosteal retrograde dissection of the muscle prevents damage to muscle fibers and to proper deep arteries and nerves. Monopolar cauterization has absolutely to be avoided during muscle dissection. Adequate muscle tension is obtained by leaving a small muscular cuff attached to the craniotomy, to which the muscle is sutured during reconstruction. The fascia temporalis is also easily reconstructed if a cuff is left attached to the craniotomy [11, 14, 33, 34]. If the zygomatic arch is mobilized, we leave it attached to the masseter muscle and perform preplating. This allows a better cosmetic reconstruction and prevents postoperative deficit in mastication. To avoid any masticatory disturbance, the temporomandibular joint also has to be left intact during drilling of the temporal floor.

Violation of the frontal and/or other paranasal sinuses is a source of harmful complications. In the event of cranialization of air sinuses by mucosal exenteration, plugging pieces of muscle and fibrin glue into the frontal ostium, eventually filling the ethmoidal and sphenoidal cavities with autologous fat grafts and covering any bone defect in the anterior fossa with a vascularized thick pericranial graft prevent CSF leakage, pneumocephalus and late mucocele formation. Infections after cranialization are avoided by resterilizing the instruments and ensuring that the surgical team redress. Enophthalmus and pulsatile exophthalmus have been described after OZ craniotomy. Respecting the integrity of the periorbita, performing osteotomies in the orbital roof in such a way as to minimize bone gaps and accurate orbit roof reconstruction avoid these complications.

Postoperative periorbital swelling is a common occurrence in patients submitted to an OZ approach, but usually resolves in a few days with no residual functional or cosmetic deficit. In rare cases massive conjunctival edema occurs, requiring temporary tarsorrhaphy. Accurate reconstruction and repositioning of the bone flap(s) with plates and screws or other rigid fixation devices avoid disfiguring sinking of the bone. Bone edges should be tightly reapproximated at least along one or two sides to favor osteointegration. Strategic placement of the craniotomy burr holes so that they will remain hidden under the reapposed muscle and the use of shaped titanium plates and bone dust to cover bony defects are useful for final good cosmetic results.

References

1. McArthur LL (1912) An aseptic surgical access to the pituitary body and its neighborhood. JAMA 58:2009-2011
2. Frazier CH (1913) An approach to the hypophysis through the anterior cranial fossa. Ann Surg 57:145-152
3. Yasargil MG (1969) Microsurgery applied to neurosurgery. Thieme, Stuttgart, pp 119-143
4. Yasargil MG, Fox JL, Ray MW (1975) The operative approach to aneurysms of the anterior communicating artery. In: Krayenbฺhl H (ed) Advances and technical standards in neurosurgery, vol. 2. Springer, Vienna New York, pp 113-170
5. Jane JA, Park TS, Pobereskin LH et al (1982) The supraorbital approach. Technical note. Neurosurgery 11(4):537-542
6. Pellerin P, Lesoin F, Dhellemmes P et al (1984) Usefulness of the orbitofrontomalar approach associated with bone reconstruction for frontotemporosphenoid meningiomas. Neurosurgery 15(5):715-718
7. Hakuba A, Liu S, Nishimura S (1986) The orbitozygomatic infratemporal approach. A new surgical technique. Surg Neurol 26:271-276
8. Al-Mefty O (1987) Supraorbital-pterional approach to skull base lesions. Neurosurgery 21(4):474-477
9. Aziz KMA, Froelich SC, Cohen PL et al (2002) The one-piece orbitozygomatic approach: the MacCarty burr hole and the inferior orbital fissure as keys to technique and application. Acta Neurochir (Wien) 144(1):15-24
10. Delashaw JB Jr, Tedeschi H, Rhoton AL Jr (1992) Modified supraorbital craniotomy: Technical note. Neurosurgery 30(6):954-956
11. Lemole GM Jr, Henn JS, Zabramski JM, Spetzler RF (2003) Modifications to the orbitozygomatic approach. A technical note. J Neurosurg 99(5):924-930
12. Pieper DR, Al-Mefty O (1999) Cranio-orbito-zygomatic approach. Oper Tech Neurosurg 2(1):2-9
13. Sekhar LN, Janecka IP, Jones NF (1988) Subtemporal-infratemporal and basal subfrontal approach to extensive cranial base tumours. Acta Neurochir (Wien) 92(1-4):83-92
14. Zabramski JM, Kiris T, Sankhla SK et al (1998) Orbitozygomatic craniotomy. Technical note. J Neurosurg 89(2):336-341
15. Hayashi N, Hirashima Y, Kurimoto M et al (2002) One-piece pedunculated frontotemporal orbitozygomatic craniotomy by creation of a subperiosteal tunnel beneath the temporal muscle: technical note. Neurosurgery 51(6):1520-1523
16. Balasingam V, Noguchi A, McMenomey SO, Delashaw JB Jr (2005) Modified osteoplastic orbitozygomatic craniotomy. Technical note. J Neurosurg 102(5):940-944

17. Miller ML, Kaufman BA, Lew SM (2008) Modified osteoplastic orbitozygomatic craniotomy in the pediatric population. Childs Nerv Syst 24(7):845-850

18. Fujitsu K, Kuwarabara T (1985) Zygomatic approach for lesions in the interpeduncular cistern. J Neurosurg 62:340-343

19. Ikeda K, Yamashita J, Hashimoto M, Futami K (1991) Orbitozygomatic temporopolar approach for a high basilar tip aneurysm associated with a short intracranial internal carotid artery: a new surgical approach. Neurosurgery 28:105-110

20. Sindou M, Emery E, Acevedo G, Ben David U (2001) Respective indications for orbital rim, zygomatic arch and orbito-zygomatic osteotomies in the surgical approach to central skull base lesions. Critical, retrospective review in 146 cases. Acta Neurochir (Wien) 143(10):967-975

21. Al-Mefty O, Anand VK (1990) Zygomatic approach to skull-base lesions. J Neurosurg 73(5):668-673

22. Uttley D, Archer DJ, Marsh HT et al (1991) Improved access to lesions of the central skull base by mobilization of the zygoma: experience with 54 cases. Neurosurgery 28(1):99-104

23. Di Rienzo A, Ricci A, Scogna A et al (2004) The open-mouth fronto-orbitotemporozygomatic approach for extensive benign tumors with coexisting splanchnocranial and neurocranial involvement. Neurosurgery 54(5):1170-1179

24. Schwartz MS, Anderson GJ, Horgan MA et al (1999) Quantification of increased exposure resulting from orbital rim and orbitozygomatic osteotomy via the frontotemporal transsylvian approach. J Neurosurg 91:1020-1026

25. Gonzalez LF, Crawford NR, Horgan MA et al (2002) Working area and angle of attack in three cranial base approaches: pterional, orbitozygomatic, and maxillary extension of the orbitozygomatic approach. Neurosurgery 50(3):550-557

26. Tanriover N, Ulm AJ, Rhoton AL Jr et al (2006) One-piece versus two-piece orbitozygomatic craniotomy: quantitative and qualitative considerations. Neurosurgery 58(4 Suppl 2):ONS229-237

27. Feneis H, Dauber W (2000) Pocket atlas of human anatomy, 4th edn. Thieme, Stuttgart New York, pp 9-34, 54-55, 78-82, 322-332

28. Rhoton AL (2002) The anterior and middle cranial base. Neurosurgery 51(Suppl 1):273-302

29. Lyons BM (1998) Surgical anatomy of the skull base. In: Donald PJ (ed) Surgery of the skull base. Lippincot-Raven Philadelphia, pp 15-30

30. Rhoton AL (2002) The orbit. Neurosurgery 51(Suppl 1):303-334

31. Chicoine MR, van Loveren HR (2000) Surgical approaches to the cavernous sinus. In: Robertson JT, Coakhan HB, Robertson JH (eds) Cranial base surgery. Churchill Livingstone, London, pp 171-185

32. Yasargil MG, Reichman MV, Kubik S (1987) Preservation of the frontotemporal branch of the facial nerve using the interfascial temporalis flap for pterional craniotomy. Technical article. J Neurosurg 67(3):463-466

33. Coscarella E, Vishteh AG, Spetzler RF et al (2000) Subfascial and submuscular methods of temporal muscle dissection and their relationship to the frontal branch of the facial nerve. Technical note. J Neurosurg 92(5):877-880

34. Oikawa S, Mizuno M, Muraoka S, Kobayashi S (1996) Retrograde dissection of the temporalis muscle preventing muscle atrophy for pterional craniotomy. Technical note. J Neurosurg 84(2):297-299

35. Shimizu S, Tanriover N, Rhoton AL Jr et al (2005) The MacCarty keyhole and inferior orbital fissure in orbitozygomatic craniotomy. Neurosurgery 57(Suppl 1):152-159

36. Noguchi A, Balasingam V, Shiokawa Y et al (2005) Extradural anterior clinoidectomy. Technical note. J Neurosurg 102(5):945-950

37. Dolenc VV (1999) A combined transorbital-transclinoid and transsylvian approach to carotid-ophthalmic aneurysms without retraction of the brain. Acta Neurochir Suppl 72:89-97

38. Kawase T, Shiobara R, Toya S (1991) Anterior transpetrosal-transtentorial approach for sphenopetroclival meningiomas: surgical method and results in 10 patients. Neurosurgery 28:869-876

39. Day JD, Giannotta SL, Fukushima T (1994) Extradural temporopolar approach to lesions of the upper basilar artery and infrachiasmatic region. J Neurosurg 81(2)230-235

Transcallosal Approaches to Intraventricular Tumors

6

Roberto Delfini and Angelo Pichierri

6.1 History

Walter E. Dandy pioneered the interhemispheric transcallosal routes to the lateral ventricles. He described, in 1921, the posterior transcallosal approach with division of the splenium for removal of pineal tumors, and followed this by reporting a series of third ventricle tumors in 1933 [1]. Busch performed the first interforniceal approach in 1944 for a malignant glioma [2]. Kempe and Blaylock reported their series of paratrigonal lesions approached through a posterior transcallosal approach in 1976 [3]. Three years later Hirsch et al. proposed coagulating the thalamostriate vein to enlarge the paraforniceal approach with a subchoroidal route [4]. In 1996, Yasargil emphasized the importance of preserving the posterior half of the corpus callosum and proposed a transprecuneus approach for trigonal lesions [5]. In 1998, Wen et al. presented an anatomical study of the choroidal fissure and of the supra- and subchoroidal surgical routes [6]. In 2001 Rosenfeld et al. reported a limited anterior forniceal splitting technique for the cure of hypothalamic hamartomas [7].

6.2 Introduction

Transcallosal approaches allow access to the deep internal structures without violating the gray matter at the

R. Delfini (✉)
Dept of Neurological Sciences, Neurosurgery
"Sapienza" University of Rome, Italy

cost of a small callosotomy [1, 3, 5, 8–13]. They permit an optimal exposure of the lateral ventricles (excluding the temporal horn), the roof of the third ventricle, and the pineal region. The following are the main possible alternatives when a callosotomy is planned (Fig. 6.1, top row):

1. Frontal paramedian craniotomy with anterior median/paramedian callosotomy
2. Posterior frontal paramedian craniotomy with middle median/paramedian callosotomy
3. Parietooccipital paramedian craniotomy with posterior callosotomy and with division of the splenium
4. Parietooccipital paramedian craniotomy with a paracallosal–transprecuneal route

The transcallosal approach is also used as first step when a superior access to the third ventricle is required [1, 2, 4–8, 13–16].

The second step is represented by one of the following routes chosen on the basis of the location/nature of the lesion (Fig. 6.1, bottom row):

- Anterior midline callosotomy: anterior/standard interforniceal route
- Middle midline callosotomy: standard interforniceal route
- Anterior paramedian callosotomy: paraforniceal/subsuprachoroidal routes
- Middle paramedian callosotomy: supra-/subchoroidal routes

Exposure and control of the third and lateral ventricles may be achieved via transcortical (middle frontal gyrus, superior parietal lobule, transtemporal, transoccipital), transbasal (subfrontal translamina terminalis, transsylvian, supracerebellar sub-/transtentorial, suboccipital supra-/transtentorial) and endoscopic routes [3, 5, 9, 10, 11, 13, 14, 16, 17].

P. Cappabianca et al. (eds.), *Cranial, Craniofacial and Skull Base Surgery*.
© Springer-Verlag Italia 2010

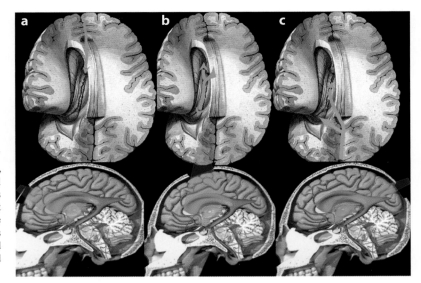

Fig. 6.1 Illustrations of the anterior (**a**), middle (**b**) and posterior (**c**) transcallosal approaches; the paracallosal route (**c**) is also depicted. The green cones represent the exposure of the ventricles possible with each callosotomy; the yellow cones represent the further exposures gained with additional steps (forniceal and choroidal approaches)

A multitude of pathological processes may develop primarily or secondarily from and into the ventricles (Tables 6.1 and 6.2) [1, 5, 8, 13, 15]. They are often harbored within the body of the lateral ventricles, the frontal horn, the roof of the third ventricle or, less frequently, the trigone, the lateral walls of the third ventricles, and the occipital or temporal horns.

Transcallosal approaches are required if the transcortical alternative implies an excessive corticotomy or a long route through the white matter and if the transbasal approaches fail to obtain an optimal exposure/control of the lesion [3, 5, 9–11, 13, 14, 16, 17]. Some specific tumors are preferably reached through the corpus callosum: ependymomas, subependymomas, intraventricular meningiomas, colloid cysts, hypothalamic hamartomas, cavernomas, and intraventricular metastases [9, 13, 16]. Subcortical lesions, such as neuroectodermal tumors, are best managed via transcortical access because of their infiltrative nature [16].

Conditions requiring direct decompression of optic structures, extraaxial lesions originating at the skull base with secondary extension into the floor of the third ventricle, such as meningiomas, craniopharyngiomas, or pituitary adenomas, may also be best accessed by transbasal approaches [13, 16]. Giant intrinsic craniopharyngiomas, central neurocytomas, teratomas, disgerminomas and many other lesions require a discus-

Table 6.1 Most common intraventricular tumors, their preferred location and frequency according to our series

Tumor	Preferred location	Frequency (%)
Meningioma	Lateral ventricle	32.50
Neurocytoma	Foramen of Monro	20.70
Ganglioglioma	Temporal horn	17.50
Oligodendroglioma	Frontal temporal horns	12.50
Astrocytoma	Middle cell	12.50
Cavernoma	Thalamus	12.50

Table 6.2 Less common intraventricular tumors and their preferred location

Lesion	Preferred location
Colloid cyst	Anterior roof of the third ventricle
Craniopharyngioma	Floor of the third ventricle
Ependymoma	Middle cell
Epidermoid/dermoid	Floor of the third ventricle
Fibrillary astrocytoma	Thalamus
Germinoma	Pineal region
Glioblastoma multiforme	Thalamus
Hypothalamic hamartoma	Lateral anterior third ventricle
Lymphoma	Periventricular
Mixed tumor	Secondary extension
Neurocysticercosis	Trigone
Papilloma	Lateral ventricle
Pinealoma	Pineal region
Primitive neuroectodermal tumor	Secondary extension
Subependymoma	Lateral ventricle
Subependymal giant cell astrocytoma	Lateral ventricle
Subependymoma	Middle cell/trigone

Table 6.3 Neuropsychological assessment tests (they take about one and a half hours)

Test	Target
London tower test	Planning
Mini mental test	General assessment of cognitive status
Phonemic verbal fluency test	Verbal skills
Raven progressive matrices	Nonverbal reasoning
Rev test	Memory (short- and long-term)
Stroop test	Attention
Trail making test	Visuospatial competence and attention
Wisconsin card sorting test	Abstract thinking
Zung scale (self-rating)	Mood

sion of the most appropriate approach on the bases of the following factors:

- Location.
- Presumed diagnosis.
- Advantages/disadvantages of the specific approach.
- Concomitant hydrocephalus (transcortical routes may be feasible if the nervous tissue thickness is reduced to 3 cm or less).
- Clinical condition of the patient (thorough neuropsychological assessment to establish baseline functional data; Table 6.3).

6.3 Surgical Technique

Both neuronavigation and endoscopy are very useful in assisting the surgeon in all the approaches [18]. Neuronavigation allows a precise planning of all the steps: craniotomy, surgical routes, location of structures and of the lesion. Pure endoscopy and endoscopically assisted surgery make it possible to reduce invasiveness of the approach as the endoscope provides outstanding visualization and magnification of the inner structures.

6.3.1 Anterior Transcallosal Approach

The patient is positioned supine with the head in a neutral pin fixation and flexed at 15°. Some authors prefer a lateral position with the sagittal plane of the head parallel to the floor and the side of the craniotomy downward [18]. This way, a natural retraction of the homolateral hemisphere and a greater horizontal working angle can be obtained. Nevertheless, the anatomy may

be less familiar and the midline distorted by gravity. Moreover, exposure of the contralateral ventricle and of the contralateral third ventricle wall could be difficult due to natural prolapse of the septum pellucidum into the surgical field. Other minor issues of this position are the extra setup time and the possibility of axillary neuropathy from prolonged surgery/inadequate padding. Standing slightly to one side of the patient allows the same horizontal working angles.

When a temporary external ventricular drainage has been placed preoperatively to resolve an acute hydrocephalus, the shunt allows relaxation of the brain during the initial steps of the approach. Nonetheless, the drainage could cause collapse of ventricular chambers, thus making deeper exploration more difficult. The drainage should therefore be closed about 18 hours prior surgery, clinical conditions permitting; wider ventricular chambers will be available.

The skin incision is L-shaped with the vertical part along the midline and with the base posterior to the coronal suture. If the patient is bald, a bicoronal (not basal) incision is the best option. Craniotomy is generally performed above the nondominant hemisphere. This is also the best choice for contralateral lesions, because the transcallosal routes offer good visualization of both the lateral ventricles. Incising the falx could be necessary for very lateral contralateral lesions. This allows a good cone of vision without the need to further retract the cerebral cortex. The craniotomy has dimensions of 6×4 cm, oversteps the midline and has a posterior limit 1 cm anterior to the coronal suture (Fig. 6.2a). The dura mater is opened in a semicircular fashion with the base along the superior longitudinal sinus (Fig. 6.2b). Complete exposure of the superior longitudinal sinus entails maximization of the dural opening and the need for minor cortical retraction. Long cotton sponges are placed between the reflected dura and the sinus to avoid strangulation of the sinus and consequent thrombosis. Attention must be paid to any veins which enter the dura before merging into the sinus. In these cases, the dura mater should be opened respecting these vessels with the consequence that the surgical field is reduced or compartmentalized. To avoid this situation it is of the utmost importance to determine the position of the parasagittal veins by venous MR angiography. The position, the size and even the side of the craniotomy may be modified on the basis of an unfavorable venous anatomy. Generally, 70% of the venous tributaries enter the sagittal sinus within the sector 2 cm posterior to the coronal suture [16]. Cotton sponges wrapped in latex (cut from surgical gloves) are employed to

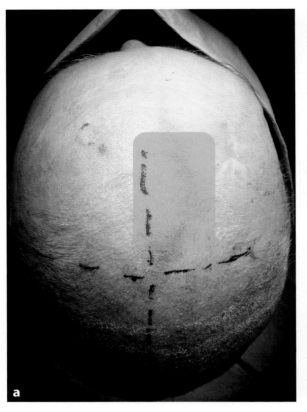

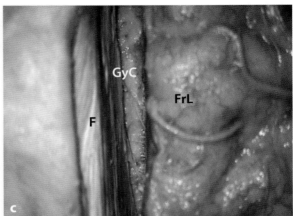

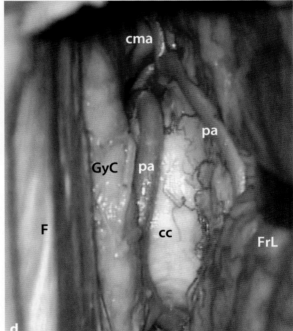

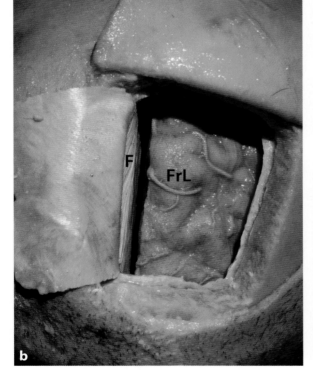

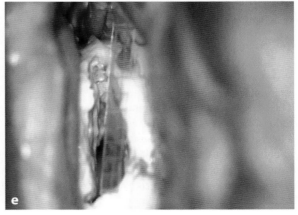

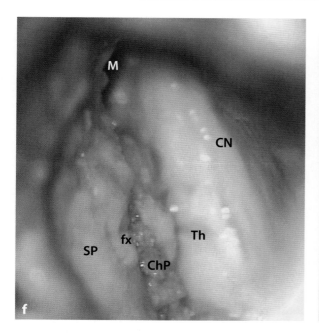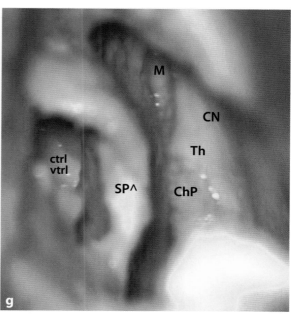

Fig. 6.2 Right anterior transcallosal approach. **a** Site of craniotomy. **b** Dural opening. **c** Magnified view of the interhemispheric space with the cingular cortex at the bottom of the surgical field. **d** Exposure of the corpus callosum with the anterior cerebral arteries lying above it. **e** Anterior callosotomy (about 1 cm). **e** Cella media of the right lateral ventricle. **f** Opening of the septum pellucidum to access the contralateral ventricle. **g** Opening of the septum pellucidum to access the contralateral ventricle. *cc* corpus callosum, *cma* callosomarginal artery, *ctrl vtrl* contralateral ventricle, *ChP* choroid plexus, *CN* caudate nucleus, *F* falx, *FrL* frontal lobe, *fx* fornix, *GyC* gyrus cinguli (cingulate gyrus), *pa* pericallosal artery, *M* foramen of Monro, *SP^* septum pellucidum (cut), *Th* Thalamus

maintain the hemisphere retracted by 3 or 4 cm. This allows the optimal cone of vision and working angles.

The gyrus of the cingulum may occasionally be mismatched with the corpus callosum: the right and left gyri can be adherent, resembling a continuous structure (Figs. 6.2c and 6.8a, b). The callosomarginal arteries pass in the cingulate sulcus while the pericallosal arteries run above the corpus callosum. They are good anatomical landmarks although they may sometimes lie on the same plane (pericallosal more superficial than expected) and can vary in number. The gray matter of the cingulum surrounded by the pia mater, however, differs sufficiently from the relatively hypovascular and pale white corpus callosum to permit a safe distinction (Fig. 6.2d).

Once the corpus callosum has been exposed, the midline is indicated by its longitudinal raphe which is bordered by two protrusions: the medial longitudinal striae or nerves of Lancisi (Fig. 6.3c). These represent the efference of a thin gray layer which coats the corpus callosum: the induseum griseum. Together they form the dorsal hippocampus whose function is unknown: it may be a rudimentary evolutionary remnant; however, it seems to be widely interconnected with the ventral hippocampus [19].

A 1-cm (maximum 2-cm) longitudinal callosotomy is adequate for accessing the lateral and third ventricles (Figs. 6.2e and 6.8c). This limited opening does not generally imply postoperative neuropsychological sequelae (see section 6.6 Limits and Disadvantages of the Transcallosal Approach). The exact position of the incision should be planned carefully to obtain an optimal exposure and control of the lesion. The anterior half of the corpus callosum is the most appropriate site. The rostrum and splenium should be preserved as they are most often associated with neurological deficits [14, 16, 20]. The individual anatomical features or the pathological distortions of the corpus callosum/septum pellucidum/fornices complex should also be taken into consideration to avoid damage to the fornices at the end of the callosotomy. It is important to evaluate any adherences of the upper forniceal surface to the corpus callosum and their points of anterior and posterior insertions by a preoperative MRI scan [21].

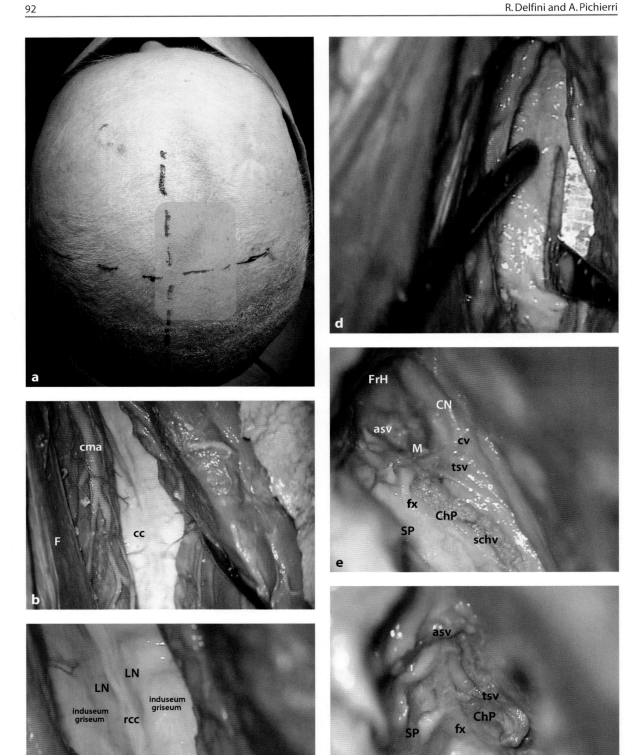

A strictly median callosotomy between the two nerves of Lancisi provides access to the cavum septi pellucidi when an interforniceal approach to the third ventricles is planned or in case bilateral control of the lateral ventricles is anticipated. Otherwise, a paramedian callosotomy allows direct access to the lateral ventricle at the acceptable cost of limited damage to the induseum griseum (not of its efferent system). Lateralization of the incision can be planned on the basis of the lateral extension of the cavum septi pellucidi. The margins of the callosotomy must be bloodless to avoid postoperative intraventricular hemorrhage.

If the chamber below the corpus callosum is bordered by smooth, vertical walls and no choroidal structure can be identified, then we have entered the cavum septi pellucidi. The pressure from the lateral ventricles results in these walls loosely sticking together, and the midline may be distorted if this pressure acts asymmetrically on the septal laminae (Fig. 6.8d). Bilateral fenestration of the septum (not less than 1 cm^2) allows access to the lateral ventricles and exposure of the septum pellucidum inserting on the body of the fornices.

If the lateral ventricles are directly accessed with a paramedian callosotomy, several landmarks can be observed (Fig. 6.2f): the septum pellucidum, the frontal horn and the middle cell containing the choroid plexus, the foramen of Monro, the thalamostriate veins, the anterior septal vein, the thalamus, and the caudate nucleus. These structures are all covered with ependyma (gray–black hue). Fenestration of the septum pellucidum is necessary in this approach too, since it will avoid a restriction of the surgical field due to its bulging, trace the midline, and allow access to the contralateral ventricle (Fig. 6.2g). Exposure of the endoventricular structures offered by this approach is depicted in Fig. 6.1a in light green.

Fig. 6.3 Right middle transcallosal approach. **a** Site of craniotomy. **b** Exposure of the corpus callosum with the callosomarginal arteries lying in the cingulate sulcus. **c** View of the middle portion of the corpus callosum with the tiny gray layer of the induseum griseum above it, the median rostrum, and the paramedian nerves of Lancisi. **d** Middle callosotomy (1 cm). **e, f** View of the anterior half (**e**) and posterior half (**f**) of the exposed lateral ventricle. *asv* anterior septal vein, *cc* corpus callosum, *ChP* choroid plexus, *cma* callosomarginal artery, *CN* caudate nucleus, *cv* caudate vein, *F* falx, *fx* fornix, *FrH* frontal horn, *is-spln* inner surface of the splenium, *LN* Lancisi's nerve, *M* foramen of Monro, *rcc* raphe corpus callosum, *schv* superior choroid vein, *SP* septum pellucidum, *Tr* trigone, *tsv* thalmostriate vein

←

6.3.2 Middle Transcallosal Approach

Patient positioning and the shape of the scalp incision are the same as in the anterior approach. The position of the incision and the craniotomy are more posterior: one-third anterior and two-thirds posterior to the coronal suture (Fig. 6.3a).

The indications for a median or paramedian callosotomy have already been discussed above (Fig. 6.3b–d). The more posterior the paramedian callosotomy is, the more lateral it should be (in terms of millimeters) because the fornices begin to diverge and the corpus callosum tends to be more adherent to these structures (individual characteristics may be studied by a preoperative MRI scan, as already mentioned) [21].

This approach allows a complete view of the lateral ventricles from the frontal horn to the anterior part of the trigone and, medially, the epithalamus (Fig. 6.3e, f). The foramen of Monro is not in the center of the surgical field. Therefore, manipulation of the lesion through this structure is not recommended. The exposure gained via this approach is shown in Fig. 6.1b in light green.

6.3.3 Posterior Transcallosal Approach

The patient is positioned prone with the head in neutral pin fixation (Fig. 6.4a). Craniotomy is performed 4–5 cm anteriorly to the torcular Herophili as the target is the posterior portion of the middle cell (Fig. 6.4a). Venous MR angiography can be referred to as a guide indicating the individual position of the craniotomy, as discussed above. Once the dura is opened and reflected toward the superior longitudinal sinus and the hemisphere is retracted, the posterior half of the corpus callosum with its splenium appears at the bottom of the surgical field.

A paramedian incision of the corpus callosum is only possible because on the midline it adheres to the choroid plexus and to the roof of the third ventricle with the psalterium fornicis and the fornices which, in turn, diverge to reach the hippocampus. These two factors make the ventricles noncontiguous at this level (Fig. 6.4b). The posterior corpus callosum is rich in valuable association fibers (see below), and the callosotomy must not exceed 1 cm. As a consequence, this approach is suitable for lesions with exclusive extension in the posterior third of the middle cella and in the trigone (Fig. 6.1c, Fig. 6.4c).

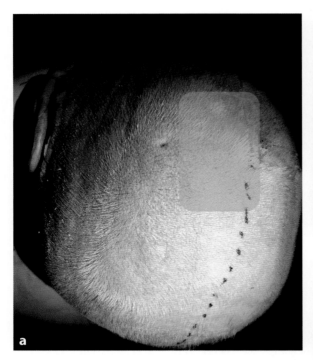

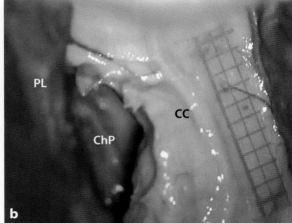

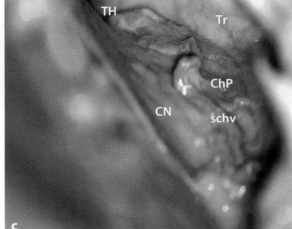

Fig. 6.4 Right posterior transcallosal approach. **a** Site of craniotomy. **b** Paramedian callosotomy (about 1 cm) and access to the trigone of the homolateral ventricle. **c** View of the trigone and of the posterior part of the temporal horn. *CC* corpus callosum, *ChP* choroid plexus, *CN* caudate nucleus, *PL* parietal lobe, *schv* superior choroid vein, *TH* temporal horn, *Tr* trigone

6.3.4 Posterior Approach with Division of the Splenium

A parietooccipital craniotomy is performed 1–2 cm anterior to the torcular Herophili (average area 4×5 cm; Fig. 6.5a). The pineal region and the posterior third of the roof of the third ventricle are the target of this approach. Once the dura has been opened and reflected toward the superior sagittal sinus, the posterior part of the cerebral falx and the upper tentorium are exposed (Fig. 6.5b). The pineal vein, the Rosenthal veins, and the internal occipital and cerebral veins merge into the vein of Galen just anterior to the falcotentorial junction (Fig. 6.5c). At this site, the arachnoid membrane anatomy is complex: the quadrigeminal cistern contains the vein of Galen and the pineal region, the ambient cistern

harbors the basal veins of Rosenthal, and the velum interpositum is crossed by the internal cerebral cistern (Fig. 6.5b,c). The splenium lies anterior to the venous complex. These structures cover the pineal gland, the epithalamus and the habenular commissure above which the third ventricle can be accessed (Fig. 6.5d–f). This entry is covered by the thela choroidea crossed by the posteromedial choroidal artery and the internal cerebral veins (Fig. 6.5g). Nevertheless, access to the third ventricle is feasible via this entrance (Fig. 6.5h).

Division of the splenium is a high-risk maneuver because postoperative visuospatial impairment is common (Fig. 6.5d) [22]. Therefore, this approach should be used for lesions that reduce the splenium to a thin layer of white matter displacing anteriorly the interhemispheric fibers.

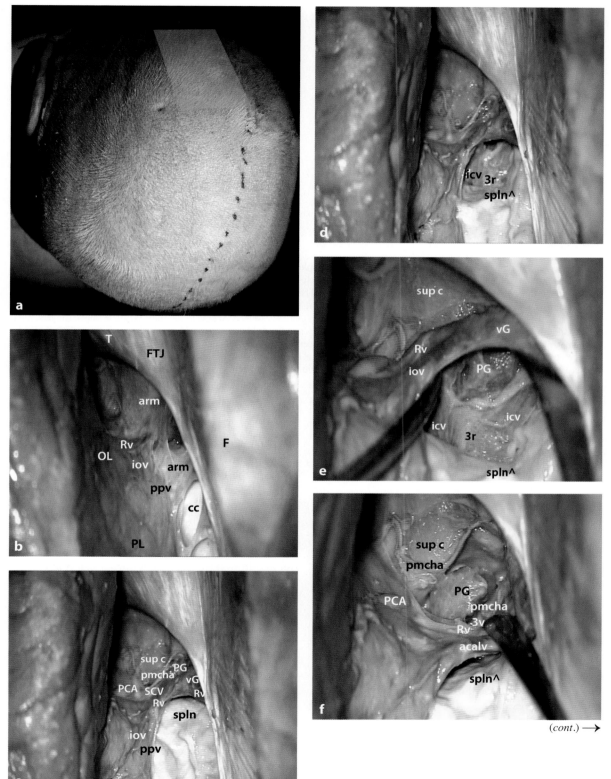

Fig. 6.5 (For legend see page 96)

(*cont.*) →

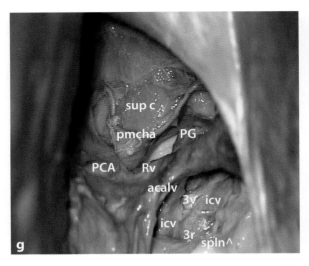
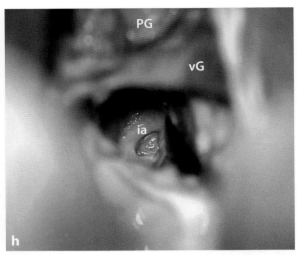

Fig. 6.5 (*cont.*) Posterior callosal approach with division of the splenium. **a** Site of craniotomy. **b** View of the falcotentorial junction above the pineal region and of the mesial aspect of the parietooccipital lobes. **c** The pineal region, the superior colliculi and the deep venous system after dissection from the arachnoid membranes. **d** The internal cerebral veins and the posterior part of the third ventricle after division of the splenium. **e, f** The pineal gland exposed displacing the veins laterally (**e**) and anteriorly (**f**). **g** View of the superior colliculi and the pineal gland and of their relationships with the regional vessels. **h** Access to the third ventricle above the habenular commissure. *3r* third ventricle roof, *3v* third ventricle, *acalv* anterior calcarine vein, *arm* arachnoid membrane, *cc* corpus callosum, *F* falx, *FTJ* falcotentorial junction, *ia* interthalamic adhesion, *icv* internal cerebral vein, *iov* internal occipital vein, *OL* occipital lobe, *PCA* posterior cerebral artery (third segment, P3), *PG* pineal gland, *PL* parietal lobe, *pmcha* posteromedial choroid artery, *ppv* posterior pericallosal vein, *Rv* Rosenthal vein, *SCV* superior cerebellar vein, *spln^* splenium (cut), *sup c* superior colliculus, *T* tentorium, *vG* vein of Galen

6.3.5 Posterior Paracallosal Transprecuneal Approach

Once the posterior region of the corpus callosum has been exposed via the aforementioned steps, a corticotomy is performed at the inferior level of the precuneal gyrus, anteriorly to the parietooccipital fissure (Fig. 6.6a, b). This route should be above and anterior to the optic pathways. The trigone is reached after a short route inside the forceps major; the choroid plexus is, once again, the most important anatomical landmark (Fig. 6.6c). The temporal horn deepens at the lateral margin of the surgical field, while the occipital horn develops superiorly and superficially from the surgeon's perspective. The medial wall of the lateral ventricle and the posterior roof of the third ventricle are exposed medially; inferomedially lies the body of the lateral ventricle (Fig. 6.6d).

The indications for this approach are limited to the rare lesions that push on the medial wall of the atrium or which involve both the epithalamus and the atrium. Interruption of some fibers that join the cingulum from the precuneus occurs during the corticotomy. These fibers are involved in complex visuospatial networks between the limbic system and the prefrontal cortex [23, 24]. Even though iatrogenic impairment due to this approach has not been reported, the route of access should be parallel to these fibers in order to minimize white matter disruption. The corticotomy and the myelotomy should be performed from superior to inferior and from posterior to anterior.

6.4 Approaches to the Third Ventricles

6.4.1 Paraforniceal Approach

The paraforniceal approach utilizes the natural communication between the third and lateral ventricles through the foramen of Monro (therefore, it can also be called the transforaminal approach) (Fig. 6.7a, b). It is useful in lesions that impinge upon the foramen or in patients in whom chronic hydrocephalus causes a dilatation of the foramina. Surgical exposure is limited posteriorly

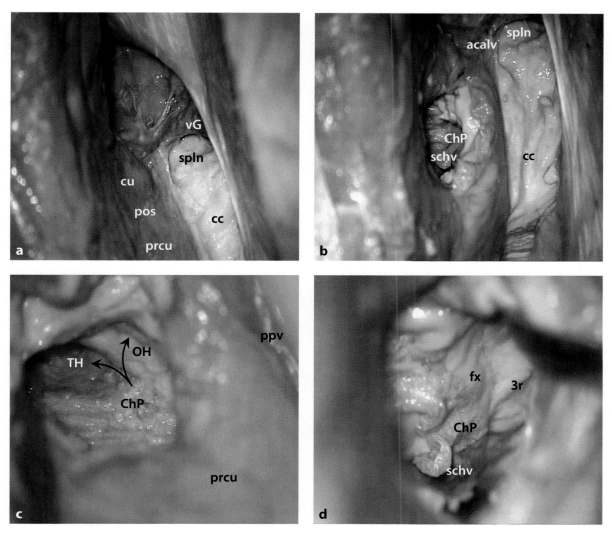

Fig. 6.6 Right paracallosal transprecuneal approach. **a** View of the falcotentorial junction, the pineal region and the mesial aspect of the parietooccipital cortex. **b** A longitudinal corticotomy is carried out anteriorly to the parieto-occipital fissure, in the inferior portion of the precuneus. **c, d** Inferolateral (**c**) and superomedial (**d**) views of the lateral ventricle accessed through its atrium. *3r* third ventricle roof, *acalv* anterior calcarine vein, *cc* corpus callosum, *ChP* choroid plexus, *cu* cuneus (gyrus), *fx* fornix, *OH* occipital horn, *pos* parietooccipital sulcus, *ppv* posterior pericallosal vein, *prcu* precuneus (gyrus), *schv* superior choroid vein, *spln* splenium, *TH* temporal horn, *vG* vein of Galen

by the interthalamic adhesion. Complete exposure (but not surgical control) of the third ventricle is gained with the assistance of an endoscope (Fig. 6.7c, d). If the foramen is too small to operate through, another approach should be chosen.

Cutting the homolateral column of the fornix is commonly described when anterior enlargement of the foramen of Monro is essential. Removal of part of the an-

terior thalamic nucleus is generally suggested for posterior enlargement of this foramen [14, 13, 16]. In the latter case, because of the tight relationship of the thalamus with the internal cerebral vein and its tributaries. these veins are at high risk of damage; in the former case, permanent short-term memory impairment will result if there is a preexisting nonfunctional contralateral fornix.

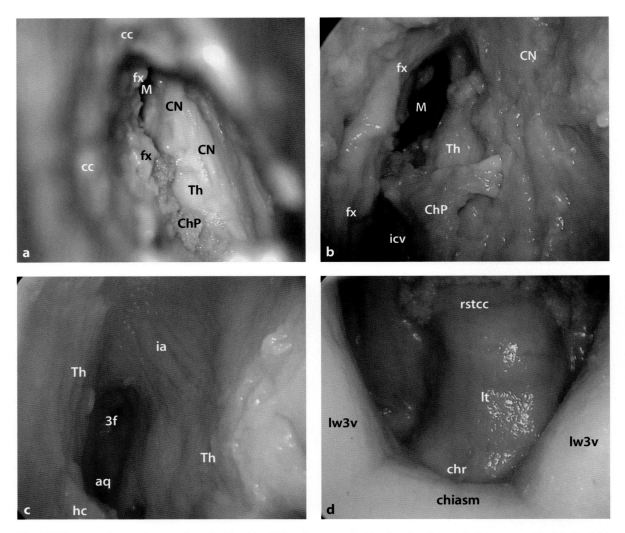

Fig. 6.7 Right paraforniceal approach. **a, b** After identifying the anatomical landmarks of the right lateral ventricle (**a**), the third ventricle is approached by dissecting the homolateral fornix from the thalamus (**b**). The space is limited anteriorly by the internal cerebral vein which still separates the access from the foramen of Monro (**b**). **c, d** Endoscopic views of the most posterior (**c**) and anterior (**d**) portions of the third ventricle visible with this approach. *3f* third ventricle floor, *aq* aqueduct of Sylvius, *cc* corpus callosum, *ChP* choroid plexus, *chr* chiasmatic recess, *CN* caudate nucleus, *fx* fornix, *hc* habenular commisure, *ia* interthalamic adhesion, *icv* internal cerebral vein, *lt* lamina terminalis, *lw3v* lateral wall of the third ventricle, *M* foramen of Monro, *rstcc* rostrum of the corpus callosum, *Th* thalamus

6.4.2 Interforniceal Approach

This approach is illustrated in Fig. 6.8. The septum pellucidum is attached inferiorly to the dorsal aspect of the fornices. There are two variations for the interforniceal technique.

The standard approach involves dissection along the midline and allows separation of the bodies of the for-

nices which are then retracted together with the underlying internal cerebral veins and posteromedial choroidal arteries. The dissection is limited posteriorly by the psalterium fornicis (about 2.5 cm posterior to the foramen of Monro) [21]. As mentioned above, a short septum pellucidum seen on the preoperative sagittal plane MRI scan implies an adhesion between the fornices and the corpus callosum; this can further limit the

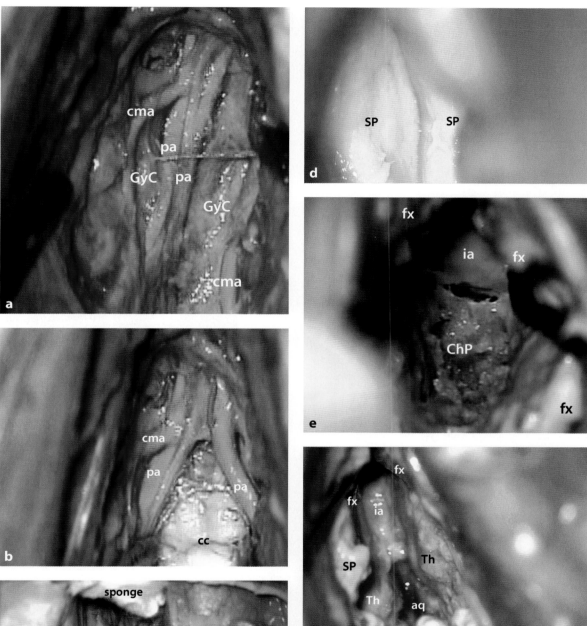

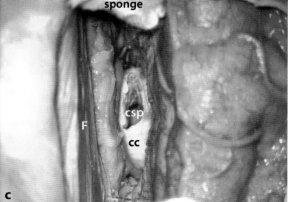

Fig. 6.8 Interforniceal approach. **a, b** Following the technique for the middle transcallosal approach, the corpus callosum is reached. **c** A longitudinal median callosotomy (about 1 cm) is made in order to access the cavum septi pellucidi. **d,** Then the fornices are divaricated to access the choroid plexus (**e**) and the third ventricle (**f**). *aq* aqueduct of Sylvius, *cc* corpus callosum, *ChP* choroid plexus, *cma* callosomarginal artery, *csp* cavum septi pellucidi, *F* falx, *fx* fornix, *GyC* gyrus cinguli (cingulate gyrus), *ia* interthalamic adhesion, *pa* pericallosal artery, *SP* septum pellucidum, *Th* thalamus

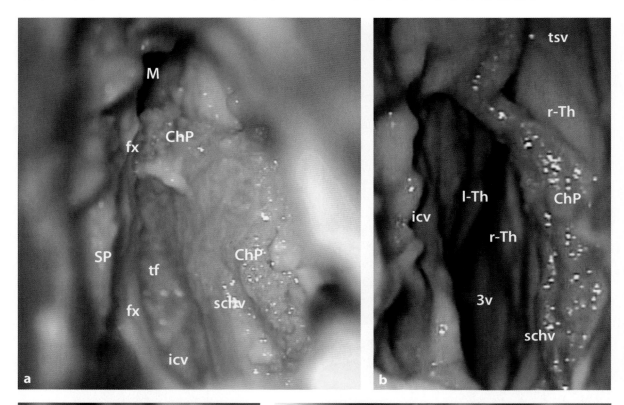

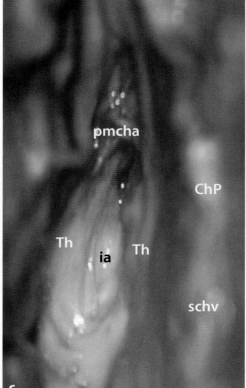

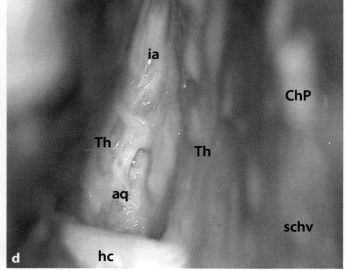

Fig. 6.9 Suprachoroidal approach. **a–c** After an anterior or middle calloso-tomy (**a**), the choroid plexus is divided from the homolateral fornix opening the tenia fornicis (**b**) exposing the third ventricle (**c**). **d** View of the posterior half of the third ventricle. *3v* third ventricle, *aq* aqueduct of Sylvius, *ChP* choroid plexus, *fx* fornix, *hc* habenular commisure, *ia* interthalamic adhe-sion, *icv* internal cerebral vein, *l-Chp* left choroid plexus, *l-Th* left thalamus, *M* foramen of Monro, *pmcha* posteromedial choroid artery, *r-Th* right thal-amus, *schv* superior choroid vein, *SP* septum pellucidum, *tf* tenia fornicis, *Th* thalamus, *tsv* thalmostriate vein

dissection, thus contraindicating this approach. However, the interforniceal route offers a wider view of the superior half of the third ventricle from its anterior wall to the pineal recess and aqueduct of Sylvius with the interthalamic adhesion in the center (Fig. 6.8f).

The anterior forniceal approach is a mini-invasive alternative which entails a limited dissection between the foramina of Monro and the anterior commissure (where also some fibers from the fornices swap). This variation translates the surgical field anteriorly [17].

6.4.3 Suprachoroidal Approach

This route passes between the fornix and choroid plexus through the tenia fornicis. The internal cerebral veins and posteromedial choroidal artery are gently pushed laterally together with the choroid plexus (Fig. 6.9a). This bends medially in proximity to the foramen of Monro in a posterior direction along the midline in a hairpin fashion, blocking surgical access anteriorly and preventing the creation of a single transforaminal–suprachoroidal corridor. The plexus itself may be coagulated and divided, but the most intimate arteriovenous relationships of the plexus are just at that site (Fig. 6.9b). This route has been proposed as a low-risk alternative to the subchoroidal approach, as the veins are not stretched [6, 15]. On the other hand, the whole third ventricle can be exposed with this approach while the visualization of its deepest portion is blocked by the interthalamic adhesion; however, the infundibular recess and the aqueduct of Sylvius are visible (Fig. 6.9c, d).

6.4.4 Subchoroidal Approach

The tenia choroidea is used for this approach. The choroid plexus is dislocated medially from the internal cerebral vein and the posteromedial choroidal artery. In this approach, the veins limit the surgical exposure, in particular the thalamostriate vein which comes from the dorsal aspect of the thalamus and adheres to the plexus prior to merging into the internal cerebral vein (Fig. 6.10a, b); the septal vein may also be stretched by surgical maneuvers at this level (Fig. 6.10c).

It may be helpful to define the junction among these veins preoperatively (venous MR angiography is adequate). If this junction is very anterior, the surgical route will suffice. If the junction is more posterior, a transforaminal route with a small anterior subchoroidal extension may be preferable. If there are multiple thalamostriate veins, the sacrifice of one of them seems safe [6]. Whether the thalamostriate and the anterior septal veins are dispensable remains controversial,– but it seems that their unilateral sacrifice may be acceptable because of profuse collateralization. We are very cautious about this topic, because the consequences of their interruption are unpredictable. Coagulation of the anterior septal and thalamostriate veins would allow a single transforaminal–subchoroidal corridor which provides a similar amount of exposure as the suprachoroidal route.

6.4.5 Removal of the Lesion

The lesion is generally debulked and then dissected peripherally [5, 8, 13, 14, 16]. Large cotton sponges must be placed into the sloping portions of the surgical field to avoid tumor particles and blood gravitating into the ventricles [14, 16].

6.5 Advantages of the Transcallosal Approach

Any transcallosal route can provide access to the lateral ventricle sparing cerebral matter and minimizing the risk of postoperative epilepsy and poroencephalic cysts [5, 7, 8, 9, 11–17].

Transcortical routes require disruption of a large amount of cortex and white matter, and maintenance of the retraction may be difficult [9]. With regard to the paracallosal approach, the transcortical route to the lesion is through a not strictly well-expressed tissue and it is often short as it is involved in lesions that develop in the trigone and in the occipitomesial cortex which is therefore already thin.

Other advantages of the transcortical routes include short, straightforward and multiple trajectories to the third ventricle, and wider flexibility of the cone of vision and of the working angles [5, 6, 7, 9, 13–16, 22]. Moreover, a bilateral exposure of the Monro foramina and of the roof of the third ventricles is possible only using these approaches; homolateral visualization of the third ventricle is problematic with the transcortical routes.

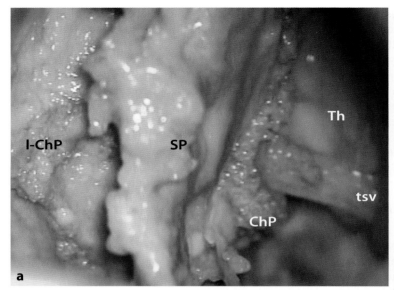

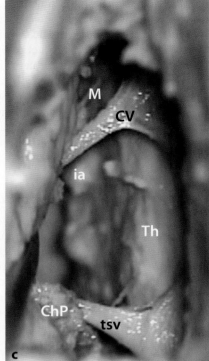

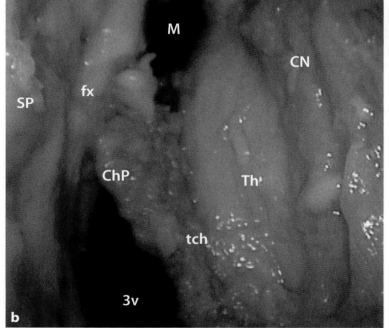

Fig. 6.10 Subchoroidal approach. A usual anterior or middle callosotomy is carried out. **a** The septum pellucidum has been opened to show the contralateral ventricle. **b** The choroid plexus is attached to the fornix through the tenia fornicis (cut in this specimen) and to the homolateral thalamus through the tenia choroidea. **c** The third ventricle is accessed opening the tenia choroidea and displacing the choroid plexus medially; note that the available corridor is narrowed by the deep venous system. *3v* third ventricle, *ChP* choroid plexus, *CN* caudate nucleus, *CV* caudate vein, *fx* fornix, *ia* interthalamic adhesion, *l-ChP* left choroid plexus, *M* foramen of Monro, *SP* septum pellucidum, *tch* tenia choroidea, *Th* thalamus, *tsv* thalmostriate vein

Compared with the translamina terminalis subfrontal approach, less retraction and manipulation of the anterior cerebral and anterior communicating arteries are required [9]. Exposure through the lamina terminalis permits only a limited view into the third ventricular chamber and, consequently, limits the extent of possible resection compared with the transcallosal approach. The use of the transcortical approach implies the risk of a specific neurological deficit according to the site of the corticotomy. In our experience, the transcortical approach is burdened by a higher incidence of motor deficits (+4.4%), speech disorders (+15.4%) and visual deficits (7.8%). The safest routes of access are through the superior parietal gyrus and the middle frontal gyrus, but these are not free from the following risks:

- Superior parietal gyrus: apraxia, acalculia, damage to the optic radiation, postoperative epilepsy
- Middle frontal gyrus: damage to the frontal ocular field, postoperative epilepsy

After the use of a transcortical route, we have observed personality change in 7.8% of patients (perifrontal horn gliomas), memory impairment in 7.8% (giant craniopharyngioma, temporal glioma), psychotic deterioration in 3.9% (temporal horn mixed glioma), and eating disorders in 3.9% (papillary glioneuronal tumor of the third ventricle). In these patients we consider that the tumor location and the surgical manipulation of adjacent deep structures were responsible for the mental disorders rather than the approach itself. Thus, we think that a transcallosal approach would not have avoided these deficits in these patients.

6.6 Limits and Disadvantages of the Transcallosal Approach

Transcallosal approaches are not suitable for lesions of the temporal horn [5, 9, 13, 16]. A direct posterior corridor should be considered in lesions that are less than 1.5 cm in size and located primarily in the posterior part of the ventricular chamber. Lesions that are primarily basal with lateral extension, presenting a restricted or narrow apex that deforms the middle and anterior fornix, may require a combined basal (for lateral access) and transcallosal midline approach.

The need of some degree of cortical retraction is common to the transcortical, transcallosal and even transbasal approaches. The real problem concerns the parasagittal veins, since their closure leads to unpredictable results ranging from absence of symptoms to cortical and subcortical deficits, seizures and, eventually, massive venous infarctions and death [1, 4, 5, 9, 11, 14, 22].

Postoperative neuropsychological deficits have been described for callosotomies of the rostrum and of the splenium. The most common disturbances are:

- Mnemonic and attentive deficits, confabulations (especially for damage to the anterior two-thirds of the corpus callosum).
- Working, retrieval and associative memory (especially for damage to the rostrum).
- Hemilexia with/without agraphia, astereognosis, motor incoordination (callosal ataxia), inability to

perform previously acquired complex motor schemes (apraxia), acalculia, agnosia for callosotomies of the posterior half.
- Hemiparesis (most related to venous impairment).
- Akinetic mutism (most related to bilateral retraction of the cingulate gyri).

The corpus callosum is made up of 300 million axons, most of which serve homotopic interconnections [20, 23]. Following the most recent topographical review we can distinguish five regions from anterior to posterior:

- Anterior half:
  - Region 1 (one-sixth): prefrontal fibers
  - Region 2 (one-third): premotor fibers
- Posterior half:
  - Region 3 (one-sixth): motor fibers
  - Region 4 (one-twelfth): primary sensory fibers
  - Region 5 (one-quarter): parietal, temporal, occipital fibers.

It is remarkable that fibers from the motor cortex cross the corpus callosum more posteriorly with respect to the traditional Witelson's scheme. Region 5 is rich in heterotopic fibers which interconnect different areas of the parietotemporooccipital lobes. This may explain why damaging the splenium often has clinical repercussions.

It should also be noted that the literature on this topic deals with epileptic patients and corpus callosum gliomas in whom the callosotomies are complete or significantly more extensive. Many reports belong to a period when microsurgical instrumentation (microscope and CUSA included) and techniques had not reached the high level of our time. In fact, more recent series show a marked reduction in these deficits [11]. Moreover, these deficits are temporary and the patients recover fully after a couple of months. Actually, it is not possible to predict the neuropsychological deficit entity after callosotomy [11, 14, 16]. In general, callosotomies of 1–2 cm hardly lead to permanent deficits, and young people and children recover more easily than adults, probably due to an intrinsically increased cerebral plasticity. Homotopic and heterotopic fibers of the corpus callosum are very useful but not essential for common daily activities; lost networks may be compensated for and recreated with specific rehabilitation techniques.

In conclusion, we consider unwarranted the fear of performing such approaches in patients who require superior interactions between left and right hemispheres (such as artists and highly specialized professionals). An overt worsening of manual performance and neuropsychological functions is possible in the immediate postoperative period. In some patients, this may impact deeply on their working, social or artistic life. Nevertheless, exercise, practice and rehabilitation can succeed in recovering these functions. To choose a transcortical approach merely because of the risk of some degree of disconnection syndrome may have a boomerang effect: cortical areas considered silent in the past are now considered to be involved in a complex network of cognition and multisensory integration (e.g. the superior parietal lobule and visuospatial integration, the middle frontal gyrus and the visual pathways integrated with cognition, awareness and behavior). Besides the corticotomy, a route through the white matter is necessary to reach the lesion. This entails the destruction of associative, inter-/intralobar and long tract fibers. The creation of an epileptic focus requires antiepileptic drugs which also reduce neuropsychological functions and creativity.

6.7 Limits and Disadvantages of the Approaches to the Third Ventricles

The transcortical and transcallosal routes require the same surgical corridors to reach the third ventricle (para-/interforniceal, supra-/subchoroidal). The advantages and the disadvantages are therefore also common to both approaches.

6.7.1 Paraforniceal Route

This route guarantees a wide and anatomic exposure of the third ventricle, especially in patients with an enlarged Monro foramen (6–10 mm) and in patients with chronic hydrocephalus. On the other hand, it can provoke mutism, lethargy, hemiplegia, mnemonic impairment following damage to the internal cerebral veins,

the choroidal artery or the fornix (if the contralateral fornix had a preexisting dysfunction) [9, 14, 16].

6.7.2 Transchoroidal Routes

Lesions stretching to the roof of the third ventricle or the posterior two-thirds of the third ventricle are best approached by this route [6]. The thalamus limits the exposure of small and very deep lesions. As discussed in section 6.3 Surgical Technique, the corridor offered by the two transchoroidal routes overlaps. Strokes and hemorrhages are most common with the subchoroidal approach because the internal cerebral veins and their tributaries course beneath the tela choroidea; thrombosis/damage may occur due to an excessive retraction or manipulation [14, 16]. The clinical sequelae of any closure of the thalamostriate and anterior septal veins are unpredictable [4]. Venous anastomoses may partially or even totally compensate for the closure, but this is not predictable in the individual patient. Venous coagulation should, in our opinion, be utilized only if absolutely necessary and if the thalamostriate veins are multiple. The suprachoroidal corridor avoids the intimate venous relationships of the subchoroidal route [6, 14, 16].

6.7.3 Interforniceal Approach

The widest access to the third ventricle can be obtained via this route [12, 14, 16, 17, 21]. Veins and arteries are gently pushed laterally together with the plexus and the fornices. The most important issue in this approach is the management of the fornices. Simple manipulation and traction often provoke temporary memory impairment, and any bilateral mechanical damage or prolonged traction will cause permanent postoperative loss of short-term memory fixation [16].

References

1. Dandy WE (1933) Benign tumors in the third ventricle of the brain: diagnosis and treatment. Charles C Thomas, Baltimore
2. Busch E (1944) A new approach for the removal of tumors of the third ventricle. Acta Psychiatr Scand 19:57–60
3. Kempe LG, Blaylock R (1976) Lateral-trigonal intraventricular tumors. A new operative approach. Acta Neurochir (Wien) 35:233–242
4. Hirsch JF, Zouanaoui A, Renier D, Pierre-Kahn A (1979) A new surgical approach to the third ventricle with interruption of the striothalamic vein. Acta Neurochir (Wien) 47:135–147
5. Yasargil MG (1996) Microneurosurgery of CNS tumors (IVB). Thieme, Leipzig
6. Wen HT, Rhoton AL Jr, de Oliveira E (1998) Transchoroidal approach to the third ventricle: an anatomic study of the choroidal fissure and its clinical application. Neurosurgery 42:1205–1217

7. Rosenfeld JV, Harvey AS, Wrennall J et al (2001) Transcallosal resection of hypothalamic hamartomas, with control of seizures, in children with gelastic epilepsy. Neurosurgery 48:108–118

8. Amar AP, Ghosh S, Apuzzo ML (2003) Ventricular tumors. In: Winn RH (ed) Youmans neurological surgery, 5th edn. Elsevier, Amsterdam, p 1237

9. D'Angelo VA, Galarza M, Catapano D et al (2005) Lateral ventricle tumors: surgical strategies according to tumor origin and development. A series of 72 cases. Neurosurgery 56:ONS36–ONS45

10. Kawashima M, Li X, Rhoton AL Jr et al (2006) Surgical approaches to the atrium of the lateral ventricle: microsurgical anatomy. Surg Neurol 65:436–445

11. Mazza M, Di Rienzo A, Costagliola C et al (2004) The interhemispheric transcallosal-transversal approach to the lesions of the anterior and middle third ventricle: surgical validity and neuropsychological evaluation of the outcome. Brain Cogn 55:525–534

12. Timurkaynak E, Izci Y, Acar F (2006) Transcavum septum pellucidum interforniceal approach for the colloid cyst of the third ventricle. Operative nuance. Surg Neurol 66:544–547

13. Yasargil MG, Abdukrauf SI (2008) Surgery of intraventricular tumors. Neurosurgery 62:SHC1029–SHC1041

14. Apuzzo ML (1998) Surgery of the third ventricle. In: Rengachary SS, Wilkins RH (eds) Neurosurgical operative atlas. Williams & Wilkins, Baltimore

15. Kasowski HJ, Nahed BV, Piepmeier JM (2005) Transcallosal transchoroidal approach to tumors of the third ventricle. Neurosurgery 57:ONS361–ONS366

16. Wen HT, Mussi ACM, Rhoton AL Jr et al (2006) Surgical approach to lesions located in the lateral, third and fourth ventricles. In: Sekhar L, Fessler R (eds) Atlas of neurosurgical techniques: brain. Thieme Verlag, Leipzig, pp 507–546

17. Siwanuwatn R, Deshmukh P, Feiz-Erfan I et al (2005) Microsurgery anatomy of the transcallosal anterior interforniceal approach to the third ventricle. Neurosurgery 56:ONS390–ONS396

18. Fronda C, Miller D, Kappus C et al (2008) The benefit of image guidance for the contralateral interhemispheric approach to the lateral ventricle. Clin Neurol Neurosurg 110:580–586

19. Di Leva A, Tschabitscher M, Rodriguez y Baena R (2007) Lancisi's nerve and the seat of the soul. Neurosurgery 60:563–568

20. Hofer S, Frahm J (2006) Topography of the human corpus callosum revisited – comprehensive fiber tractography using diffusion tensor magnetic resonance imaging. Neuroimage 32:989–994

21. Ozer MA, Kayalioglu G, Ert M (2005) Topographic anatomy of the fornix as a guide for the transcallosal-interforniceal approach with a special emphasis on sex differences. Neurol Med Chir (Tokyo) 45:607–613

22. Lozier AP, Bruce JN (2003) Surgical approaches to posterior third ventricular tumors. Neurosurg Clin N Am 14:527–545

23. Fernández-Miranda JC, Rhoton AL Jr, Alvarez-Linera J et al (2008) Three-dimensional microsurgical and tractographic anatomy of the white matter of the human brain. Neurosurgery 62(6 Suppl 3):989–1026

24. Ghaem O, Mellet E, Crivello F et al (1997) Mental navigation along memorized routes activates the hippocampus, precuneus, and insula. Neuroreport 8:739–744

Subtemporal Approach

Pasqualino Ciappetta and Pietro I. D'Urso

7.1 Introduction

The subtemporal approach is historically known as the standard approach for the treatment of tumoral, vascular and inflammatory lesions of the middle cranial fossa, the tentorium, the anterior and middle tentorial incisura, the upper-third of the clivus and the petroclival region.

This approach had been recognized universally for many years as the best way to treat basilar artery (BA) apex, P1 and P2 posterior cerebral artery (PCA) and superior cerebellar artery (SCA) aneurysms until the introduction of the pterional approach in 1976 by Yasargil et al. [1].

Continual advances in surgical anatomical studies of the skull base in the last 15 years have led to the technical evolution of this approach, allowing its extension towards adjacent areas and permitting the development of extended subtemporal approaches, obtained by zygomatic, orbital, temporal or frontotemporoorbital osteotomies and petrous apex resections. Knowledge of the topographic anatomy of the cranial region, where the varying surgical corridors described in this chapter must be prepared, is as fundamental as continual practice by cadaver dissection.

For a more detailed anatomical study of the middle cranial fossa, study of the anatomical works of Rhoton is recommended [2].

The discussion in this chapter of the surgical techniques of the subtemporal approach includes a section describing the anterior subtemporal approach, which can be used to expose the anterior portion of the middle cranial fossa and the anterior and middle incisural space lesions, a section describing the posterior subtemporal approach, which is used to reach lesions of the posterior portion of the middle cranial fossa and the middle incisural space until the conjunction with its posterior portion, corresponding to the ambient cistern, and sections describing variants of the extended subtemporal approach that deal with specific pathologies, their topographic location and their extension from the middle cranial fossa towards adjacent areas.

7.2 Surgical Pathology

7.2.1 Meningiomas

The standard subtemporal approach and its variations are most frequently requested for sphenoidal wing meningiomas, followed by Yasargil's T1- and T2-type tentorial tumors arising from the inner ring of the tentorium [3] (Fig. 7.1). The subtemporal approach can be used for petroclival meningiomas that do not extend below the upper clivus. For lesions extending above and below the tentorium situated on the tentorial edge or in the petroclival area, only those with a small infratentorial component can be removed by the subtemporal approach.

Meningiomas originating from Meckel's cave (MC) are uncommon and account for approximately 0.5% of all intracranial tumors and 1% of all intracranial meningiomas. Samii et al. [4] classified these tumors into four distinct types according to extension and involvement

P. Ciappetta (✉)
Dept of Neurological Sciences
University of Bari Medical School, Bari, Italy

P. Cappabianca et al. (eds.), *Cranial, Craniofacial and Skull Base Surgery*.
© Springer-Verlag Italia 2010

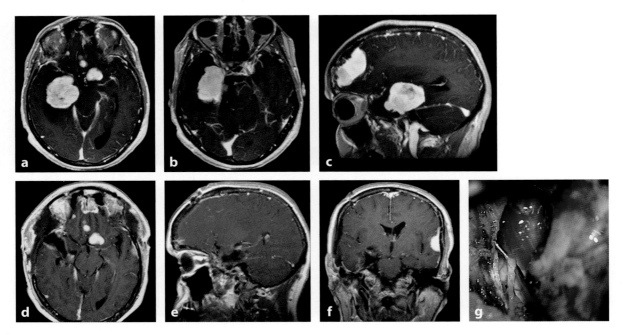

Fig. 7.1 **a, b** Axial T1-weighted MR images after gadolinium injection show multiple meningiomas with a large right tentorial meningioma in part extending into the lateral incisural space. **c** Same patient. Sagittal T1-weighted MR image after gadolinium injection of the tentorial meningioma. In the frontal region a large frontal meningioma is evident. **d–f** Postoperative axial, sagittal and coronal T1-weighted MR images after gadolinium injection show complete removal of the frontal and tentorial tumors. **g** Intraoperative photograph after tumor removal shows the preserved trochlear nerve; the integral nerve is lifted from the surface of the brainstem, against which it was previously compressed by the tumor. Histological diagnosis: atypical meningioma

of the surrounding structures of MC: type I includes tumors mainly confined to MC; type II includes MC meningiomas with major extension into the middle fossa with or without extension to the cavernous sinus (CS); type III includes MC meningiomas with major extension into the cerebellopontine angle (CPA); and type IV includes MC meningiomas with extension both into the middle fossa and into the CP angle with or without infiltration of the CS.

Meningiomas affecting MC may extend in different directions and may therefore show distinct surgical problems.

In the surgical decision-making process, the following factors must be considered: (1) tumor mass extension into the neighboring structures, principally into the CPA and middle fossa; (2) the presence of CS infiltration and carotid artery encasement; (3) typical images of en plaque tumor growing; and (4) petrous apex erosion and involvement of the petrous bone. Cranial nerve (CN) impairment, especially of III, IV and VI CNs, can provide additional information about tumor invasion of the CS [4].

7.2.2 Schwannomas

Schwannomas arising from the intracranial portion of the trigeminal nerve are rare, accounting for 0.07–0.33% of intracranial tumors and 0.8–8% of intracranial schwannomas [5]. These tumors may arise from the trigeminal nerve root, the gasserian ganglion (GG), or one of the three peripheral branches, indicating that trigeminal schwannomas may grow into one, two, or all three distinct compartments: the subdural (CPA), interdural (lateral wall of the CS and MC) and epidural or extracranial (orbit, pterygopalatine fossa and infratemporal fossa) spaces. These tumors are often seen extending into multiple cranial fossae: the posterior, middle and infratemporal fossa and the orbit. Yoshida and Kawase classified these tumors into three types in relation to the compartment involved: type M (14.8%) including middle fossa tumors originating from the GG or the peripheral branch at the lateral wall of the CS (Fig. 7.2); type P (18.5%) including posterior fossa tumors originating from the root of the trigeminal nerve; and type E (3.7%) including tumors arising from the ex-

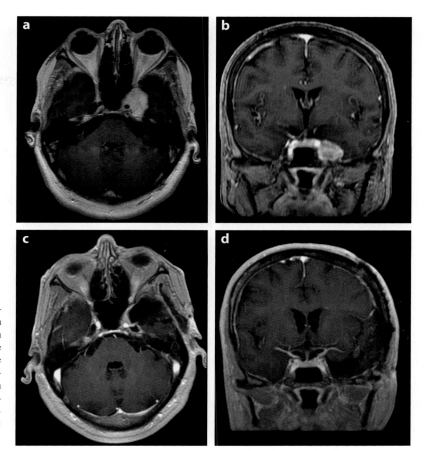

Fig. 7.2 a, b Axial and coronal T1-weighted MR images after gadolinium injection show an apparently benign tumor of the medial portion of the middle cranial fossa extending in part into the cavernous sinus. **c, d** Postoperative T1-weighted MR images after gadolinium injection confirm complete tumor removal through the subtemporal interdural approach. Histological diagnosis: schwannoma Antoni type A

tracranial peripheral branches of the trigeminal nerve. The only type E tumor in the series was located in the infratemporal fossa, indicating that the origin of this tumor was the third branch of the trigeminal nerve. The remaining three complex types consist of tumors extending into multiple compartments: type MP (37%) include dumbbell-shaped tumors located in both the posterior and middle fossae (Fig. 7.3); type ME (18.5%) include dumbbell-shaped tumors located in the middle fossa and the extracranial space (the orbit, pterygopalatine fossa, or infratemporal fossa); and type MPE (7.4%) include tumors located in all three compartments, the posterior and middle cranial fossae and the extracranial space (the orbit, pterygopalatine fossa, or infratemporal fossa). In the two MPE cases of the series, the tumor extended along the second branch of the trigeminal nerve into the pterygopalatine and infratemporal fossa (Fig. 7.4) [6].

Facial nerve schwannomas (FNSs) are uncommon tumors arising from anywhere along the course of the facial nerve, from the CPA to the neuromuscular junc-

tion; however, there is a predilection for the geniculate ganglion. From the geniculate ganglion, a facial nerve schwannoma may extend to involve the tympanic and/or labyrinthine portion of the facial nerve. Uncommonly, FNSs extend to involve the middle cranial fossa by means of direct upward spread through the roof of the temporal bone or anterior spread through the facial hiatus towards the greater superficial petrosal nerve (GSPN) [7] (Fig. 7.5). In the series of Wiggins et al. the involved portions of the facial nerve included the following seven segments: cerebellopontine angle and internal auditory canal (50%), labyrinthine (54%), geniculate fossa (83%), GSPN (25%), tympanic (54%), and mastoid (33%) [8]. Lesions arising from the geniculate ganglion can have a "bulbous" enlargement at the geniculate fossa. FNSs emanating from the GSPN scallop the anterior margin of the geniculate fossa and the adjacent bony petrous apex. Schwannomas of the oculomotor nerve and trochlear nerve are very uncommon especially when not associated with neurofibromatosis (Fig. 7.6).

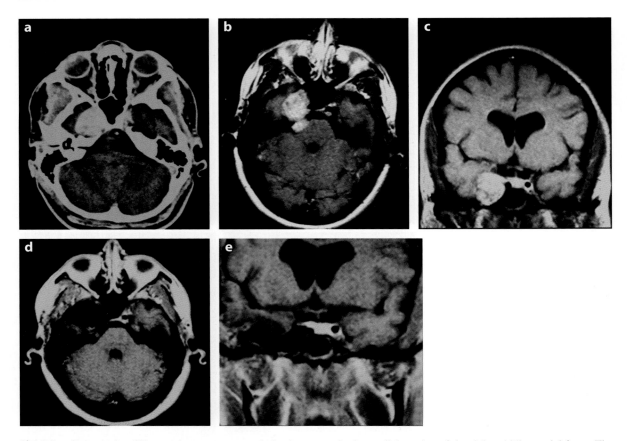

Fig. 7.3 a Preoperative CT scan shows an apparently benign tumor in the medial portion of the right middle cranial fossa. The erosion of the right petrous apex is suggestive of a trigeminal neurinoma. **b** Axial T1-weighted MR image after gadolinium injection shows the tumor slightly extending from the middle cranial fossa into the posterior cranial fossa and the lateral surface of the pons. **c** Coronal T1-weighted MR image after gadolinium injection shows partial involvement of the right cavernous sinus. **d, e** Postoperative axial and coronal T1-weighted MR images after gadolinium injection show complete tumor removal through the subtemporal interdural approach. Histological diagnosis: schwannoma Antoni type A

Fig. 7.4 Drawing showing developmental patterns of trigeminal nerve schwannomas. Type M: middle fossa tumors originating from the GG or the peripheral branch at the lateral wall of the CS; Type P: posterior fossa tumors originating from the root of the trigeminal nerve; Type E: extracranial tumors in the epidural space (E1 in the orbit and E2 in the pterygopalatine fossa and infratemporal fossa)

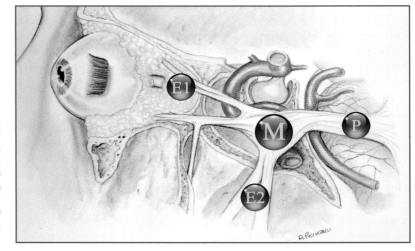

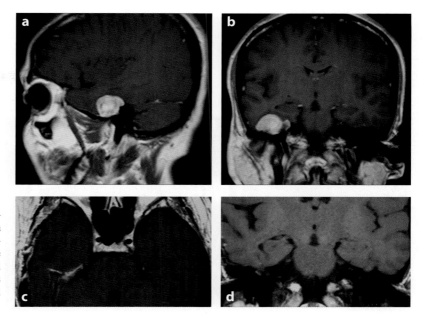

Fig. 7.5 a, b Sagittal and coronal T1-weighted MR images after gadolinium injection show a likely benign tumor arising from the skull base at the level of the tegmen timpani. **c, d** Postoperative axial and coronal T1-weighted MR images after gadolinium injection. Histological diagnosis: schwannoma Antoni type A

Trochlear nerve schwannomas were classified by Celli et al. [9] into three groups according to the classification of Jefferson [10] for the trigeminal variety: cisternal, cisternocavernous, and cavernous. Trochlear nerve schwannomas almost always occur in the cisternal position (88%) and less frequently in the cisternocavernous (8%) and cavernous positions (4%). Almost all schwannomas originating from the trochlear nerve occupy the ambient cistern, ventrolateral to the mesencephalon and pons. These tumors are usually located just beneath the tentorium edge, partially adhering to the tentorium and compressing the midbrain medially. The trochlear nerve is usually identified in the posterior or posteroinferior aspect of the tumor. Only 33 cases of oculomotor nerve neurinomas have been published in the literature: 44% of these are cisternal, 39% involve the CS and 17% extend from the CS to the cistern [11].

7.2.3 Cavernous Sinus Pathology

Several pathological entities involve the CS. Some arise as intrinsic CS pathologies and others spread into the sinus from adjacent areas. Lesions of the CS can be classified into benign and malignant [12]. The benign lesions involving the CS include neoplastic lesions such as meningiomas, trigeminal and abducens schwannomas, pituitary adenomas and granular cell tumors [13–

16]. The nonneoplastic benign lesions include vascular lesions such as intracavernous carotid artery aneurysms, cavernous malformations and carotid cavernous fistulas [17–19]. Other benign processes involving the CS include cholesterol granuloma and inflammatory diseases [16, 20]. These last lesions can include infectious inflammatory processes, such as CS thrombophlebitis and mycotic infections and noninfectious inflammatory processes such as Tolosa-Hunt syndrome, inflammatory pseudotumors and giant cell granulomas [21]. Malignant lesions involving the CS mostly spread to the CS from adjacent compartments. Adenoid cystic carcinomas are notorious in spreading along CNs to the CS region. Chordomas can involve the region of the CS arising from adjacent notochord remnants. Malignancies of the paranasal sinuses can also spread into the CS.

7.2.4 Pituitary Adenomas

Pituitary adenomas represent a significant proportion (up to 13%) of all intracranial tumors.

A subgroup of pituitary adenomas (5–10%) invade the lateral parasellar structures and the CS and pose obvious problems for the surgical strategy, since transsphenoidal removal of these adenomas can be incomplete [22]. Goel et al., reporting on a series of 118 cases of giant pituitary adenomas, introduced a classification that includes four grades of giant pituitary ade-noma: grade I in which the tumors are confined under the diaphragma sellae; grade II in which there is evi-dence of encroachment into the CS; grade III in which the superior wall of the CS is elevated and there is ex-tension of this elevation into the surrounding structures;

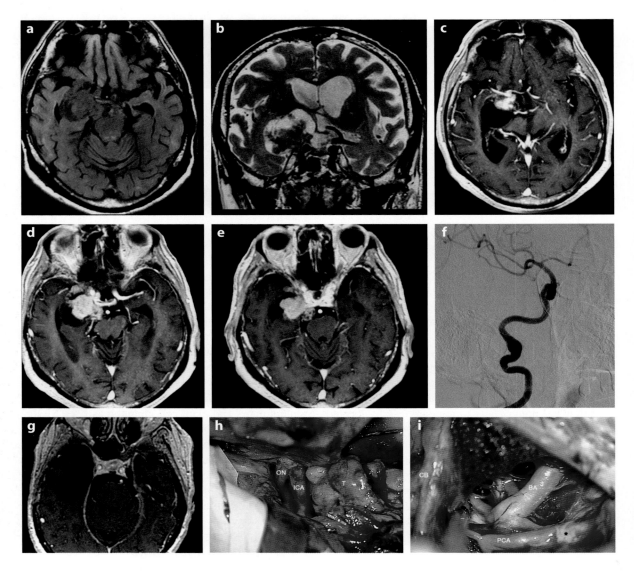

Fig. 7.6 a, b Axial T1-weighted and coronal T2-weighted MR images show a tumor occupying the right mesial temporal region and extending into the crural cistern in front of the brainstem. **c–e** Axial T1-weighted MR images after gadolinium injection of three dif-ferent layers show the tumor extending from the tentorial incisura to the supraclinoid region; on the superior tumor pole a cystic component may be seen. The tight relationship with the supraclinoid ICA and its bifurcation is also evident. **f** Selective right carotid angiogram shows the pulling and uncoiling of the ICA and its branches caused by the underlying tumor. **g** Postoperative axial T1-weighted MR image after gadolinium injection shows complete tumor extirpation. **h** Intraoperative photograph; pretemporal approach. In the operative field the tumor (*T*), right optic nerve (*ON*) and right supraclinoid ICA are evident. **i** Intraoperative photograph of the surgical field at the end of the operation shows the carotid bifurcation (*CB*) and basilar artery (*BA*) quadrifurcation after complete tumor resection. The asterisk indicates the residual portion of cranial nerve III because its anterior portion was completely substituted by the tumor. Histological diagnosis: schwannoma Antoni type A

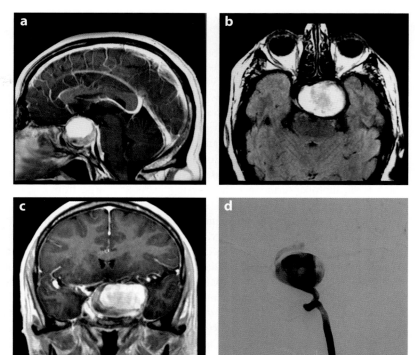

Fig. 7.7 a Sagittal T1-weighted MR image after gadolinium injection shows a giant intrasellar aneurysm extending into the suprasellar region in great part thrombosed. **b, c** Axial and coronal T1-weighted MR images after gadolinium injection show extension into the left parasellar region as well. **d** Selective internal carotid angiography confirms the diagnosis of a giant aneurysm of the intracavernous portion of the ICA

and grade IV in which all of the surrounding structures are breached and there is invasion into the subarachnoid space with encasement of arterial structures [23].

Giant aneurysms projecting into the sellar region and with extension into the CS and medial portion of the middle cranial fossa can mimic a giant pituitary tumor (Fig. 7.7), since they have similar clinical, endocrinological and neurological symptoms.

An aneurysm extending into the sellar region with chiasmal compression was found as early as 1889 by Mitchell and in 1912 by Cushing [24]. Raymond found that 1.4% to 5% of all intracranial aneurysms referred to neurosurgeons projected into the sella [25]; these can account for up to 10% of the lesions causing parasellar syndrome. On the other hand, there is a coexisting aneurysm in 6.7% of pituitary adenomas. This is of particular interest since the differential diagnosis from pituitary tumors may be difficult.

7.2.5 Chordomas and Chondrosarcomas

Chordomas are malignant tumors arising from the remnants of the notochord, originating from the sphenooc-

cipital synchondrosis and then the midline; however, lateral extension is not uncommon. Chordomas can extend from the clivus to the CS, sphenoid sinus, ethmoid sinus, sella turcica, suprasellar cistern, orbits, nasopharynx, infratemporal fossa, parapharyngeal space, hypoglossal canals, jugular foramen and prevertebral space. The parasellar region is most frequently involved (23–60%), followed by the prepontine (36–48%) and the nasopharyngeal (10–25%) regions. Meyer et al. found extension into the middle cranial fossa in 32.1% of cases [26]. Chordomas of the petrous apex region have also been reported in the literature and in one series the petrous apex was involved in 15% of cases [27].

Chondrosarcomas develop mainly in the bones of the skull base and temporal bone because they mature predominantly by endochondral ossification. The areas of petrooccipital, sphenooccipital and sphenopetrosal synchondrosis, as well as a large part of the petrous portion of the temporal bone, are sites in the mature skull that have undergone endochondral development. Kveton et al. reported that chondrosarcomas accounted for 6% of all skull-base lesions [28]. The most common skull-base sites vary among studies, with common sites of involvement including the temporooccipital junction and the middle cranial fossa.

7.2.6 Inflammatory Lesions

Regarding inflammatory lesions, cholesterol granulomas represent the foreign-body giant cell reaction to cholesterol with associated fibrosis, vascular proliferation, hemosiderin-laden macrophages, and round cells. They can be found throughout the temporal bone and are usually seen in conjunction with serous otitis media, chronic otitis media, with or without cholesteatoma, seen in prior otological surgery or local trauma. Past terms for these lesions have included epidermoid cyst, which is an improper term since there is no squamous or epithelial lining, mucosal cyst, and giant cholesterol cyst. They were first reported in the mastoid and middle ear in the later part of the 19th century, but petrous apex cholesterol granuloma (Fig. 7.8) was not recognized as a distinct entity until the late 1980s. Giant cell reparative granuloma (GCRG) is a reactive inflammatory process related to trauma and intraosseous hemorrhages. GCRG and giant cell tumor (GCT) are two of the many bone lesions containing giant cells. GCRG has frequently been misdiagnosed as GCT. GCT is a neoplastic process with the potential to metastasize even though it is histologically benign. GCRG arises from the periosteal connective tissue, whereas GCT originates in the connective tissue of the bone marrow. The senior author (P.C.) reported in 1990 a GCRG mimicking an intracranial tumor in the middle cranial fossa. The tumor presented as a large extradural mass starting from the sphenoid bone (great wing) and occupying the middle cranial fossa, displacing the right temporal lobe upward [29].

Petrous apex cholesteatomas are congenital or acquired. The congenital cholesteatomas are thought to arise from a squamous epithelial rest, found in the normal pneumatized bone, and acquired cholesteatoma is caused by hypoventilation of the middle ear with resultant retraction of the tympanic membrane. Deep penetration into the petrous apex is relatively rare, but can occur through a variety of routes, usually the supralabyrinthine or subcochlear route. Both forms usually involve the anterior portion of the petrous apex. Pathologically, congenital and acquired cholesteatomas are identical. They are keratin-filled, epithelial-lined cysts that demonstrate linear growth patterns characteristic of ordinary skin.

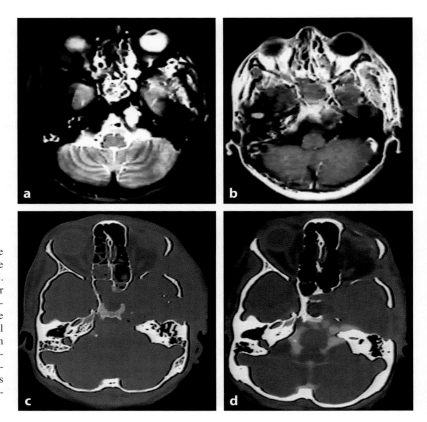

Fig. 7.8 a Axial T2-weighted MR image shows an osteolytic area involving the petrous apex and superolateral left clivus. **b** Axial T1-weighted MR image after gadolinium injection shows inhomogeneous enhancement in the same area. The patient was submitted to a subtemporal petrous apex resection and the was lesion removed. **c** Postoperative CT scan confirms petrous apex resection. **d** Same examination with cisternography confirms total tumor removal. Histological examination: cholesterol granuloma

7.2.7 Aneurysms

Nearly 95% of saccular arterial aneurysms arise within the anterior incisural space. The aneurysms arise from the part of the circle of Willis located anterior to Liliequist's membrane, from the internal carotid, middle cerebral artery and from the various segments of the anterior cerebral artery. Aneurysms located behind Liliequist's membrane arise at the basilar apex in the interpeduncular cistern (Fig. 7.9) and may be located above or below the dorsum sellae or in the prepontine cistern. The infrequent aneurysms arising in the middle incisural space are usually located on the PCA at the origin of its first major cortical branch or on the SCA at its bifurcation into the rostral and caudal trunks.

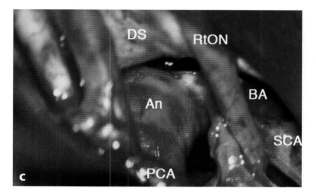

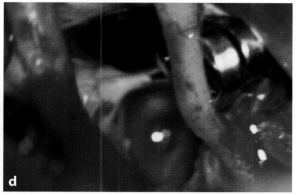

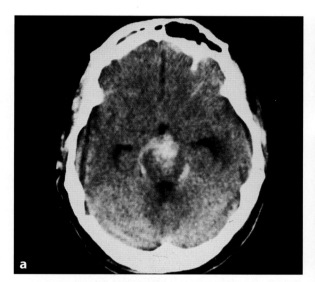

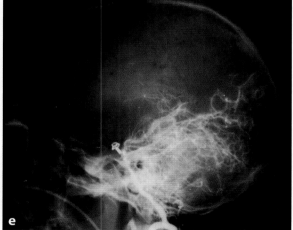

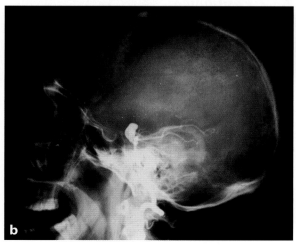

Fig. 7.9 a CT scan on admission shows a subarachnoid hemorrhage and a clot in the interpeduncular cistern, with initial ventricular system dilatation. **b** Same patient. Vertebrobasilar angiogram shows a basilar apex aneurysm. The neck of the aneurysm is on a level with the dorsum sellae base. **c** Same patient. Intraoperative photograph; frontotemporal craniotomy with orbitozygomatic osteotomy; pretemporal approach. **d** Intraoperative photograph shows the clipped aneurysm. **e** Postoperative angiogram confirms closure of the aneurysm neck. *An* aneurysm, *BA* basilar artery, *DS* dorsum sellae, *PCA* posterior cerebral artery, *RtON* right oculomotor nerve, *SCA* superior cerebellar artery

7.3 Anterior Subtemporal Approach

This approach was described by Sano in 1980 and called the "temporopolar approach" [30]. It essentially consists of a pterional approach with a more extensive exposure of the temporal lobe. The temporal lobe is pulled back, exposing the space between the oculomotor nerve and the free edge of the tentorium, creating an anterolateral view to the interpeduncular fossa (halfway between the straight view obtained in the pterional approach and the lateral view obtained in the subtemporal approach).

In the 1990s, de Oliveira et al. described this approach in detail with the term "pretemporal approach" directed toward the interpeduncular fossa and the petroclival region [31]. The rationale for the pretemporal approach is to combine into one approach the advantages offered in the above-mentioned approaches (the pterional, temporopolar and subtemporal; Fig. 7.10). The pretemporal approach offers the possibility to enhance the angles of view of the interpeduncular region according to intraoperative needs, ranging from the straight downward view of the pterional approach to the strictly lateral view of the subtemporal approach. The pretemporal approach offers access to

the floor of the middle fossa and CS (parasellar and middle fossa components) by retracting the temporal lobe posteriorly (Fig. 7.10).

7.3.1 Indications

The anterior subtemporal approach is used for skull-base lesions including extrinsic lesions, such as meningiomas of the middle fossa, tentorial meningiomas (T1–T2 of Yasargil) [3], chondrosarcomas, chordomas, craniopharyngiomas, neurinomas of the trigeminal nerve and other lesions within MC.

Intra- and extradural temporopolar approaches have also been reported as effective techniques for attempting to remove giant pituitary adenomas invading the CS and parasellar region. However, complications are relatively frequent and permanent sequelae are not negligible. Supra- and infratentorial lesions, such as tentorial and petroclival meningiomas and trigeminal nerve schwannomas, can be removed with this approach if the dominant component is supratentorial. In the opposite case, the infratentorial approach must be used. If the two components are of similar volume, a combined supra-/infratentorial approach may be necessary.

An anatomical study was performed by Ulm et al. comparing six approaches to the perimesencephalic cisterns with emphasis on exposure of the PCA and its branches. The PCA origin and the P1 and P2a were exposed in all cases with this approach. In addition, the authors were able to expose the origin and most of the cisternal segment of the anterior choroidal artery [32].

7.3.2 Positioning

The positioning of the patient is basically the same as for the pterional approach consisting of elevating the head, contralateral rotation by approximately 20° and extension of the neck, which depends on the aim of the surgery. For the basilar apex, PCA (P2–P2a) aneurysms and for lesions located in the ambient cistern we use a 30° extension (Fig. 7.11).

7.3.3 Skin Incision

The incision starts in front of the tragus, slightly lower than for the pterional approach, and extends above the

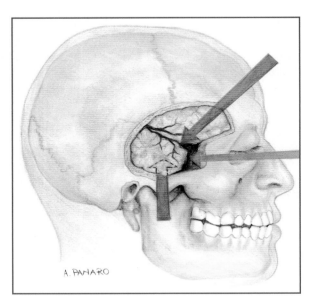

Fig. 7.10 Illustration showing the different angles of sight obtained with the pterional approach (*red arrow* transsylvian corridor), orbitozygomatic approach (*blue arrow* temporopolar corridor) and subtemporal approach (*purple arrow* subtemporal corridor)

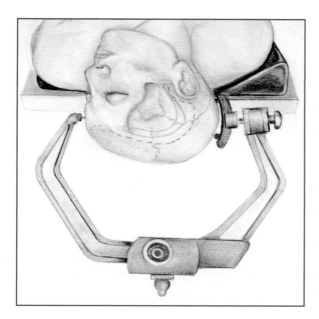

Fig. 7.11 Drawing showing the patient position, head fixation, skin incision (*red broken line*) and possible craniotomy extensions (*blue solid lines*)

ear, making a gentle curve to arch toward the midline behind the hairline (Fig. 7.11).

7.3.4 Interfascial Dissection

The interfascial dissection follows the same principles as for the pterional approach; however, as for any surgical approach aimed at exposing the entire extent of the temporal pole, it is advisable to expose the entire zygomatic bone and zygomatic arch during the craniotomy. The zygomatic bone and its frontal process constitute the lateral rim of the orbit, and the zygomatic arch is the horizontal component that passes externally to the temporalis muscle and is directed toward the external acoustic meatus.

A subfascial dissection of the temporalis muscle aponeurosis avoids injury to the frontalis branch of the facial nerve and facilitates closure. A small myofascial cuff is left attached to the superior temporal line before dissection of the temporalis muscle. The temporalis muscle has to be detached from the entire zygomatic bone and reflected over the horizontal portion of the zygomatic arch. Posteriorly the temporalis muscle is retracted until the posterior root of the zygomatic arch is exposed.

7.3.5 Craniotomy

The standard burr holes used for the classic pterional approach are made: one just lateral to the orbital rim in the keyhole region, one posteroinferiorly in the temporal squama, and the third just in front of the superior temporal line in the frontal bone (Fig. 7.12a). In elderly patients, a fourth burr hole posterosuperiorly in the temporal bone may allow better dural separation before the craniotomy. The bone flap differs from the standard pterional bone flap in that it extends more posteriorly and inferiorly in the temporal region. After cutting the bone flap with the craniotome, it can be fractured low at the pterion. Removal of the anteroinferior portion of the temporal squama down to the floor of the temporal fossa anteriorly with rongeurs follows. With rongeurs and a high-speed air drill, the pterion and lesser wing of the sphenoid are thoroughly removed with particularly aggressive removal of the posterior aspect of pterion and part of the greater sphenoid wing to completely expose the dura over the anterior aspect of the temporal pole.

This procedure creates an unobstructed corridor along the anterior aspect of the temporal pole (temporopolar corridor) and another along the floor of the middle fossa, under the temporal lobe (subtemporal corridor) (Fig. 7.10). The dura mater is opened as shown in Fig. 7.12b and reflected over the edges of the craniotomy. The pretemporal approach proceeds by opening the basal cisterns to release cerebrospinal fluid (CSF) and splitting the sylvian fissure. The lesion can be inspected and approached initially through the pterional corridor. If this is sufficient, there is no need to proceed with the retraction of the temporal pole. If the temporopolar corridor is necessary, the dissection proceeds with coagulation and sectioning of the superficial sylvian veins draining toward the sphenoparietal sinus and any veins draining the basal surface of the temporal lobe toward the floor of the middle fossa. At this stage, it is mandatory to separate the anteromedial surface of the uncus from the oculomotor nerve, tentorial edge, and brainstem by cutting the arachnoidal adhesions. After releasing the anteromedial surface of the uncus, the pole of the temporal lobe is lifted and pulled backward, creating an unobstructed view of the interpeduncular fossa, ahead of the temporal pole (Fig. 7.13).

Various authors have reported that the temporal lobe withstands anterior to posterior retraction much better than lateral to medial retraction. First the spatula is adjusted to the contour of the temporal pole, and is then gently applied against the floor of the middle fossa. The well-adjusted spatula along with the temporal pole is

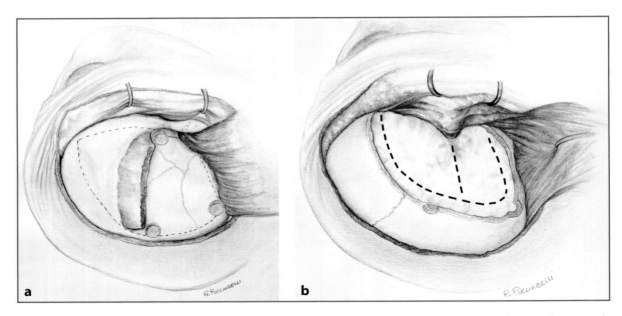

Fig. 7.12 Positioning and skin incision for the pretemporal approach. **a** The detachment begins at the angle between the zygomatic bone and the zygomatic arch. After leaving a cuff over the superior temporal line, the temporalis muscle is reflected over the zygomatic arch. Three burr holes are made: one just lateral to the orbital rim in the keyhole region, one posteroinferiorly in the temporal squama, and the third just in front of the superior temporal line in the frontal bone. In elderly patients, a fourth burr hole (not shown) postero-superiorly in the temporal bone may allow better dural separation before the craniotomy. **b** After bone flap removal, the roof of the orbit and the wings of the sphenoid are extensively drilled out

lifted away from the floor of the middle fossa, then pulled backward, creating the temporopolar corridor. The surgical views offered by the temporopolar corridor are shown in Fig. 7.13. At this stage, if the posterior communicating artery (PComA) blocks access to the interpeduncular region, as long as it is not of the fetal type, it can be sectioned. Most of the perforators, including the arteries perforating the anterior thalamus, arise from the proximal half of the PComA. By sectioning it proximal to the distal third, the blood flow to most of the perforators can be preserved (Fig. 7.14). Dividing the PComA allows greater maneuverability, especially when the it is short. This also moves its perforator out of the surgical trajectory, as the main working field is medial and lateral to the oculomotor nerve. The PComA is cut in a perforator-free zone; this is close to the junction of the PComA and the PCA in more than 80% of patients, as reported by Krayenbühl and Krisht. In their experience, deciding whether it is safe to cut the PComA is based on its relative size compared to the P1 segment of the PCA. This decision was made irrespective of the actual size of the PComA itself. In patients with a fetal-type PComA the authors avoided its

resection [33]. The subtemporal route, as described by Drake et al., can be used as well, depending on the intraoperative needs [34].

Oculomotor nerve palsy, although temporary in most cases, is a problem for subtemporal and temporopolar routes to the interpeduncular region, because in these two approaches the third nerve stays in the center of the surgical view, blocking access to the interpeduncular region. Whenever necessary, the space between the oculomotor nerve and the tentorial edge can be enhanced by retracting the tentorial edge laterally using sutures or even by cutting the tentorial edge. Before cutting the tentorial edge, it is essential to check the location of the trochlear nerve. It can be located by lifting the tentorial edge, where its entry site into the tentorial edge can be easily seen. The tentorial edge is then cut and coagulated laterally.

The pretemporal approach is a variation of the pterional approach that combines the advantages of the pterional, temporopolar, and subtemporal routes. The anterior subtemporal or pretemporal approach is therefore one of the options to consider when dealing with lesions located in the interpeduncular region, upper

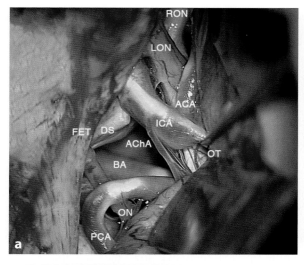

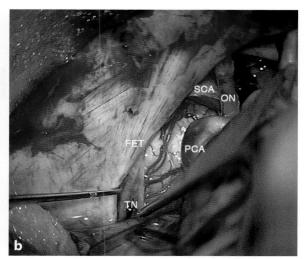

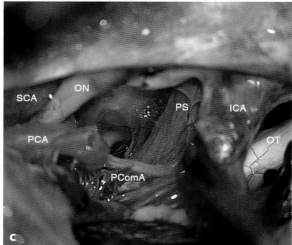

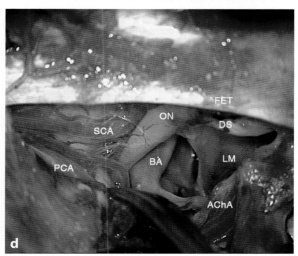

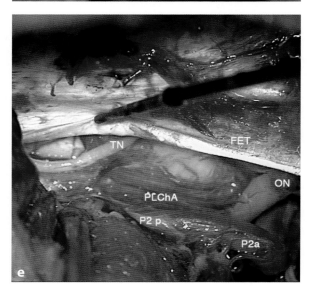

Fig. 7.13 a Intraoperative photograph shows good exposure of the left tentorial anterior and middle incisura obtained through the pretemporal and subtemporal corridors. In this patient the basilar apex is well above the superior margin of the dorsum sellae. **b** Same patient. A more lateral exposure showing the pontomesencephalic junction surface and the neurovascular structures in the ambient cistern. **c** Intraoperative photograph of another patient showing structures in the left lateral incisural space from the subtemporal corridor. **d** Same patient. More lateral view. **e** Same patient. More posterior exposure. The lifting of the free edge of the tentorium shows the trochlear nerve entering the tentorium. The junction between the P2a and P2p segments (*P2a, P2p*) of the posterior cerebral artery is shown. *ACA* anterior cerebral artery, *AChA* anterior choroidal artery and tiny perforating vessels, *BA* basilar artery, *DS* dorsum sellae, *FET* free edge of tentorium, *ICA* internal carotid artery, *LM* Liliequist's membrane, *LON* left optic nerve, *ON* oculomotor nerve, *OT* optic tract, *PCA* posterior cerebral artery, *PComA* posterior communicating artery, *PLChA* posterolateral choroidal artery arising from the P2a–P2p junction, *PS* pituitary stalk, *RON* right optic nerve, *SCA* superior cerebellar artery, *TN* trochlear nerve in the arachnoidal covering

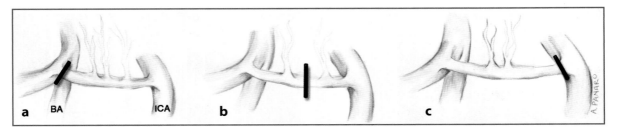

Fig. 7.14 Three options for dividing the PComA: cut close to the P1/P2 junction **a**; cut in its middle segment **b**; cut close to its take-off from the ICA **c**. *BA* basilar artery, *ICA* internal carotid artery

petroclival region, middle fossa, sellar region, parasellar region, and the anterior portion of the tentorial incisura (Figs. 7.1 and 7.6).

In 1994, Day et al. described an extradural temporopolar approach, called the anterolateral transcavernous approach, which is more versatile in exposing skull-base areas than the previous approach, but is characterized by extensive bone removal and an extradural dissection minimizing retraction of the frontal and temporal lobes. The advantages of this technique include preservation of the anterior temporal venous drainage, a wide operative field allowing the microscope to be maneuvered through an arc of at least 90° and minimal brain retraction (Fig. 7.15). The main highlights of this route are: (1) extradural removal of the sphenoid wing and exposure of the superior orbital fissure and foramen rotundum; (2) extradural removal

of the anterior clinoid process; (3) decompression of the optical canal; (4) extradural retraction of the temporal tip; (5) transcavernous mobilization of the carotid artery and oculomotor nerve; and (6) removal of the posterior clinoid process [35]. The fundamental difference from the preceding approach consists of an extensive dissection of the middle cranial fossa dura mater, associated with extradural removal of the anterior clinoid process. The dura is incised over the sylvian fissure, the incision is extended to the optic nerve sheath dura, and an L-shaped incision is made by medially extending the incision along the frontal base for 2–3 cm (Fig. 7.15).

In the approach Day et al., the transcavernous exposure is extradural and lateral instead of extradural and subdural, as described by Dolenc [36] and Yonekawa et al. [37]. The dural fibrous ring of the internal carotid

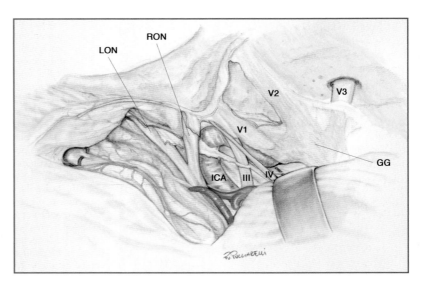

Fig. 7.15 Drawing showing an extradural temporopolar approach: the dural incision over the sylvian fissure with extension over the optic nerve sheath dura; an L-shaped incision is made by medially extending the incision along the frontal base for 2–3 cm. *GG* gasserian ganglion, *ICA* internal carotid artery, *LON* left optic nerve, *RON* right optic nerve

artery (ICA) may be laterally opened to release it from its dural attachment. Then, the frontal lobe is separated medially and the temporal lobe posterolaterally in such a way as to preserve the temporal veins.

7.4 Extension of the Pretemporal Approach (Intra- and Extradural) with Orbitozygomatic Osteotomies

The inclusion of additional osteotomies to the pretemporal approach has greatly improved surgical exposure. Basal exposure of the middle cranial fossa also allows treatment of lesions that arise from or extend to the extradural compartment of this region.

This approach can access the components of the orbit, the CS, the infratemporal fossa, the petrous apex, the intrapetrous ICA and the remainder of the middle cranial fossa.

7.4.1 Positioning

The positioning is the same as for the previously described approach.

7.4.2 Skin Incision

The scalp incision starts 1 to 2 cm below the zygomatic arch, just in front of the tragus, and behind the superficial temporal artery, anatomically the artery is usually located posterior to the frontalis branch of the facial nerve. The incision proceeds behind the hairline in a curvilinear fashion to the opposite side, to end at the superior temporal line (Fig. 7.23a). In some cases, a bicoronal incision can also be used. The pericranium is usually reflected anteriorly along with the scalp flap.

7.4.3 Interfascial Dissection

An interfascial flap is performed, taking care to extend the inferior part of the incision in the superficial temporal fascia toward the posterior root of the zygomatic arch to preserve the frontalis branch of the facial nerve. The external layer of the temporalis fascia, which is contiguous with the external parotid fascia, is pushed

anteriorly with the aid of a periosteal elevator. After the fascia is reflected anteriorly, the zygomatic process of the temporal bone and the zygomatic bone with its frontal and temporal process are well exposed.

7.4.4 Craniotomy and Orbitozygomatic Osteotomy

First, the zygomatic osteotomy is performed. The zygomatic arch is cut in an oblique fashion, first posteriorly at its root and in front of the glenoid process, then anteriorly at the junction of the arch and the zygomatic bone. The zygomatic bone (malar eminence) is cut obliquely anteriorly at the level of the zygomaticofacial foramina (Fig. 7.23a). At this point, the temporalis muscle is dissected from the temporal fossa and reflected inferiorly with the zygomatic arch toward the infratemporal fossa. A pretemporal craniotomy is performed flush with the floor of the middle fossa. The orbitozygomatic osteotomy can also be obtained in one piece containing the craniotomic flap and zygomalar bone. The orbitozygomatic craniotomy provides unhindered extradural exposure of the elements of the anterior and middle cranial fossae. With the orbitozygomatic craniotomy, the entire CS can be exposed through its lateral wall by peeling off its outer dural layer. The dural tent over the superior orbital fissure is incised and gently peeled from the anterior portion of the lateral wall of the CS. This maneuver exposes the oculomotor, trochlear, and first and second divisions of the trigeminal nerve. The spaces between the divisions of the trigeminal nerve can be used to gain access or follow tumor extensions into the sphenoidal sinus and infratemporal fossa.

For the extradural exposure of the remainder of the trigeminal nerve and of the intrapetrous ICA, the dura is peeled from the temporal bone to reach the foramen spinosum and expose the middle meningeal artery, which is coagulated and cut. The course of the GSPN along the petrosphenoidal fissure can be well seen medial to the middle meningeal artery and posterior to V3. According to the pathology, the extradural exposure can be started anteriorly and worked posteriorly or vice versa. The intrapetrous carotid artery can be exposed in the petrous bone coursing parallel and inferior to the GSPN. At times, the intrapetrous carotid lacks any bony covering at this location. To expose the petrous apex, the dura is separated from the lateral wall of the CS along the posterior border of V3. The petrous apex can be removed to improve exposure of the petro-clival region.

7.5 Subtemporal Approach in Trigeminal Neurinomas

7.5.1 General Considerations

Trigeminal nerve root schwannoma (TNRS) is the parasellar tumoral lesion with the most varied sites and extensions (Fig. 7.3). These tumors may arise from the trigeminal nerve root, the GG, or one of the three peripheral branches, indicating that TNRS may grow into one, two, or all three distinct compartments: the subdural (CPA), interdural (lateral wall of the CS and MC), and epidural or extracranial (orbit, pterygopalatine fossa, and infratemporal fossa) spaces.

The exact location and extension pattern of TNRS, which are often seen extending into multiple cranial fossae, are: the posterior fossa, the middle fossa, the infratemporal fossa and the orbit. Neuroimaging technologies, including magnetic resonance imaging, provide information on the precise anatomy of the trigeminal nerve and its surrounding structures and the preoperative diagnosis of the extension pattern, essential for the complete and safe removal of TNRS.

Yoshida and Kawase classified the trigeminal neurinomas of his series into three basic types (see section Schwannomas, and Fig. 7.4). The authors considered that extracranial regions should be divided into two subgroups on the basis of surgical strategy: the orbit and the infratemporal and pterygopalatine fossae. Their series included three tumors involving the orbit, but did not include any tumors localized only in the orbit. Two tumors were dumbbell-shaped and extended into the orbit from the middle fossa via the superior orbital fissure and another was a dumbbell-shaped tumor extending from the middle fossa into the orbit via the pterygopalatine fossa and the inferior orbital fissure along the second division of the trigeminal nerve branch [6].

The anterior subtemporal interdural approach can be used in tumors localized exclusively in the middle cranial fossa, but can be extended toward the posterior cranial fossa, with an anterior transpetrosal approach and toward the orbit and infratemporal fossa with an orbitozygomatic and infratemporal approach, respectively. When a posterior fossa tumor is large, the tentorium must be cut using the same anterior transpetrosal

technique. Thus, tumors involving the three fossae can be totally removed by a single-stage operation performed via a single trajectory.

7.5.2 Subtemporal Interdural Approach

The rationale for this intervention is based on the anatomical observation that the dura mater of the CS and the GG consists of two layers: an outer periosteal layer and an inner meningeal layer, called the dura propria [38].

These two layers are tightly fused together, except where they are separated to provide space for the dural venous sinuses, venous plexi, and CNs that pass through the parasellar region. The periosteal layer of the dura remains tightly attached to the inner surface of the cranium and is considered to be the internal periosteum of the cranial bone. The periosteal layer of the dura is continuous with the outer periosteum, which covers the external surface of the cranial bone through the suture lines and nerve and vessel foramina. The dura propria faces the brain surface covered by the arachnoid. The dura propria and the arachnoid typically follow CNs for varying distances as they leave the cranial cavity (Fig. 7.15). The dura propria that follows each CN becomes the epineurium, whereas the pia-arachnoid continues as the perineurium that invests each nerve fascicle.

The trigeminal nerve passes from the posterior fossa over the trigeminal impression of the petrous apex between the periosteal and meningeal (dura propria) layers of the middle fossa dura, carrying with it the arachnoid and dura propria from the posterior fossa. MC is a cleft-like dural pocket that originates from the dura propria of the posterior fossa, between the two layers of the middle fossa dura. The contents of MC are the sensory and motor roots of the trigeminal nerve, GG, and the arachnoid layer (Fig. 7.16). The cleavage plane between these two layers of dura propria continues distally as the cleavage plane between the epineural sheaths of the trigeminal nerve divisions and the dura propria of the middle fossa. This cleavage plane serves as the anatomic basis for the interdural exposure of the contents of MC (Fig. 7.16).

7.5.2.1 Surgical Technique

Positioning and craniotomy are the same as those described for the anterior subtemporal approach. The zy-

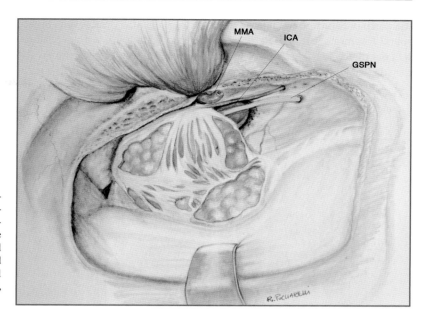

Fig. 7.16 Illustration showing the extradural middle fossa view of a dumbbell-shaped trigeminal schwannoma with exposure of the petrous carotid artery, three divisions and ganglion of the fifth cranial nerve, and entry into the expanded Meckel's cave. *GSPN* greater superficial petrosal nerve, *ICA* internal carotid artery, *MMA* middle meningeal artery

gomatic osteotomy is advised since it allows a more tangential approach to the middle cranial fossa base.

7.5.2.2 Dura Elevation and Peeling of the Meningeal Dura of the Middle Fossa

Youssef et al. believe the elevation of the dura of the middle fossa floor in a posterior to anterior direction protects the GSPN, which enters the middle fossa epidural space through the facial hiatus [39]. The arcuate eminence is identified. The middle meningeal artery is cauterized and cut at the foramen spinosum. The cleavage plane between the dura propria and the periosteal dura, which contains this artery, is identified and developed by dissection. The dura propria layer is peeled from the periosteal layer in an anterior direction toward the foramen ovale. This cleavage plane continues as the plane between the dura propria of the middle fossa and the epineural sheath of V3 at the foramen ovale. The V2 division is exposed by incising the periosteal layer of dura that covers the anterior margin of the foramen rotundum and by peeling the dura propria of the middle fossa from the epineural sheath of the V2 division. Continued peeling of the dura propria superomedially toward the superior orbital fissure exposes the V1 invested by its epineural sheath, which is continuous with the inner membranous layer of the CS lat-

eral wall. The dura propria is then progressively peeled from the epineural sheath of each division of the trigeminal nerve back toward MC. The periosteal layer of the dura is cut along the posterior aspect of V3 and MC. Peeling the dura propria of the middle fossa from the dorsolateral wall of MC is stopped short of the opening of the superior petrosal sinus (SPS), which lies within the end of that cleavage plane.

7.5.3 Extension into the Posterior Cranial Fossa with an Anterior Transpetrosal Approach

"Dumbbell" trigeminal neurinomas usually consist of two components: the body of the tumor in MC and a posterior extension through the porous trigeminus into the subarachnoid space of the posterior fossa.

The early stage of this approach consists of the subtemporal epidural approach. Following a temporal skin incision, the temporal fascia is dissected from the temporal muscle and reflected inferiorly. The pedicle of the temporal fascia is used for closure of the dural defect. The temporal muscle itself is reflected anteroinferiorly. After temporal craniotomy, the middle cranial fossa is exposed epidurally to the anterior portion of the petrous edge and the lateral edges of the oval and round foramina. The middle meningeal artery should be coagulated and cut at the foramen spinosum, and the superficial greater petrosal nerve should be sharply detached, together with the periosteal dura from the meningeal dura of the temporal base to avoid facial nerve injury at the geniculate ganglion. Incising the periosteal dura covering the superior orbital fissure and

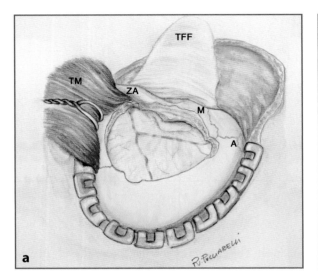

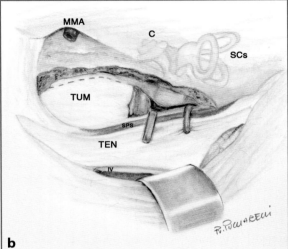

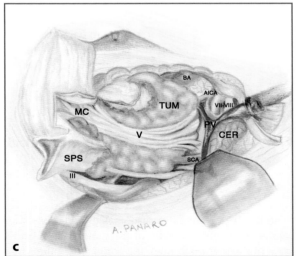

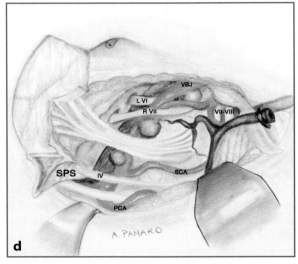

Fig. 7.17 a Craniotomy site. The temporal fascia is separated from the muscle. The craniotomy is extended under the zygomatic arch and adjacent to the external auditory meatus. **b** Epidural view of the anterior pyramid. Intraosseous structures (auditory organs and the carotid artery) have been drawn as a superimposed layer. The broken line shows the margin of bone resection. The SPS is clipped. **c** In the removal of larger posterior fossa tumors, the SPS should be ligated and cut, and the tentorium should be incised to obtain a wide operative field. **d** An anterior transpetrosal approach is indicated for basilar trunk aneurysms located between the level of the pituitary floor and the internal carotid canal on a lateral angiogram, anterior inferior cerebellar artery aneurysms, and vertebrobasilar junction aneurysms. *A* asterion, *AICA* anterior inferior cerebellar artery, *BA* basilar artery, *C* cochlea, *CER* cerebellum, *M* mastoid, *MC* Meckel's cave, *MMA* middle meningeal artery, *PCA* posterior cerebral artery, *PV* petrosal vein, *SCA* superior cerebellar artery, *SCs* semicircular canals, *SPS* superior petrosal sinus, *TEN* tentorium, *TFF* temporal fascia flap, *TM* temporal muscle, *TUM* tumor, *V* trigeminal nerve, *VBJ* vertebrobasilar junction, *ZA* zygomatic arch

the round and oval foramina can expose a middle fossa tumor, which is located in the interdural space. Such a tumor is usually wrapped in trigeminal nerve fibers that in most cases can be carefully dissected from the tumor. The first stage in accessing posterior fossa tumors is an anterior petrosectomy, which consists of drilling the petrous apex medial to the superficial greater petrosal nerve and anterior to the arcuate eminence (Fig. 7.8c, d). Small posterior fossa tumors with a diameter of less than 10 mm can be exposed and removed by extension of the dural incision at the lateral wall of MC toward the internal auditory meatus, without tentorial incision. For removal of larger posterior fossa tumors, the middle fossa dura should be incised, the SPS should be ligated and cut, and the tentorium should be incised to obtain a wide operative field (Fig. 7.17a–c). Tumors in MC are usually wrapped in the plexiform portion of the trigeminal nerve (Fig. 7.16).

Posterior fossa tumors are sometimes cystic and soft, and internal decompression allows total removal of large tumors via this approach. The fourth and sixth CNs, which are located inferiorly and medially to the tumor, respectively, should be carefully preserved during removal of a posterior fossa tumor. The dural defect around the SPS can be repaired after removal of the tumor using a pedicle of the temporal fascia and fibrin glue.

This approach has also been used in other nonneoplastic petrous apex lesions, described in the pathology section (petrous apex cholesterol granulomas, chordomas and chondrosarcomas).

7.5.4 Extension into the Infratemporal Fossa

Following a temporal craniotomy combined with a zygomatic or orbitozygomatic osteotomy, the lateral portion of the middle cranial fossa is resected to expose the tumor extending into the infratemporal fossa. In cases in which the tumor extends into the orbit, the superior and lateral wall of the orbit should be removed following the orbitozygomatic osteotomy. The middle fossa floor is resected until the enlarged oval or round foramen adjacent to the tumor is opened. Tumors in the extracranial space can be exposed by incision of the membrane, which continues to the periosteal dura covering middle fossa tumors.

Using this epidural–interdural approach tumors extending into the extracranial space from the middle

fossa can be entirely removed without exposing the temporal lobe or CNs other than the fifth CN. The subdural space may be opened only when the posterior margin of the tumor is removed from MC. Following removal of the tumor, the dural defect at MC should be repaired using a pedicle of the temporal fascia to avoid CSF leakage.

7.5.5 Subtemporal Interdural Approach in Other Skull-Base Tumors

The subtemporal interdural approach has also been described in dumbbell-shaped chordomas of the skull base [40]. These tumors, which usually occur in the axial skeleton, may extend into the subdural space when they originate from the skull base. The subtemporal interdural approach with zygomatic osteotomy and anterior petrosal approach may permit a one-stage removal of a tumor located in two distinct compartments. The parasellar component is in the CS, which is in the interdural space between the meningeal dura and the periosteal dura. The CS tumor can be approached via the pretemporal epidural approach. The zygomatic osteotomy added to this approach allows a wide operative field especially in large parasellar tumors with upward extension. The posterior fossa component is located between the pyramidal apex and the upper clivus (petroclival region) and the anterior transpetrosal approach is one of the best methods to access this deep-seated area.

The surgical technique, in part, has been previously described for trigeminal neurinomas.

The petrous apex and the lateral aspects of the superior orbital fissure, foramen rotundum and foramen ovale have been exposed. The petrous apex, which is medial to the superficial greater petrosal nerve and the arcuate eminence, is drilled off. The superior and anterior wall of the internal auditory canal may be opened. The cochlear and the superior semicircular canal in the arcuate eminence should not be drilled to preserve the patient's hearing. The periosteal dura is cut from the superior orbital fissure to the foramen ovale via the foramen rotundum and peeled off from the lateral wall of the CS. The three peripheral branches of the trigeminal nerve and GG, trochlear nerve, and oculomotor nerve are exposed. The parasellar tumor covered by a thin fibrous membrane is observed between these CNs. The spaces between these CNs have been identified as anterolateral (Mullan; V1–V2), lateral (V2–V3), paramedial (III–IV), and superolateral (Parkinson; VI–IV) triangles. The dura of the middle cranial base is incised into a T-shape toward the SPS (Fig. 7.18a). The dura of the posterior fossa is also incised into a T-shape just below the SPS (Fig. 7.18a). The SPS is ligated and cut, and the tentorium is incised to the medial edge with careful attention to the trochlear nerve.

After incision of the lateral wall of MC, the posterior fossa tumor is exposed (Fig. 7.18b). The parasellar component of this tumor is removed carefully from the

various triangles described previously. The thin fibrous membrane covering the tumor should be left behind to preserve the function of the CNs. Careful attention should be directed toward the ICA, which courses inferomedially to the tumor. The tumor protruding into the sphenoid sinus can be removed under the mucosa of the sinus.

After removal of the CS tumor, the posterior fossa component, located medial to the trigeminal nerve root, is removed. Because the trigeminal nerve root has been

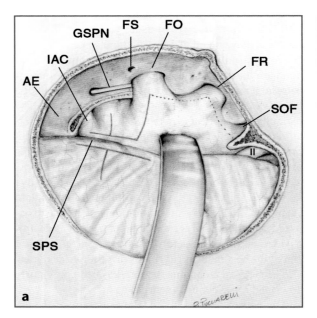

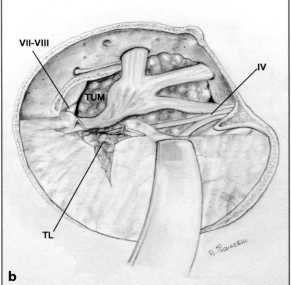

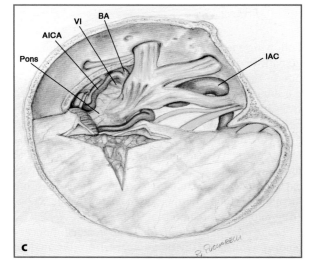

Fig. 7.18 a Interdural approach to the cavernous sinus and for anterior petrosectomy. The solid lines indicate the dural incision for resection of the superior petrosal sinus and tentorium. The broken line indicates the incision of the periosteal dura to enter the cavernous sinus. The GSPN and AE are the landmarks for anterior petrosectomy. The petrous apex medial to these landmarks is drilled to expose the posterior fossa dura. **b** Parasellar and posterior fossa components of the lesion (chordoma) exposed by the zygomatic transpetrosal approach. **c** Operative field after tumor removal. *BA* basilar artery, *AE* arcuate eminence, *AICA* anterior inferior cerebellar artery, *FO* foramen ovale, *FR* foramen rotundum, *FS* foramen spinosum, *GSPN* greater superficial petrosal nerve, *IAC* internal auditory canal, *SOF* superior orbital fissure, *SPS* superior petrosal sinus, *TL* temporal lobe, *TUM* tumor

mobilized by resection of the pyramidal apex, the petroclival region tumor can be removed working above and below the trigeminal nerve root. This tumor adheres to the ventral surface of the pons, which can be observed directly by this approach. The tumor is dissected carefully from the pons, abducens nerve, the BA, and its branches. The ultrasonic aspirator is beneficial in reducing the tumor bulk after dissection of the tumor from the adjacent structures to a certain extent. The operative field after tumor removal is shown schematically (Fig. 7.18c).

The cavities in the CS after tumor removal and the anterior petrosectomy are filled with subcutaneous fat from the lower abdomen and fixed with fibrin glue to prevent postoperative CSF leakage.

7.6 Posterior Subtemporal Approach

7.6.1 Indications

The posterior subtemporal approach is used for posterolateral tentorial tumors, posterolateral middle cranial fossa meningiomas (Fig. 7.19), trigeminal neurinomas, and dorsolateral brainstem lesions.

7.6.2 Positioning

Under general anesthesia, the patient is placed in the lateral position with the side of the planned craniotomy

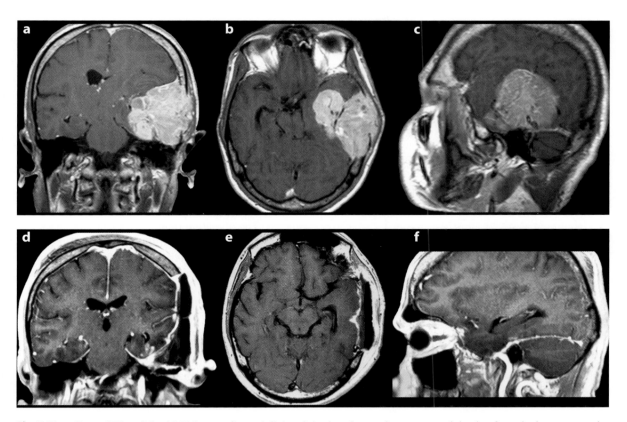

Fig. 7.19 a Coronal T1-weighted MR image after gadolinium injection shows a huge tumor originating from the lower convexity in the posterior temporal region and causing osteolysis of the temporoparietal bone. The tumor lies on the middle cranial fossa with compression and contralateral dislocation of the ventricular system. **b** Same patient. Axial T1-weighted MR image after gadolinium injection clarifies the posterior extension into the middle cranial fossa of the tumor with mesencephalon warping. **c** Sagittal T1-weighted MR image after gadolinium injection. The tumor portion lying on the posterior region of the middle cranial fossa (on the tegmen tympani) is tightly adjacent to the transverse sinus. **d–f** Postoperative coronal, axial and sagittal T1-weighted MR images after gadolinium injection show complete tumor resection. Histological diagnosis: meningeal hemangiopericytoma

upwards. To facilitate the approach, the patient's head is tilted below the horizontal position by approximately 10–15°. To approach brainstem tumors, the neck is rotated toward the floor 15° off the horizontal plane, with the patient's nose pointing downwards. For posterolateral tentorial or middle fossa tumors, the neck must be rotated to achieve a head position parallel to the floor. The patient's back is slightly flexed, and all pressure points, including the axilla, are padded. The three-point head-rest is applied for head fixation (Fig. 7.20).

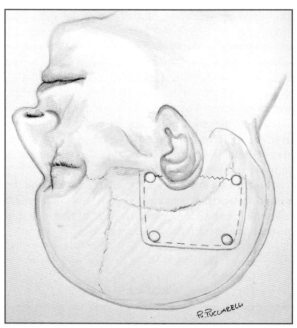

Fig. 7.21 Drawing illustrating the skin incision and the craniotomy margins

7.6.3 Skin Incision

A horseshoe-shaped incision is created, offset slightly posterior to the ear, starting at the root of the zygoma, extending superiorly to the supratemporal line and posteriorly approximately 2.5 cm behind the mastoid process. The operative field includes provision for extension of the incision into the suboccipital region to allow access to the posterior fossa, should a combined subtemporal–suboccipital approach prove to be necessary (Fig. 7.21).

7.6.4 Craniotomy

Craniotomy is performed such that the inferior margin of the craniotomy is at the level of the floor of the middle fossa. The dura is then opened exposing the posteroinferior temporal region and the exact location of the entry of the vein of Labbé into the transverse sinus is identified. The microscope is used to view the temporal lobe while it is retracted until the medial tentorial edge is visualized. Retractors are then placed far posteriorly under the deep temporal lobe. Gently working

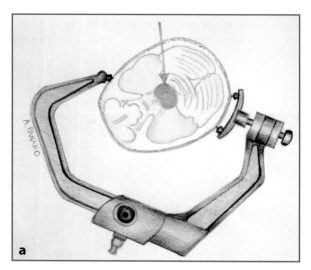

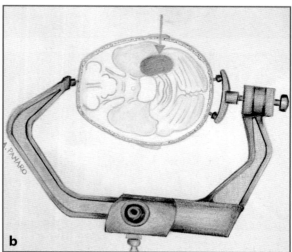

Fig. 7.20 Drawing illustrating patient head positioning. **a** To approach brainstem lesions, the patient's head is tilted below the horizontal position by approximately 10–15°. **b** To approach posterolateral tentorial or middle cranial fossa lesions, the patient's head is parallel to the floor

the retractors further posteriorly and increasing the amount of mediotemporal retraction can visualize the posterolateral aspect of the brainstem. Sharp dissection is used to open the arachnoid planes anteriorly, allowing identification of the oculomotor nerve, the cerebral peduncle and the basilar, posterior cerebral, and superior cerebellar arteries. As the lateral brainstem is visualized, a right-angle hook can be used to elevate the tentorium laterally, exposing the course of the trochlear nerve around the lateral brainstem. The nerve can be followed posteriorly to the point of origin from the dorsal brainstem. Stay sutures are placed in the tentorial edge to retract it laterally, taking care to remain posterior to the insertion of the trochlear nerve into the tentorial edge. The tentorium can then be opened laterally, allowing a wide view of the lateral and posterolateral brainstem. The removal of the petrous apex can be accomplished as previously described.

As the posterolateral aspect of the pontomesencephalic junction is encountered, the folia of the superior vermis are visualized. With the use of a small tapered blade retractor, the vermis can be elevated posterolaterally providing full visualization of the trigeminal root fibers as they enter the brainstem. As the retractors are deepened, the microscope is gradually rotated to a more posterior position, allowing visualization of the posterolateral brainstem. The brainstem can then be entered for the resection of intraparenchymal lesions.

Goel and Nadkarni described a posterior subtemporal approach centered on the external auditory meatus very similar to the previous technique for the surgical treatment of trigeminal neurinomas of the middle cranial fossa mainly located in the posterior part of the middle cranial fossa [41]. The possible tumor extension in the posterior cranial fossa is treated with a basal extension of the approach or adding a petrosal approach.

The main surgical difficulty encountered in any posterior subtemporal approach is the sacrifice of the Labbé vein or other bridging veins which leads to significant postoperative morbidity. Sugita et al. [42] described a method for preserving large bridging veins by stripping them from the brain surface. Koperna et al. [43] described a technique for preserving the Labbé vein by dissecting it from its dural bed and shifting its fixation point to the dura. These techniques do not, however, alter the entry point of the vein into the dura, which is the most vulnerable point for causing avulsion or torsion injury during retraction of the brain.

Thus, Kyoshima et al. have come up with an extremely useful technique to preserve the subtemporal bridging veins, avoiding placing tension on the bridg-

ing veins at their entry point. When a larger bridging vein from the temporal lobe enters the dura attached to the bone of the temporal base before it empties into the transverse or tentorial sinus, the dura is dissected widely from the bone and is cut vertically toward the medial side of the temporal base in front of the entrance of the vein into the dura. The dura, which includes part of the entrance and interdural course of the vein, is then reflected and retracted over the brain without exerting increasing tension on the bridging segment. The addition of a transverse dural incision extending posteriorly to the medial side of the interdural segment of the vein results in easier mobilization of the temporal lobe [44]

7.7 Transtemporal–Transchoroidal Fissure Approach

This approach is a valid alternative to the preceding if the Labbé vein or other draining veins of the temporal lobe impede its retraction. The approach was created for the removal of lesions of the ambient cistern area (Fig. 7.22). The ambient cistern is not easily accessible. The pterional approach, the subtemporal approach, and the occipital interhemispheric transtentorial approaches have been used with difficulty to treat lesions in this region (e.g., the P2 segment of the PCA) [45]. Occasional reports have appeared describing the transtemporal–transchoroidal fissure approach to treat vascular lesions in the ambient cistern, but have not provided details regarding the technique [45]. The subtemporal approach can be used for lesions located in the inferior part of the ambient cistern but is unsuitable for lesions located more superiorly because of the risk of injury to the Labbé vein and temporal lobe.

In terms of the transcortical approach, the shortest and straightest axis to the temporal horn and choroidal fissure is through the middle temporal gyrus and subsequently through the lateral wall of the temporal horn. However, this route is associated with a high risk of neurological deficits.

Ebeling and Reulen [46] studied 50 temporal lobes and found that the optic radiation at the tip of the temporal horn lies in the roof of the ventricle. In the middle portion of the temporal horn, the optic radiation courses along the roof and lateral ventricular wall, whereas in the atrium, the optic radiation courses along the wall of the lateral ventricle only. Gonzalez and Smith [47] recommended that the surgical approach to the temporal horn target the floor or the lower lateral wall of the tem-

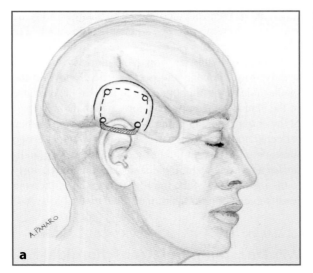

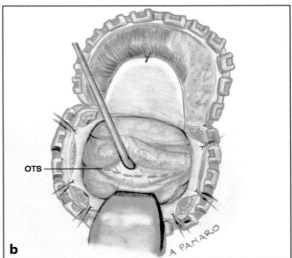

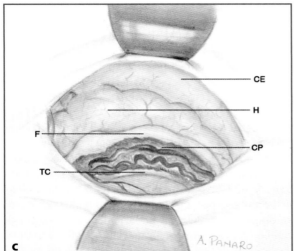

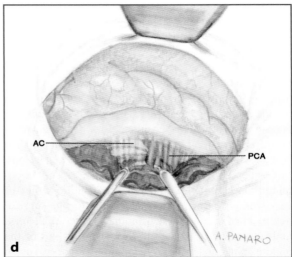

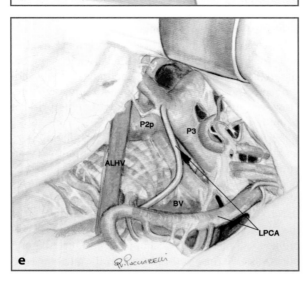

Fig. 7.22 Posterior subtemporal approach to the higher portion of the ambient cistern. **a** Right temporal scalp (*solid line*) and bone flap (*broken line*). The bone removal (*red cross-hatched area*) at the lower margin of the bone flap gives access to the floor of the middle fossa. **b** U-shaped dura; opening. The temporal horn is approached through a cortical incision (*broken line*) in the occipitotemporal sulcus between the inferior temporal and occipitotemporal gyri. **c** Temporal horn opening to expose the choroid plexus, collateral eminence, fimbria, hippocampus, and the tail of the caudate nucleus. **d** Choroidal fissure opening by dissection of the tenia fimbriae to expose the ambient cistern. **e** The hippocampus and the tenia fimbria are retracted caudally, exposing the distal portion of P2 and the P2–P3 junction of the posterior cerebral artery. *AC* ambient cistern, *ALHV* anterior longitudinal hippocampal vein, *BV* basal vein, *CE* collateral eminence, *CP* choroid plexus, *F* fimbria, *H* hippocampus, *LPCA* lateral posterior choroidal arteries, *OTS* occipitotemporal sulcus, *PCA* posterior cerebral artery, *TC* tail of caudate

poral horn. The sensory speech cortex is located at the posterior aspect of the superior and middle temporal gyri in the dominant hemisphere.

Various routes can be used to expose the temporal horn to avoid potential neurological deficits from damage to Meyer's loop and Wernicke's area. Heros [48] used a cortical incision through the inferior temporal gyrus as a corridor to the temporal horn for the treatment of arteriovenous malformations in the mesial temporal lobe. Nagata et al. [49] recommended approaching the temporal horn through an incision along the occipitotemporal sulcus. Ikeda et al. [50] also suggested an inferior temporal gyrectomy as a corridor for the transchoroidal approach to treat aneurysms, arteriovenous malformations, and meningiomas in the ambient cistern without inflicting additional neurological deficits. Because the optic radiation courses primarily in the roof and lateral wall of the temporal horn, most authors have suggested approaching the temporal horn through its floor or lower lateral wall [45, 47–50].

To avoid deficits related to injuries to Wernicke's area, a cortical incision in the inferior part of the temporal lobe has been recommended [45, 48–50]. The disadvantage of accessing lesions from the inferior temporal gyrus or below is that the axis of this approach is not straight; thus a greater retraction of the hippocampus is necessary [51]. However, Yasargil et al. reported that in their anatomical and clinical experience the anterior portion of Meyer's loop completely covers the entire lateral wall of the temporal horn; for this reason, they believe that the pterional transsylvian approach allows better and safer access to the temporal horn and the ambient cistern [52]. Anteromedial access into the temporal horn is gained by entering through the middle portion of the periinsular sulcus (basal portion of the superior temporal gyrus) while staying posterior to the uncinate fasciculus and the anterior white commissure. This corridor into the temporal horn followed by opening the tenia fimbria would allow access to the distal portion of the P2 segment of the PCA. For lesions involving the cerebral peduncle, the latter corridor can be used to gain access to P2/P3 PCA aneurysms as well as ventral and ventrolateral peduncular region gliomas and cavernomas.

7.8 Subtemporal Approach in Posterior Circulation Aneurysms

Posterior fossa aneurysms are more frequently located at the basilar bifurcation. They occur where the BA divides into the PCAs. The neck of the aneurysm is usually located in the basilar bifurcation, but it can extend laterally to include the PCA and its perforators. They usually project superiorly, following the direction of the blood flow in the BA. They may also project anteriorly, posteriorly or laterally. The direction of projection of aneurysms is important because it gives an idea as to the relationship of the aneurysm to the perforating branches of the basilar bifurcation and the P1 segment of the PCAs (posterior thalamoperforating arteries).

Basilar bifurcation aneurysms are divided into three groups according to their position in relation to the upper portion of the dorsum sellae. Anatomical studies have shown that the top of the BA is located within 1 cm of the level of the dorsum sellae in 87% of patients. The apex of the bifurcation is below the tip of the dorsum sellae in 19% of patients, at about the same height in 51%, and superior to the tip in 30%. Although the BA is typically considered to bifurcate at the pontomesencephalic junction, the bifurcation of the PCA into P1 segment may be located as far caudally as 10 mm below the pontomesencephalic junction and as far rostrally as the mamillary bodies. The location of the basilar bifurcation with respect to the dorsum sellae is inversely related to the patient's height. With age, the tortuosity of the intracranial vessels increases and tends to push the basilar bifurcation rostrally [53].

Among factors to be considered in the selection of the most adequate surgical approach to deal with BA aneurysms including the exact origin of the sac and its projection and size, the relative height of the basilar bifurcation is most important in determining the preferred approach. Aneurysms arising from a bifurcation located above the posterior clinoid process are best dealt with by a pterional approach, while aneurysms arising from a low bifurcation (below the floor of the sella) are better handled via a subtemporal approach.

For many years the subtemporal route popularized by Drake was the universally used approach for aneurysms of the basilar bifurcation, P1-PCA and proximal portion of the SCA. This approach should be reserved for patients in whom the carotid artery is short, the PComA is dominant and the basilar bifurcation is below the dorsum sellae and above the internal auditory canal [54].

Ordinarily, the right side (86% in the series of Drake) has been used unless the projection or complexity of the aneurysms, left oculomotor palsy, left-sided blindness or a right hemiparesis demand an approach under the dominant temporal lobe [34]. The patient is positioned in lateral decubitus and a small temporal bone flap above and in front of the ear is turned out. The temporal squama is removed with rongeurs or drills down to the level of the zygomatic root so that the bony opening is as flush with the middle fossa floor as possible. With time and great experience (1,767 posterior circulation aneurysms) this flap has been substituted by Drake and coworkers for a small subtemporal craniectomy through a linear incision similar to the Frazier-Spiller operation for tic douloureux, which can easily be converted to a frontotemporal or posterior temporal bone flap if necessary [34].

The prospective of the subtemporal approach is ordinarily perpendicular to the sagittal plane (lateral view of the brainstem and anterior and middle incisural space) with a good view of the ipsilateral P1 and contralateral P1 hidden behind a large sac with its perforators. The appropriate maneuver suggested by Drake to expose the contralateral P1 is to angle the retractor forward a few degrees under the temporal pole and then displace the waist of the sac posteriorly. This approach has also permitted the authors to treat omolateral carotid artery aneurysms by only moving the retractor tip forward under the temporal pole. For treatment of associated aneurysms of the middle cerebral artery, carotid bifurcation and the anterior communicating artery, the frontotemporal transsylvian approach is the standard option. The Labbé vein, well posterior, has never been a problem in Drake's experience.

The next steps are visualization of the tentorial free edge and the "disengagement of uncus from its position inside the edge of the tentorium." Elevation of the uncus by the retractor tip exposes the opening to the inerpeduncular cistern covered by Liliequist's membrane crossed by the oculomotor nerve. Retraction of the uncus usually elevates the oculomotor nerve permitting one to work underneath the nerve to clip the aneurysm except in the case of a high basilar bifurcation or a giant sac, when it may be necessary to separate the third nerve from the uncus.

The opening into the interpeduncular cistern can be widened significantly by the maneuver of placing a suture at the edge of the tentorium just in front of, but free of, the insertion and intradural course of the fourth nerve. This maneuver obviates the need for dividing the tentorium for most aneurysms at the basilar bifurcation including those arising at the origin of the SCA. However, Drake has stated that in one-third of patients with a low-lying basilar bifurcation aneurysm, tentorium division remained necessary. He also affirmed not to have ever needed to remove the posterior clinoid process, because the lateral perspective obtained with this approach

does not obstruct the view of the aneurysm sac. The PComA was rarely divided in Drake's series. This artery should be preserved in case of injury to the P1 or if it becomes necessary to include P1 in the clip, an event that has rarely happened in the author's experience.

7.8.1 Differences from the Pterional Approach

Yasargil et al. described the pterional approach in 1976 to offer an anterior anatomical perspective on the basilar bifurcation [1]. Drake affirmed that this approach "gives excellent, though narrow, visualization of the anterior aspect of most basilar bifurcation aneurysms and particularly the opposite P1 origin and its perforators" and in his series it was used only occasionally because the author found it "narrow and confining with less visualization of the aneurysm, especially posteriorly in the interpeduncular fossa."

This is an approach for use preferably in normal or high-lying aneurysms, in the latter even if technical difficulties have been recorded because the surgical corridor courses above the ICA bifurcation.

Yamamura described a radiographic method for determining the exposure of basilar bifurcation aneurysms. A baseline is established between the anterior and posterior clinoid processes. The height of the ICA bifurcation and the height of the aneurysm's neck above the baseline determines the working space during a transsylvian approach. From this analysis, a high basilar bifurcation associated with a low ICA bifurcation would be the hardest configuration to expose a basilar bifurcation aneurysm via a transsylvian approach [55]. Another aspect to consider before deciding to use the pterional approach is the degree of posterior displacement of the basilar tip from the posterior clinoid process as described by Samson et al. A displacement of more than 10 mm (>13% of patients) may be associated with increased operative morbidity [56].

There are three osseous obstacles to the BA apex with this approach: the anterior clinoid process, the posterior clinoid process, and the dorsum sellae. Resection of these three obstacles partially or totally makes the classic pterional approach more difficult.

Notwithstanding the described problems, the treatment of BA bifurcation aneurysms performed by Yasargil offered good results well before the discovery and evolution of skull-base approaches, which confirms the masterly nature of his work.

7.8.2 Role of the Pretemporal Approach

This approach has already been described in clarifying the advantages characterizing the pterional approach. In aneurysms of the basilar apex (Fig. 7.9) and P1/P2a artery specifically, exposure of the anterior and middle incisural space is excellent (Fig. 7.13) and may be increased with tentorial incision, to obtain a wider workspace than the classic single pterional and subtemporal approaches of Drake. This approach may be further amplified with the association of an orbitozygomatic osteotomy for a high basilar bifurcation aneurysm or a transcavernous transsellar approach for a low-lying lesion. The latter approach is used also for complex and giant BA aneurysms. The orbitozygomatic resection allows a better view of the lesion from a basal perspective. In such cases, it is very useful to decompress the optic nerve canal, remove the anterior clinoid process and open the proximal and distal dural ring (Fig. 7.23). This technique lengthens the subarachnoid segment of the ICA and makes it more flexible.

A main advantage of the pretemporal transcavernous approach is that it involves widening the operative field depth by creating windows between the carotid artery and CNs III and IV. However, anatomic variations among patients may continue to hinder the full potential benefit that might be derived from such an approach. Such variations include: (1) the course of the oculomotor nerve; (2) a prominent posterior clinoid process; and (3) the course, length, and diameter of the PComA [11].

There are strategies for overcoming the disadvantages associated with such variations. For example, the oculomotor nerve can be fully exposed along its subarachnoidal and intracavernous portions and thus can be easily mobilized to achieve better exposure [57]. The

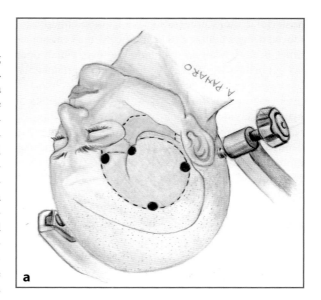

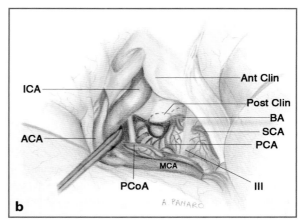

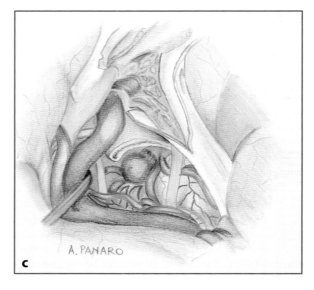

Fig. 7.23 a Orbitozygomatic transcavernous approach. Head position and site of cranioorbitozygomatic osteotomies. A pterional bone flap (*blue*) is elevated as the first piece and the orbitozygomatic osteotomy (*green*) is elevated as the second piece. **b** Operative exposure of a low-lying basilar apex aneurysm. The exposure is directed between the carotid artery and oculomotor nerve. The PComA has been elevated. The neck of the aneurysm is located behind the dorsum sellae and posterior clinoid process. **c** The transcavernous exposure is completed with exposure of the clinoid segment of the ICA and unroofing of the optic canal and dorsum sellae resection. *ACA* anterior cerebral artery. *Ant Clin* anterior clinoid, *BA* basilar artery, *ICA* internal carotid artery, *MCA* middle cerebral artery, *PCA* posterior cerebral artery, *PCoA* posterior communicating artery, *Post Clin* posterior clinoid, *SCA* superior cerebellar artery

posterior clinoid process can be trimmed and/or removed using a high-speed drill. The PComA can sometimes be long with an undulating course, which does not get in the way of its exposure. However, frequently, the PComA is short and has a course that is almost in the middle of the field of view. In these situations, it may also create a tension-band effect by pulling the ICA posteriorly and thus additionally reducing the depth of the field of exposure. Because the PComA has blood flow from more than one source (the ICA and PCA), it makes sense to consider cutting the PComA as a potentially safe step that can help widen the exposure at its depth (Fig. 7.14). Dividing the artery is especially helpful and safe in situations in which a short, adult-type PComA exists with the longest perforator-free zone closest to the PCA [34]. In this case, small hemoclips are placed as far apart as possible from one another at the longest perforator-free zone. The artery in-between is coagulated and cut, and the cut ends retract as a result of the elastic tension within the artery. The main disadvantage of this approach is the almost inevitable postoperative palsy of the oculomotor nerve.

7.8.3 Role of th5e Anterior Transpetrosal Approach

This approach is indicated for basilar trunk aneurysms located between the level of the pituitary floor and the internal carotid canal on a lateral angiogram (upper basilar trunk aneurysms, anterior inferior cerebellar artery aneurysms, and vertebrobasilar junction aneurysms) (Fig. 7.17d). This approach is highly indicated for aneurysms projecting to the brainstem because the perforating arteries around the aneurysm can be better observed and carefully dissected from the neck of the aneurysm.

A recent anatomical study performed on cadavers compared the two techniques, the transcavernous approach and anterior petrosectomy, used to manage retrosellar and upper clival BA aneurysms. Although this was a purely anatomical study, it clearly showed the real entity of the surgical exposure and the possible complications related to both surgical approaches [58].

Surgical approaches to manage basilar bifurcation aneurysms often have focused on the expansion of the deep windows of exposure [59]. However, the expansion of the surgical window may imply a risk to certain anatomic structures. In the transcavernous approach, the carotidooculomotor window may be expanded by

drilling the anterior and posterior clinoid processes, unroofing the optic nerve, opening the CS, and mobilizing the ICA (cutting proximal and distal dural rings) [45, 59]. The surgical view is unobstructed, and no vital structures, such as CNs, become interposed between the lesion and the surgeon's view. However, there are some drawbacks. Retracting the temporal lobe posteriorly often necessitates the sacrifice of temporal veins. Extensive manipulation of CN III and the mobilization of the ICA are necessary to augment the carotid oculomotor window. Potential injury to CN IV (as it crosses over CN III at the apex of the orbit) may follow the drilling of the anterior clinoid process or the unroofing of the optic canal. In some cases, the PComA must be sacrificed to ensure adequate surgical access to the interpeduncular and prepontine cisterns. Unroofing the optic canal carries the potential risk of injuring the optic nerve and violating the sphenoidal sinus. Bleeding that may occur from the basilar venous plexus and CS is a major risk during this procedure. For this reason, a complete resection of the posterior clinoid may be not performed in patients with a well-developed basilar plexus, and in such patients, the transcavernous approach would be difficult and/or impossible. The anterior petrosectomy, in turn, may provide a more caudal exposure of the BA and allows working space between CN III to IV (retrosellar BA), IV to V (retrosellar BA), and V to VII windows (upper clival segment of the BA) [60]. Therefore, the anterior petrosectomy provides access to the BA that is actually upper clival rather than just retrosellar [60] and allows access to a greater segment of the BA for proximal control; however, the surgical exposure is hampered by the interposed CNs. All of these neural structures along with CN VI are at risk when performing the anterior petrosectomy. In addition, retraction of the temporal lobe may damage the vein of Labbé, and drilling of the petrous bone may result in injury to the petrous carotid artery and cochlea.

7.8.4 Role of the Transtemporal– Transchoroidal Approach

This approach is used mainly for exposing the P2-PCA and aneurysms arising along its course or arteriovenous malformations localized in the ambient cistern. The P2 segment begins at the PComA, lies within the crural and ambient cisterns, and terminates lateral to the posterior edge of the midbrain. The P2 segment is divided into anterior and posterior parts because the surgical approaches to the anterior and posterior halves of this segment often differ, and because it is helpful in identifying the origin of the many branches that arise from P2. The anterior part is designated as the P2A or crural or peduncular segment because it courses around the cerebral peduncle in the crural cistern. The posterior part is designated as the P2P or the ambient or lateral mesencephalic segment because it courses lateral to the midbrain in the ambient cistern. Both segments are approximately 25 mm long.

The P2A segment begins at the PComA and courses between the cerebral peduncle and uncus that forms the medial and lateral walls of the crural cistern, and inferior to the optic tract and basal vein that crosses the roof of the cistern, to enter the proximal portion of the ambient cistern. The P2P segment commences at the posterior edge of the cerebral peduncle at the junction of the crural and ambient cisterns. It courses between the lateral midbrain and the parahippocampal and dentate gyri, which form the medial and lateral walls of the ambient cistern, below the optic tract, basal vein, and geniculate bodies and the inferolateral part of the pulvinar in the roof of the cistern, and superomedial to the trochlear nerve and tentorial edge.

As has already been described in the general description of this surgical approach, lesions located along the upper surface of the parahippocampal gyrus are hidden from the subtemporal view by the medial surface of the para-hippocampal gyrus and the surgical exposure cannot be improved by elevation of the temporal lobe [32]; for this reason, to treat P2p aneurysms, the transtemporal–transchoroidal approach is preferable because it is safer and offers better exposure of the upper portion of the ambient cistern.

References

1. Yasargil MG, Antic J, Laciga R et al (1976) Microsurgical pterional approach to aneurysms of the basilar bifurcation. Surg Neurol 6:83–91
2. Rhoton AL (2002) The supratentorial cranial space: microsurgical anatomy and surgical approaches. Neurosurgery 51(4):S1-1–S1-410
3. Yasargil MG (1996) Microneurosurgery of CNS tumors. Thieme, New York
4. Samii M, Carvalho GA, Tatagiba M, Matthies C (1997) Surgical management of meningiomas originating in Meckel's cave. Neurosurgery 41:767–774
5. Al-Mefty O, Ayoubi S, Gaber E (2002) Trigeminal schwannomas: removal of dumbbell-shaped tumors through the expanded Meckel cave and outcomes of cranial nerve function. J Neurosurg 96:453–463
6. Yoshida K, Kawase T (1999) Trigeminal neurinomas extending into multiple fossae: surgical methods and review of the literature. J Neurosurg 91:202–211
7. Ginsberg LE, DeMonte F (1999) Diagnosis please. Case 16: facial nerve schwannoma with middle cranial fossa involvement. Radiology 213:364–368
8. Wiggins RH 3rd, Harnsberger HR, Salzman KL et al (2006) The many faces of facial nerve schwannoma. AJNR Am J Neuroradiol 27:694–699
9. Celli P, Ferrante L, Acqui M et al (1992) Neurinoma of the third, fourth, and sixth cranial nerves: a survey and report of a new fourth nerve case. Surg Neurol 38:216–224
10. Jefferson G (1955) The trigeminal neurinomas with some remarks on malignant invasion of the gasserian ganglion. Clin Neurosurg 1:11–54
11. Tanriover N, Kemerdere R, Kafadar AM et al (2007) Oculomotor nerve schwannoma located in the oculomotor cistern. Surg Neurol 67:83–88
12. Krisht AF, Kadri PA, Raja A et al (2003) Pathology of the cavernous sinus. Techn Neurosurg 8:204–210
13. Sekhar LN, Sen CN, Jho HD et al (1989) Surgical treatment of intracavernous neoplasm. A four year experience. Neurosurgery 24:18–30
14. Sekhar LN, Ross D, Sen C (1993) Cavernous sinus and sphenocavernous neoplasms. In: Sekhar LN, Janecka IP (eds) Surgery of cranial base tumors. Raven Press, New York, pp 521–604
15. Al-Mefty O (1998) Operative atlas of meningioma. Lippincott-Raven, Philadelphia, pp 67–208
16. Eisenberg MB, Al-Mefty O, De Monte F et al. (1999) Benign nonmeningeal tumor of the cavernous sinus. Neurosurgery 44:949–954
17. Linskey ME, Sekhar LN, Hirsch WL Jr et al (1990) Aneurysms of the intracavernous carotid: natural history and indications for treatment. Neurosurgery 26:933–938
18. Debrum G, Vinuela F, Fox AJ et al (1988) Indications for treatment and classification of 132 carotid cavernous fistulas. Neurosurgery 22:285–289
19. Linskey ME, Sekhar LN (1992) Cavernous sinus hemangiomas: a series, review and an hypothesis. Neurosurgery 30:101–108
20. Eisenberg M, Haddad G, Al-Mefty O (1997) Petrous apex cholesterol granuloma: evolution and management. J Neurosurg 86:822–829
21. Harrison JM, Eisenberg MB (2000) Inflammatory lesions of the cavernous sinus. In: Eisenberg MB, Al-Mefty O (eds) The cavernous sinus: a comprehensive text. Lippincott Williams and Wilkins, Philadelphia, pp 339–355
22. Dolenc VV (1997) Transcranial epidural approach to pituitary tumors extending beyond the sella. Neurosurgery 41:542–550
23. Goel A, Nadkarni T, Muzumdar D et al (2004) Giant pituitary tumors: a study based on surgical treatment of 118 cases. Surg Neurol 61:436–445
24. Cushing H (1912) The pituitary body and its disorders: clinical states produced by disorders of the hypophysis cerebri. Lippincott, Philadelphia

25. Raymond LA, Tew J (1978) Large suprasellar aneurysms imitating pituitary tumor. J Neurol Neurosurg Psychiatry 41:83–87

26. Meyer JE, Oot RF, Lindorfs KK (1986) CT appearance of clival chordomas. J Comput Assist Tomogr 10:34–38

27. Kendall BE, Lee BC (1997) Cranial chordomas. Br J Radiol 50:687–698

28. Kveton JF, Brackmann DE, Glasscock ME 3rd et al (1986) Chondrosarcoma of the skull base. Otolaryngol Head Neck Surg 94:23–32

29. Ciappetta P, Salvati M, Bernardi C et al (1990) Giant cell reparative granuloma of the skull base mimicking an intracranial tumor. Case report and review of the literature. Surg Neurol 33:52–56

30. Sano K (1980) Temporopolar approach to aneurysms of the basilar artery at and around the distal bifurcation: Technical note. Neurol Res 2:361–367

31. de Oliveira E, Tedeschi H, Siqueira MG et al (1995) The pretemporal approach to the interpeduncular and petroclival regions. Acta Neurochir (Wien) 136:204–211

32. Ulm AJ, Tanriover N, Kawashima M et al (2004) Microsurgical approaches to the perimesencephalic cisterns and related segments of the posterior cerebral artery: comparison using a novel application of image guidance. Neurosurgery 54:1313–1327

33. Krayenbühl N, Krisht AF (2007) Dividing the posterior communicating artery in approaches to the interpeduncular fossa: technical aspects and safety. Neurosurgery 61:392–396

34. Drake CG, Peerles S, Hernesniemi JA (1996) Surgery of vertebro-basilar aneurysms. London, Ontario experience on 1767 patients. Springer, Vienna New York

35. Day JD, Giannotta SL, Fukushima T (1994) Extradural temporopolar approach to lesions of the upper basilar artery and infrachiasmatic region. J Neurosurg 81:230–235

36. Dolenc VV (1985) A combined epi- and subdural direct approach to carotid-ophthalmic artery aneurysms. J Neurosurg 62:667–672

37. Yonekawa Y, Ogata N, Imhof HG et al (1997) Selective extradural anterior clinoidectomy for supra- and parasellar processes. Technical note. J Neurosurg 87:636–642

38. Kawase T, van Loveren H, Keller JT et al (1996) Meningeal architecture of the cavernous sinus: clinical and surgical implications. Neurosurgery 39:527–534

39. Youssef S, Kim EY, Aziz KM et al (2006) The subtemporal interdural approach to dumbbell-shaped trigeminal schwannomas: cadaveric prosection. Neurosurgery 59:ONS270–ONS277

40. Yoshida K, Kawase T (2002) Zygomatic Transpetrosal approach for dumbbell-shaped parasellar and posterior fossa chordoma. Oper Tech Neurosurg 5:104–107

41. Goel A, Nadkarni T (1999) Basal lateral subtemporal approach for trigeminal neurinomas: report of an experience with 18 cases. Acta Neurochir (Wien) 141:711–719

42. Sugita K, Kobayashi S, Yokoo A (1982) Preservation of large bridging veins during brain retraction. Technical note. J Neurosurg 57:856–858

43. Koperna T, Tschabitscher M, Knosp E (1992) The termination of the vein of "Labbé" and its microsurgical significance. Acta Neurochir (Wien) 118:172–175

44. Kyoshima K, Oikawa S, Kobayashi S (2001) Preservation of large bridging veins of the cranial base: technical note. Neurosurgery 48:447–449

45. Seoane ER, Tedeschi H, de Oliveira EP et al (1997) Management strategies for posterior cerebral artery aneurysms: a proposed new surgical classification. Acta Neurochir (Wien) 139:325–331

46. Ebeling U, Reulen HJ (1988) Neurosurgical topography of the optic radiation in the temporal lobe. Acta Neurochir (Wien) 92:29–36

47. Gonzalez LF, Smith KA (2001) Meyer's loop. BNI Q 18:4–7

48. Heros RC (1982) Arteriovenous malformations of the medial temporal lobe. Surgical approach and neuroradiological characterization. J Neurosurg 56:44–52

49. Nagata S, Rhoton AL Jr, Barry M (1988) Microsurgical anatomy of the choroidal fissure. Surg Neurol 30:3–59

50. Ikeda K, Shoin K, Mohri M et al (2002) Surgical indications and microsurgical anatomy of the transchoroidal fissure approach for lesions in and around the ambient cistern. Neurosurgery 50:1114–1119

51. Siwanuwatn R, Deshmukh P, Zabramski JM et al (2005) Microsurgical anatomy and quantitative analysis of the transtemporal-transchoroidal fissure approach to the ambient cistern. Neurosurgery 57:228–235

52. Yasargil MG, Türe U, Yasargil DC (2004) Impact of temporal lobe surgery. J Neurosurg 101:725–738

53. Wascher TM, Spetzler RF (1995) Saccular aneurysms of the basilar bifurcation. In: Carter P, Spetzler RF (eds) Neurovascular surgery. McGraw-Hill, New York, pp 729–752

54. Gonzalez LF, Amin-Hanjani S, Bambakidis NC et al (2005) Skull base approaches to the basilar artery. Neurosurg Focus 19:E3

55. Yamamura A (1988) Diagnosis and treatment of vertebral aneurysms. J Neurosurg 69:345–349

56. Samson D, Batjer HH, Kopitnik TA Jr (1999) Current results of the surgical management of aneurysms of the basilar apex. Neurosurgery 44:697–702

57. Seone E, Tedeshi H, de Oliveira E et al (2000) The pretemporal transcavernous approach to the interpeduncular and prepontine cisterns: microsurgical anatomy and technique application. Neurosurgery 46:891–898

58. Figueiredo EG, Zabramski JM, Deshmukh P et al (2006) Comparative analysis of anterior petrosectomy and transcavernous approaches to retrosellar and upper clival basilar artery aneurysms. Neurosurgery 58:ONS13–ONS21

59. Youssef AS, Aziz KA, Kim EY et al (2004) The carotid-oculomotor window in exposure of upper basilar artery aneurysms: a cadaveric morphometric study. Neurosurgery 54:1181–1189

60. Kawase T, Toya S (1994) Anterior transpetrosal approach for basilar trunk aneurysms: further experience. In: Pasqualin A, Da Pian R (eds) New trends in management of cerebrovascular malformations. Springer, Vienna, pp 255–260

Suboccipital Lateral Approaches (Presigmoid)

8

Luciano Mastronardi, Alessandro Ducati and Takanori Fukushima

8.1 Introduction

The goal of presigmoid approaches is to expose the posterior cranial fossa via partial or complete petrosectomy and division of the tentorium. The presigmoid approaches are an anterior extension of the common suboccipital lateral approach, and provide excellent exposure of cerebellopontine angle and pons. We generally distinguish three types of presigmoid approaches, namely the retrolabyrinthine, the translabyrinthine and the transcochlear, that represent three progressive steps of the petrosectomy.

In particular, the retrolabyrinthine approach involves a presigmoid partial mastoidectomy that preserves the structures of the inner ear. Its major benefits are that hearing and facial nerve function are preserved and only minimal brain retraction is required. Combined with middle fossa exposure (combined petrosal approach) [1–5], this approach is very useful for lesions involving the petroclival junction, including petroclival meningiomas, trigeminal schwannomas, epidermoids, and large chondrosarcomas or chordomas with intradural components [1–7].

In order to carry out this approach, a detailed knowledge of mastoid anatomy is mandatory. Skull-base surgeons have to be able to perform a mastoidectomy via several presigmoid exposures:
1. Retrolabyrinthine
2. Translabyrinthine
3. Transcochlear

4. Combined petrosal (combination with middle fossa approach)
5. ELITE (extreme lateral infrajugular tanscondylar-transtubercular exposure)
6. Infralabyrinthine transjugular-infrajugular.

8.2 Transpetrosal Approaches

According to Ammirati and Samii [6]:

> The presigmoid sinus approaches to the petroclival region shortens the distance to the clivus, permits a multiangled exposure of this difficult surgical area, minimizes the amount of temporal lobe retraction, preserves the integrity of the transverse sinus, and allows for better preservation of the neurovascular structures. These factors translate into a high percentage of total tumor removal and a low incidence of permanent morbidity.

The retrolabyrinthine, translabyrinthine, and transcochlear approaches, which constitute the three major transpetrosal approaches, are typically used to treat lesions located in front of the brainstem, such as tumors or midbasilar aneurysms, following the principle of removing bone rather than retracting neural tissue. The difference between these approaches is the gradually increasing amount of resection of the mastoid process. Progressive drilling of the petrous bone, and removing the labyrinth and the cochlea exposes the anterior aspect of the brainstem, minimizing retraction and leaving the surgeon closer to the target, but causes permanent loss of hearing [1–7].

Owing to the need for a wide exposure of the sigmoid and transverse sinuses, cerebral angiography with venous phase and/or an angio-MRI scan is always advisable before surgery [1–7].

L. Mastronardi (✉)
Dept of Neurosurgery, Sant'Andrea Hospital
"Sapienza" University of Rome, Italy

The translabyrinthine and transcochlear exposures are dependent on and are a progression of the retrolabyrinthine approach. They are described in more detail in Chapter 12.

8.2.1 Retrolabyrinthine Approach: Surgical Technique and "Tricks"

Retrolabyrinthine mastoid drilling was designed for the treatment of vestibular neurectomies (for which the retrolabyrinthine approach was developed); its application in other settings is limited [1–7]. Among transpetrosal approaches, the retrolabyrinthine approach involves the smallest amount of bone resection.

For the position of the patient on the operating table we suggest the Fukushima' lateral position (Fig. 8.1) [3, 4]. The table is positioned in 15–20° reverse Trendelenburg position. The body of the patient should lie in an oblique line, with the upper arm at 45° and the lower one at 90°. Silicone pads are positioned in the lower axilla and between the legs. The leg on the table is flexed more than the other. The shoulder ipsilateral to the operative field should be the more external part of the body, in line with the limit of the table [3, 4]. The head is held in a three-pin Mayfield device. A soft roll is placed under the ipsilateral shoulder to facilitate rotation. The head should be: (1) flexed slightly on the neck, (2) declined with the vertex down, and (3) rotated toward the floor. The shoulder is taped caudally to increase the surgeon's working room. If the position is

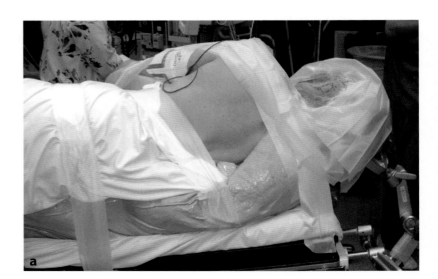

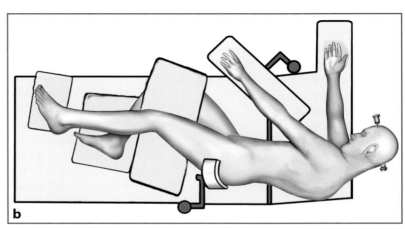

Fig. 8.1 Fukushima's lateral position. **a** Surgical position. **b** Artistic drawing

correct, the shoulder creates an edge between the neck and the chest and the mastoid is the highest structure in the operative field [3, 4] (Fig. 8.1).

In patients with a habitus precluding adequate depression of the shoulder and in patients with a short and wide neck, the park bench or the supine position can be used, with the head rotated to the opposite side, parallel to the floor, and moderately flexed and declined [1, 2, 5].

Optionally, a lumbar CSF drainage catheter can be placed, in order to minimize brain retraction [3, 4].

The skin incision begins 1 cm over and anterior to the ear and continues in a gentle curve around the ear to reach a point just 1 cm below the mastoid tip in a C-shaped fashion (Fig. 8.1). In the combined petrosal approach the incision starts from the root of the zygoma anterior to the ear and extends in a curvilinear fashion behind the ear to reach a point 2 cm below the mastoid tip, two transverse fingers posterior to the mastoid body [1–5]. In a two-layer dissection technique, the subcutaneous tissue is separated from the fascia and preserved for final reconstruction [3, 4]. The temporalis muscle is detached from the bone by sharp dissection and retracted anterior with blunt hooks, taking care to elevate the skin flap and the muscle on a plane at 45°, avoiding their prolonged compression (Fig. 8.2)

The mastoid cortex is scored and cut with a high-power drill, starting with a "large" cutting bar (5 or 6 mm in diameter) [1–5, 7]. The area to be drilled is a wide triangle, whose apexes are the root of the zygoma, the asterion and the mastoid tip (Fig. 8.6). A common mistake is to start with too-small a triangle that precludes the possibility to adequately expose the deeper structures. During this step it is necessary to gradually expose the sigmoid sinus (from the transverse-sigmoid sinus junction to the jugular bulb), the dura covering the basal part of the temporal lobe (after drilling the so-called *tegmen tympani*), and the sinodural angle (Fig. 8.3). This drilling opens the "antrum" (just deep to the superoanterior corner of the triangle), a bone cavity of the mastoid communicating with the tympanic cavity and the mastoid cells. The lateral semicircular canal (LSC) becomes clearly visible with its compact bone, and close to it the incus appears. These are critical landmarks for identification of the facial nerve (see below).

When retrolabyrinthine mastoidectomy is combined with a far-lateral or retrosigmoid approach the entire sigmoid sinus is skeletonized. The mastoid emissary vein is usually located 2 cm above the inferior nuchal line and 2 cm below the superior nuchal line in the lateral border of the mastoid bone, and inserts into the sig-

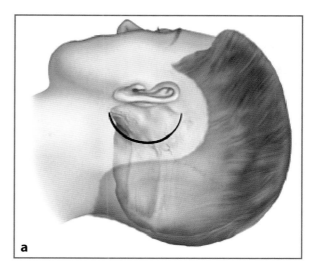

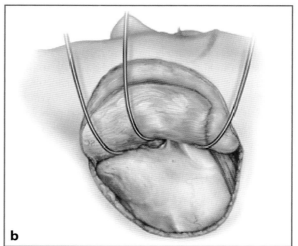

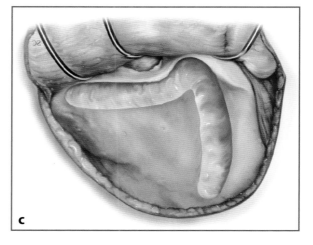

Fig. 8.2 a Incision, **b** double-layer flap elevation and **c** start drilling.

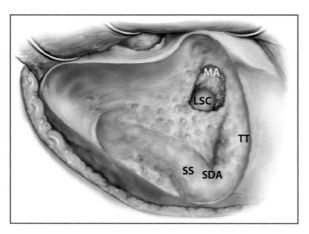

Fig. 8.3 Skeletonization of the sigmoid sinus (*SS*), the transverse sinus, the tegmen tympani (*TT*), the sinodural angle (*SDA*), the mastoid antrum (*MA*), and the lateral semicircular canal (*LSC*)

moid sinus approximately half way between the transverse sigmoid sinus junction and the jugular bulb [3, 4]. This vein is an important landmark for location of the internal auditory canal during the translabyrinthine approach [6]. Maximal attention is necessary to locate and protect the vein of Labbé at its insertion into the sigmoid sinus [1–5].

The retrolabyrinthine approach only compromises the bone anterior to the sigmoid sinus and posterior and inferior to the semicircular canals: LSC, posterior (PSC) and superior (SSC), including the *common crus* connecting the PSC and SSC (Fig. 8.4). Thus, in this exposure the mastoid is drilled posterior and inferior to

the labyrinth and cochlea, which are skeletonized but not opened so that hearing is preserved. The canals should be maximally "cleaned" by cancellous bone of mastoid cells until a blue line is visualized (that is their membranous content in transparency). Care is necessary when drilling over the PSC. The canal is sometimes covered by a large sigmoid sinus, the wall of which may be damaged. In order to prevent this complication, it seems advisable to leave a thin layer of bone (egg-shell technique) over the sigmoid sinus [3, 4] and gently retract it with a self-retaining spatula. Recognition of the deep (anterior) wall of the sigmoid sinus canal into the mastoid is another "trick" to identify the posterior border of cancellous bone posterior to the PSC that can be safely removed.

Care is taken to locate and preserve the facial nerve (Fig. 8.4) in the tympanic segment (close to the incus), genu (close to the LSC), and vertical (fallopian canal) segment. The fallopian canal should be followed from the genu as far as the digastric point on the digastric line (the intramastoid attachment of the digastric muscle) and the stylomastoid foramen [1–5]. In cadaver dissection, it is possible to recognize the bony canal of the facial nerve when a pink line appears during drilling [3, 4]. Anyway, for location, identification, and preservation of the facial nerve in its segments inside the mastoid process there are well-established landmarks (Table 8.1). First, the *mastoid antrum* indicates the depth of the labyrinth and the depth at which the facial nerve can be located (and damaged!) at the level of the tympanic segment and the genu [3, 4]. Therefore, special care is necessary when the aditus ad antrum is opened and the incus and the LSC visualized. Among the other landmarks (Table 8.1), before drilling it is advisable to identify the position of the spine of Henle (Fig. 8.2) in the posterior border of the external auditory canal. In fact, at a depth of 15–16 mm from the spine of Henle, the genu of the facial nerve is usually located [3, 4]. In clinical practice, electrical stimulation and registration of the nerve is always a fundamental adjunct for obtaining a safe procedure [3, 4, 7].

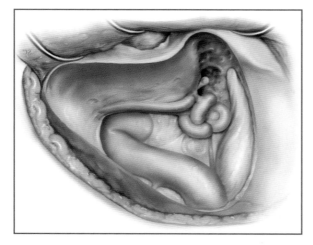

Fig. 8.4 Retrolabyrinthine mastoidectomy: final exposure

Table 8.1 Landmarks for location of facial nerve

Segment	Landmark
Descending segment (Fallopian canal)	Digastric ridge, inferiorly LSC, superiorly
Genu (close to LSC)	15–16 mm deep to the spine of Henle LSC
Tympanic segment (in the mastoid antrum)	Incus Parallel to LSC

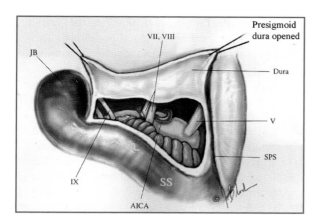

Fig. 8.5 Opening of the posterior fossa presigmoid dura mater after retrolabyrinthine mastoidectomy. *AICA* anterior inferior cerebellar artery, *JB* jugular bulb, *SPS* superior petrosal sinus, *SS* sigmoid sinus, *V VII VIII IX* cranial nerves

After retrolabyrinthine mastoid drilling it is possible to expose the presigmoid dura mater and the endolymphatic sac (Fig. 8.4). Care must be taken to avoid injury to the endolymphatic sac, which runs medial to the sigmoid sinus and inferior to the PSC. Damage to this structure can cause hearing loss as a result of endolymphatic fluid leakage [3, 4]. After opening of the presigmoid dura it is possible to expose the cranial nerves (from the 3rd to the 12th), the superior cerebellar artery, the ante-

rior-inferior cerebellar artery the posterior inferior cerebellar artery, the anterior and lateral aspect of the brainstem, and the lateral surface of the cerebellar hemisphere (Fig. 8.5). Ligation and division of the sigmoid sinus provides additional exposure by opening a wider angle between the cerebellum and the petrous bone [2], especially in combination with a traditional retrosigmoid craniotomy (for this approach see Chapter 9). In any case, in agreement with Fukushima et al. [3, 4], it is usually better to preserve the sigmoid sinus, in this way avoiding the feared venous complications, especially when the sinus is divided close to the insertion of the vein of Labbé.

As an aid to remembering all the necessary landmarks for a correct retrolabyrinthine mastoidectomy, Fukushima et al. [3, 4] identified three triangles in three different planes of depth (Fig. 8.6). The points of the outer triangle of Fukushima et al. are: the root of the zygoma, the asterion, and the mastoid tip. The points of the inner triangle are: the aditus ad antrum, the sinodural angle, and the digastric point. The points of Macewen's (deeper) triangle are: the aditus ad antrum, the half-way point between the aditus ad antrum and the sinodural angle, and the half-way point between the aditus ad antrum and the digastric point. The last triangle encloses the labyrinth [3, 4].

The following are some key landmarks that should be born in mind during mastoid dissection:

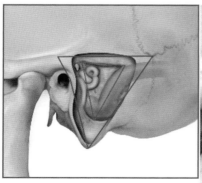
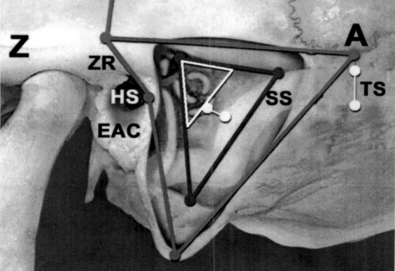

Fig. 8.6 Fukushima's triangles. *Z* root of the zygoma, *HS* spine of Henle, *EAC* external auditory canal, *SS* sigmoid sinus, *A* asterion, *TS* transverse sinus

- Trigeminal point: 1–2 cm posterior to the superior–posterior mastoid limit (along the superior nuchal line).
- Mastoid emissary vein: 2 cm above the inferior nuchal line and 2 cm below the superior nuchal line; landmark for the cochlear nerve.
- Digastric line/point: landmark for the descending facial nerve (mastoid dissection); landmark for the occipital condyle (high cervical dissection).
- Trautmann's triangle: above the jugular bulb and under the PSC; the route of access to the foramen lacerum.

8.3 Conclusions

When performed properly, this technique provides a solid adjunct to treating many petroclival lesions, mainly in combination with other approaches. Although the anatomical landmarks of the skull base are well known, acquiring the practical knowledge of neurosurgical anatomy, especially temporal bone anatomy, is a very long and tortuous process involving many visits to the cadaver laboratory.

The transpetrosal routes, especially when combined with temporal craniotomy, the middle fossa approach, the retrosigmoid approach, and/or high cervical exposure are the best option for approaching many posterior fossa lesions deeply located around the brainstem and in the cerebellopontine angle. The main advantages of these approaches are the minimal retraction of brain and the wide exposure they allow.

The retrolabyrinthine route is the first step in mastoidectomy. Indeed, translabyrinthine and transcochlear exposures are dependent on and are a progression of the retrolabyrinthine approach. Therefore, a knowledge of mastoid anatomy and of retrolabyrinthine dissection is fundamental for any skull-base surgeon, representing one of the most important "weapons" in the armamentarium against skull-base tumors.

References

1. Bambakidis NC, Gonzalez F, Amin-Hanjani S et al (2005) Combined skull base approaches to the posterior fossa. Technical note. Neurosurg Focus 19:E6
2. Erkmen K, Pravdenkova S, Al-Mefty O (2005) Surgical management of petroclival meningiomas: factors determining the choice of approach. Neurosurg Focus 15:E7
3. Fukushima T, Sameshima T, Friedman A (2006) Manual of skull base dissection, 2nd edn. AF Neurovideo, Raleigh
4. Sameshima T, Mastronardi L, Friedman A, Fukushima T (eds) (2007) Fukushima's microanatomy and dissection of the temporal bone for surgery of acoustic neuroma, and petroclival meningioma, 2nd edn. AF Neurovideo, Raleigh, pp 84–114
5. Tummala RP, Coscarella E, Morcos JJ (2005) Combined skull base approaches to the posterior fossa. Neurosurg Focus 19:E6
6. Ammirati M, Samii M (1992) Presigmoid sinus approach to petroclival meningiomas. Skull Base Surg 2:124–128
7. Aristegui M, Canalis RF, Naguib M et al (1997) Retrolabyrinthine vestibular nerve section: a current appraisal. Ear Nose Throat J 76:578–583

Suboccipital Lateral Approaches (Retrosigmoid)

9

Madjid Samii and Venelin M. Gerganov

9.1 Introduction

The lateral suboccipital or the retrosigmoid approach (RSA) was developed by Fedor Krause and utilized for the first time by him in 1898. During the following decades it was developed and became one of the main and most frequently applied operative approaches in neurosurgery [1–5]. Various pathological entities located in the cerebellopontine angle (CPA), the internal auditory canal (IAC), the petroclival area, and the lateral or anterior foramen magnum area, can be adequately accessed via the classical RSA or some of its modifications. Refinements of the operative technique led to a significant decrease in the initially high procedure-related complication rate, and nowadays the RSA is safe and relatively easy to perform. Due to the wide panoramic view offered by the approach, all stages of surgery may be performed under direct visual control, which is particularly important during dissection in proximity of the brainstem. Further, in patients with a large vestibular schwannoma (VS), the RSA is the only hearing-sparing technique.

The introduction of highly sensitive techniques for intraoperative neurophysiological monitoring added considerably to the safety of the procedure [6–8]. Nowadays we perform such monitoring whenever the RSA is used. It is done throughout the whole of the procedure: from positioning of the patient to skin closure. Monitoring of the somatosensory evoked potentials is especially important if the patient is in the semisitting position in order to prevent spinal cord compression. Preoperative functional X-rays of the cervical spine could identify patients at risk, such as those with severe degenerative spine disease or spinal instability [4].

The facial nerve is monitored continuously by electromyography transferred by loudspeakers [9, 10]. Bipolar recording needle electrodes are fixed at the eyebrow for the orbicularis oculi muscle and at the mouth angle for the orbicularis oris muscle. Electrical activation by 1–4 mA is applied during the course of surgery for difficult nerve identification or for testing the reactivity of the nerve to mechanical stimulation. Monitoring of brainstem auditory evoked potentials is essential for avoiding hearing deficit, e.g. in every case when the cerebellum is retracted. In VS surgery it allows control and prediction of the cochlear nerve function and provides instant feedback information on the functional status of the cochlear nerve. The waves I, III, and V are functional correlates of the cochlea, the nucleus cochlearis, and the colliculus inferior; the main parameters that are observed are the waves latency, amplitude, and loss. The parameter that most closely predicts deafness is loss of wave V [7]. The loss of any wave may be prevented by early recognition of its deterioration, and the surgeon's actions should be modified accordingly. The abducent and the caudal cranial nerves are monitored if necessary according to the particular tumor extension and clinical presentation.

9.2 Positioning of the Patient

The patient can be placed on the operating table in the semisitting, lateral, park-bench, or supine position with

M. Samii (✉)
International Neuroscience Institute
Hannover, Germany

P. Cappabianca et al. (eds.), *Cranial, Craniofacial and Skull Base Surgery*.
© Springer-Verlag Italia 2010

the head rotated to the contralateral side [8, 11]. Despite the risks related to the semisitting position [12] — such as venous air embolism, paradoxical air embolism, tension pneumocephalus, or circulatory instability — we prefer it for neoplastic or vascular lesions, while for microvascular decompression the supine position with the head rotated contralaterally is sufficient.

The main advantage of the semisitting position is that there is no need for constant suction so the surgeon can perform the dissections bimanually. Secondly, there is no need for frequent coagulation during the procedure because the assistant continuously irrigates the operative field.

In experienced hands the potential complications related to this position can be avoided [10, 13]. The source of major air embolism is usually the venous sinuses that, due to their bone attachments, do not collapse. Air may also enter via emissary veins or via diploic veins. The most specific and sensitive method for detection of air embolism is transesophageal echocardiography. Nevertheless, the combined monitoring of end-tidal carbon dioxide and precordial Doppler echocardiography yields similar results [14]. If immediate measures are carried out at the first sign of venous air embolism, the related morbidity is insignificant. The morbidity due to venous air embolism is similar in both the semisitting and supine position.

The head of the patient is fixed to the operating table with a three-point head fixation frame, flexed and rotated approximately 30° to the involved side (Fig. 9.1). Importantly, any occlusion of venous jugular outflow or hyperflexion of the cervical spine should be avoided.

9.3 Craniotomy

A slightly curved skin incision 2–2.5 cm medial to the mastoid process is performed and the underlying muscles are incised in line with the skin (Fig. 9.2). If the foramen magnum area has to be approached, however, the caudal end of the incision has to be extended further towards midline. The question as to whether to perform a craniectomy or craniotomy is a matter of individual preference and institutional tradition. According to our experience, the one-piece craniotomy is a more dangerous procedure in regard to the safety of venous sinuses and the risk of a dural tear. After the initial burr hole is made, the craniectomy is extended with bone rongeurs and a high-speed drill. Traditionally the position of the burr hole was determined in relation to the asterion as the point where the transverse sinus merges into the sigmoid sinus [8]. However, some recent studies have shown that the asterion is not an absolutely reliable

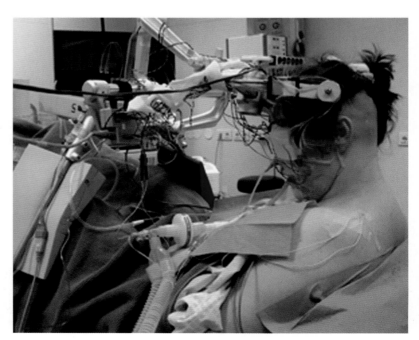

Fig. 9.1 Semisitting position of the patient with the head flexed anteriorly and rotated to the side of the approach

anatomic landmark and is variable both in the cranial–caudal and in the anterior–posterior plane [15–17]. The superior nuchal line usually overlies the transverse sinus, but is also unreliable. The course of the sigmoid sinus is less variable: it descends along an axis defined by the mastoid tip and the squamosal-parietomastoid suture junction or over the mastoid groove.

We prefer to place the burr hole 2–2.5 cm below the superior nuchal line, two-thirds behind and one-third in front of the occipitomastoid suture. Importantly, the location of the emissary vein has to be also considered. For CPA tumors, the size of the craniotomy is similar and not related to the tumor type or size. Only the borders of the sigmoid and transverse sinuses should be exposed, as more extensive exposure of these sinuses is unnecessary and might lead to their laceration or desiccation, with the risk of subsequent thrombosis (Fig. 9.3). The bone opening should extend to the floor of the posterior fossa, thus allowing access to the lateral cerebellomedullary cistern. Special care should be directed toward preservation of the mastoid emissary vein/veins. Excessive traction on the vein could lead to sinus laceration and increases the risk of venous air embolism. Its location should be studied on the thin-slice bone window CT scan of the occipital bone. During the craniotomy, the vein should be freed from any bony encasement with a diamond drill until it can be safely coagulated. For microvascular decompression a smaller craniotomy is sufficient; however it should be precisely positioned [3]. On the other hand, the foramen magnum may need to be opened to expose adequately lesions in the foramen magnum area [18].

All subsequent stages are performed with microscopic visualization. The dura is incised in a curvilinear manner just medial to the sigmoid and inferior to the transverse sinus (Fig. 9.4). This allows a primary watertight dural closure and avoids the need to use dural substitute in almost all cases. The lateral cerebellomedullary cistern is then opened and the cerebrospinal fluid is drained. Thus, the cerebellum relaxes away from the petrous bone and the self-retaining retractor supports and protects the cerebellar hemisphere, instead of compressing it.

The later steps of surgery depend upon the underlying pathological entity. In cases of VS, the intrameatal tumor portion is exposed initially [10, 13]. Careful study of high-resolution CT scans with thin slices and bone window is essential for the safe opening of the IAC. The dura is excised circularly around the posterior lip of the IAC and stripped off. The posterior and superior walls of the IAC are then drilled using decreasing sizes of di-

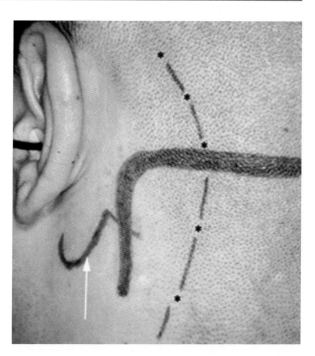

Fig. 9.2 Slightly curved skin incision is made 2–2.5 cm behind the mastoid process (*arrow*)

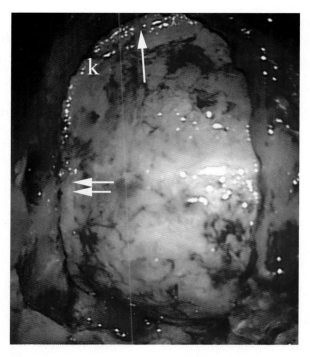

Fig. 9.3 The craniotomy exposes the margins of the transverse sinus (*single arrow*) and of the sigmoid sinus (*double arrow*). *k* sinus knee

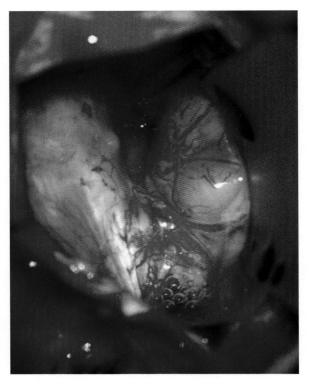

Fig. 9.4 The dura is incised along the sinuses and retracted with two sutures. The cerebellopontine angle is exposed. Both the posterior pyramid and the vestibular schwannoma are well visualized

amond drills under constant irrigation. The canal is unroofed at least over 180° of its circumference (Fig. 9.5). Less radical exposure of the IAC leads to a greater risk of either incomplete removal of the most lateral part of the tumor or a worse functional outcome. The extent of IAC opening is tailored to the extent of lateral tumor extension. In order to preserve hearing, the inner ear structures should not be damaged. Therefore, the last 2–3 mm of the bony plate next to the fundus is usually left intact. The meatal dura is then incised and the intrameatal tumor is exposed. The most lateral tumor portion is carefully mobilized out of the IAC with a microdissector. The facial and vestibulocochlear nerves can be identified laterally in the region of the fundus due to their constant relation to the bony structures. Once the nerves are exposed, the tumor is removed piecemeal. If the tumor is of highly increased consistency, primary intrameatal mobilization might be difficult.

The extrameatal part of the tumor is initially debulked with a Cavitron ultrasonic aspirator or platelet-shaped knife. After sufficient internal decompression has been achieved, the tumor capsule is dissected from the surrounding neural structures. The dissection is performed by carefully gripping the tumor capsule and dissecting in the level of the arachnoid plane. Stretching of neural structures in one direction for a long time has to be avoided. The medial segment of the facial nerve

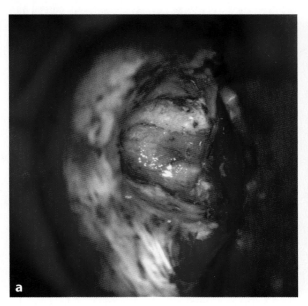

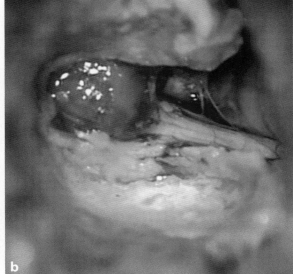

Fig. 9.5 a The IAC is opened widely with a high-speed diamond drill. **b** Following incision of the IAC dura, the VS and the cranial nerves are seen as they enter the CPA cistern (different patient)

is identified medially along the brainstem. Pulling the rest of the capsule medially and upward allows visualization of the middle and the most lateral segments of the nerve (Fig. 9.6). Once the tumor has been completely removed, the continuity of the facial nerve can be confirmed by electrical stimulation of the nerve from the brainstem to the intrameatal portion.

In meningioma surgery, the location of the tumor determines the extent of exposure [4, 5, 19, 20]. If the tumor is located retromeatally, the pure retrosigmoid suboccipital approach is sufficient; in tumors that originate anterior to the IAC and extend into Meckel's cave and/or the posterior cavernous sinus, the suprameatal extension of the retrosigmoid approach is required. Petroclival meningiomas are located medially to the Vth, VIIth, and VIIIth cranial nerves and should be removed through one of the CPA levels: the upper level (defined by the tentorium and the trigeminal nerve), the second level (between the trigeminal and the VIIth—VIIIth nerve complex), the third level (between the VIIth and VIIIth nerves and the caudal nerves), or the lowest level (between the caudal nerves and the foramen magnum). The anatomical space between the cranial nerves may be relatively narrow; however the tumor usually widens it sufficiently to allow safe manipulations. The removal should start at the level that is most widely expanded by the meningioma. Initial in-

ternal decompression is performed using an ultrasonic surgical aspirator at the appropriate levels and—in a manner similar to the procedure for VS—the tumor capsule is dissected only after sufficient internal decompression has been achieved. If the pia mater of the brainstem is infiltrated, a small part of the tumor capsule may be left (10–20% of cases).

Larger meningiomas have already displaced the brainstem, so the RSA may provide adequate access even to the contralateral side or supratentorially. If necessary, however, the petrous apex may be resected. In 1982 the senior author introduced the technique of intradural resection of the petrous apex via the retrosigmoid route – the so-called retrosigmoid suprameatal approach or RSMA [21, 22]. Later anatomical studies have shown that the exposure may be thus extended anterior by as much as 13.0 mm [23]. The degree of bone removal is determined by the individual anatomical characteristics and tumor expansion. The opening of Meckel's cave allows mobilization of the trigeminal nerve, which further increases the working space. The abducent nerve may be identified early at its brainstem exit zone and followed during tumor removal up to Dorello's canal which allows its preservation. In tumors extending supratentorially into the middle cranial fossa, additional resection of the tentorium is needed. Hence, the RSMA provides access to Meckel's cave, the petroclival area, and the middle fossa including the posterior cavernous sinus. Moreover, the risks associated with alternative approaches, such as extensive petrous bone resection or retraction of the temporal lobe with the associated risks of damage to neural and vascular structures are avoided.

In more extensive meningiomas that engulf the optic nerve and carotid artery, staged surgery may be indicated. In the first stage, the tumor part in the CPA, clivus, and/or Meckel's cave is removed via a RSMA and the brainstem is decompressed, and the risk of severe neurological deterioration is thus prevented. In the second stage, the supratentorial portion is removed via the frontotemporal route.

Intradural lesions, located in the lateral or anterior foramen magnum area can be successfully approached via the lateral suboccipital route, which combines a retrosigmoid craniectomy and a C1 hemilaminectomy/laminectomy [18]. In these cases, the craniectomy is similar to the one described above. In addition, lateral removal of the C1 lamina and wide opening of the foramen magnum are required. Thus, sufficient lateral exposure is gained, circumventing the risky dissection and/or transposition of the vertebral artery.

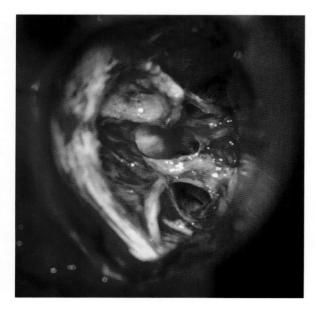

Fig. 9.6 Complete tumor removal. The facial and cochlear nerves are preserved

9.4 Dural Closure and Reconstruction of the Posterior Skull Base

The drilled area of the pyramid is sealed with multiple pieces of fat tissue that are fixed with fibrin glue (Fig. 9.7). The fat plug has specific characteristics on different MRI sequences and should not be mistaken for residual or recurrent tumor on the follow-up studies (Fig. 9.8). Prior to dural closure, the jugular veins should be compressed to make any opened veins visible for hemostasis. The compression is applied while the retractor is still in place, which allows inspection of the CPA. After the retractor has been removed and the cerebellum has reexpanded, the jugular veins are compressed again. Any torn and bleeding supracerebellar bridging veins are detected. If some mastoid air cells have been opened, they also have to be occluded with fat and fibrin glue. The dura is sutured watertight; if needed, a piece of fat may be applied over the suture line. The fat is harvested from the appropriate subcutaneous layer at the incision site. Bone wax is avoided, except for hemostasis if there is significant bleeding from the bone edges.

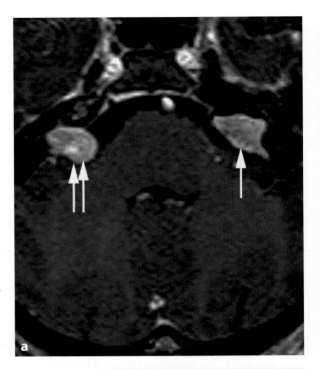

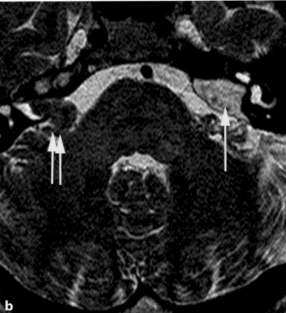

Fig. 9.8 In this patient with NF-2 and bilateral VS, the larger tumor on the left side has been removed and the IAC has been sealed with fat (*single arrows*). The smaller tumor on the right side was followed as this was the only hearing side (*double arrow*). On the postoperative T1-weighted contrast-enhanced MR image (**a**), the signal intensity on both sides appears similar and the radiologist suspected a recurrence. However, the T2-weighted image (**b**) clearly shows the fat plug

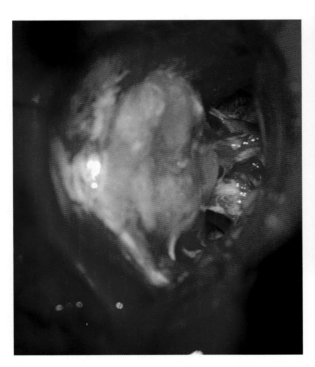

Fig. 9.7 The IAC is sealed with multiple pieces of fat and fixed with fibrin glue

Reconstruction of the posterior skull base with methyl methacrylate is necessary to avoid postoperative complications, such as pseudomeningocele, or poor a cosmetic result (Fig. 9.9). It also prevents the formation of adhesions between the dura and the neck muscles, and thus may prevent the occurrence of suboccipital headache [13, 24].

Significant suboccipital headache may be produced by the formation of scar tissue around the occipital nerves or by a posttraumatic scar neuroma. Careful examination of the area around the operative incision usually reveals a small trigger point, which corresponds to the area of the scar neuroma. Infiltration with local anesthesia usually ameliorates the symptoms. If the pain is persistent and resistant to medication, operative excision of the scar and the neuroma through a limited skin incision can be performed with immediate beneficial effect [10].

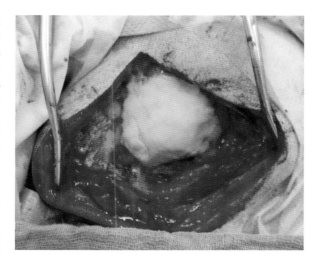

Fig. 9.9 The posterior skull base has been reconstructed with methyl methacrylate

References

1. Bennett M, Haynes DS (2008) Surgical approaches and complications in the removal of vestibular schwannomas. Neurosurg Clin N Am 19:331–343
2. Cohen NL (2008) Retrosigmoid approach for acoustic tumor removal. Neurosurg Clin N Am 19:239–250
3. Rhoton AL Jr (2000) The cerebellopontine angle and posterior fossa cranial nerves by the retrosigmoid approach. Neurosurgery 47:S93–S129
4. Samii M, Gerganov VM (2008) Surgery of extra-axial tumors of the cerebral base. Neurosurgery 62 (Suppl 3):1153–1166
5. Little AS, Jittapiromsak P, Crawford NR et al (2008) Quantitative analysis of exposure of staged orbitozygomatic and retrosigmoid craniotomies for lesions of the clivus with supratentorial extension. Neurosurgery 62 (Suppl 2):318–323
6. Romstock J, Strauss C, Fahlbush R (2000) Continuous electromyography monitoring of motor cranial nerves during cerebellopontine angle surgery. J Neurosurg 93:586–593
7. Samii M, Matthies C (1997) Management of 1000 vestibular schwannomas (acoustic neuromas): hearing function in 1000 tumor resections. Neurosurgery 40:248–262
8. Ciric I, Zhao JC, Rosenblatt S et al (2005) Suboccipital retrosigmoid approach for vestibular schwannomas: facial nerve function and hearing preservation. Neurosurgery 56:560–570
9. Ojemann RG (2001) Retrosigmoid approach to acoustic neuroma (vestibular schwannoma). Neurosurgery 48:553–558
10. Samii M, Gerganov V, Samii A (2006) Improved preservation of hearing and facial nerve function in vestibular schwannoma surgery via the retrosigmoid approach in a series of 200 patients. J Neurosurg 105:527–535
11. Yasargil MG, Smith RD, Gasser JC (1977) The microsurgical approach to acoustic neuromas. Adv Tech Stand Neurosurg 4:93–128
12. Porter JM, Pidgeon C, Cunningham AJ (1999) The sitting position in neurosurgery: a critical appraisal. Br J Anaesth 82:117–128
13. Samii M, Matthies C (1997) Management of 1000 vestibular schwannomas (acoustic neuromas): surgical management and results with an emphasis on complications and how to avoid them. Neurosurgery 40:11–21
14. Von Goesseln HH, Samii M, Sur D et al (1991) The lounging position for posterior fossa surgery: anesthesiological considerations regarding air embolism. Childs Nerv Syst 7:368–374
15. Avci E, Kocaogullar Y, Fossett D et al (2003) Lateral posterior fossa venous sinus relationships to surface landmarks. Surg Neurol 59:392–397
16. Bozbuga M, Boran BO, Sahinoglu K (2006) Surface anatomy of the posterolateral cranium regarding the localization of the initial burr-hole for a retrosigmoid approach. Neurosurg Rev 29:61–63
17. Day JD, Tschabitscher M (1998) Anatomic position of the asterion. Neurosurgery 42:198–199
18. Samii M, Klekamp J, Carvalho G (1996) Surgical results for meningiomas of the craniocervical junction. Neurosurgery 39:1086–1095
19. Bassiouni H, Hunold A, Asgari S et al (2004) Meningiomas of the posterior petrous bone: functional outcome after microsurgery. J Neurosurg 100:1014–1024
20. Nakamura M, Roser F, Dormiani M et al (2005) Facial and cochlear nerve function after surgery of cerebellopontine angle meningiomas. Neurosurgery 57:77–90
21. Samii M, Carvalho GA, Tatagiba M et al (1997) Surgical management of meningiomas originating in Meckel's cave. Neurosurgery 41:767–775
22. Samii M, Tatagiba M, Carvahlo GA (2000) Retrosigmoid intradural suprameatal approach to Meckel's cave and the

middle fossa: surgical technique and outcome. J Neurosurg 92:235–241

23. Chanda A, Nanda A (2006) Retrosigmoid intradural suprameatal approach: advantages and disadvantages from an anatomical perspective. Neurosurgery 59:1–6

24. Schaller B, Baumann A (2003) Headache after removal of vestibular schwannoma via the retrosigmoid approach: a long-term follow-up-study. Otolaryngol Head Neck Surg 128:387–395

Suboccipital Median Approach

10

Rüdiger Gerlach and Volker Seifert

10.1 Patient Preparation and Positioning

After orotracheal intubation of the patient, a central line is inserted usually via the right internal jugular or subclavian vein with the tip position just before (lateral and prone positions) or within the right atrium (semisitting position, SSP). Invasive blood pressure monitoring is performed throughout the entire procedure via a radial artery line. Routine monitoring includes electrocardiography, pulse oxymetry, invasive arterial blood pressure, and urine output. Indications for intraoperative electrophysiological monitoring (IOM) are large cerebellar lesions extending towards the pineal region as well as lesions close to or infiltrating the fourth ventricle or the medulla oblongata. IOM consists of standard somatosensory, motor, and brainstem auditory evoked potentials and cranial nerve monitoring. Direct intraoperative stimulation is performed during resection of lesions of the floor of the fourth ventricle.

10.1.1 Semisitting Position

The major concern in the use of the SSP for many neurosurgeons is venous air embolism or paradoxical air embolism with associated hemodynamic compromise. Other complications associated with the SSP are tension pneumocephalus, spinal cord damage with paraplegia, compressive peripheral neuropathy and cardiac arrest. However, complications related to positioning are rare and the authors preferred position for the majority of lesions in the posterior fossa is the SSP. In the authors' institution in all patients a standardized protocol is applied to prevent air embolism during surgery [1]. The protocol includes preoperative transesophageal echocardiography examination (TEE), intraoperative TEE monitoring, catheterization of the right atrium and a combination of fluid input, positive end-expiratory pressure (PEEP) ventilation and standardized positioning aiming at a positive pressure in the transverse and sigmoid sinus. Preoperative TEE studies have been performed with the patient in the supine position including Valsalva maneuver with intravenous echo-contrast medium to rule out a persistent foramen ovale (PFO). We then leave the probe in place and place the patient in the SSP.

Positioning is best achieved by a combination of adjustments of the different parts of the operating table and special cushions. During a first step the legs are elevated to obtain an angle of about 45° between the lower abdomen and hip. The knees are slightly flexed (30°) but the lower legs still course upwards. The upper part of the body and the head of the patient are then elevated aiming for flexing of the hip to a maximum of 90°. The inclination of the whole operating table can now be finally adjusted taking care to lower head and raise the legs such that the feet of the patient are as high as the vertex (Fig. 10.1). As mentioned above, this maneuver is performed to optimize the position such that venous pressure is increased to ultimately achieve a continuous positive venous pressure at the operation site together with other measures such as fluid input and PEEP ventilation.

R. Gerlach (✉)
Dept of Neurosurgery, Johann Wolfgang Goethe University
Frankfurt am Main, Germany

P. Cappabianca et al. (eds.), *Cranial, Craniofacial and Skull Base Surgery*.
© Springer-Verlag Italia 2010

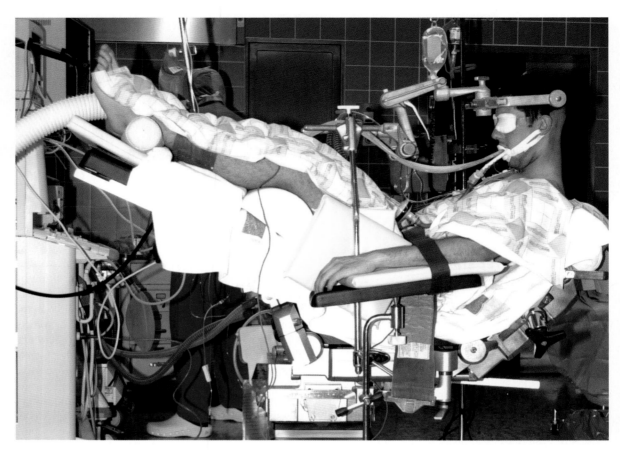

Fig. 10.1 Semisitting position

The head is anteflexed and fixed in the head clamp in a straight position. To avoid venous outflow obstruction a distance of about 2 cm is left between the chin and the sternal notch. Care is taken to prevent obstruction of the airways and ensure access to the epigastric region. During elevation of the upper part of the body the anesthesiologist should administer sufficient intravenous fluid to prevent systemic hypotension.

After final positioning of the patient the cardiac ultrasound probe is turned to give a four-chamber view and TEE position is checked with intravenous injection of 0.5 mL air. Fluid input and urine output is monitored aiming at a 5–12 cm water pressure in the right atrium. Mechanical ventilation is adjusted to achieve a PEEP of 5 to 10 mmHg which should be maintained during the surgical procedure and is adjusted in relation to occult venous bleeding or in the event of a venous air embolism. A 20-mL syringe is prepared to aspirate air

from the right atrium if venous air embolism occurs. IOM scalp electrodes can now be placed.

Routine monitoring includes electrocardiography, pulse oxymetry, invasive arterial pressure, right atrial pressure and urine output. End-tidal carbon dioxide is continuously monitored throughout the operation to detect clinically significant venous air embolism. End-tidal carbon dioxide in combination with TEE is used as the most sensitive parameter.

Usually a 2–2.5 cm strip is shaved from the inion to the upper cervical spine and the operative field is prepared and draped.

10.1.2 Lateral Position

Only in patients with a PFO, which is an exclusion criterion for SSP, is a prone or lateral position used. Pa-

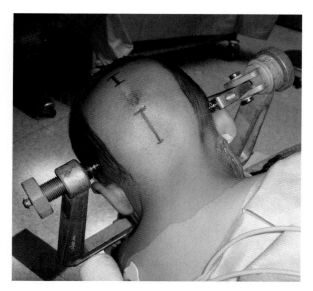

Fig. 10.2 Lateral positioning of a 15-month-old child with a dermoid of the posterior fossa

tients with a PFO are turned to a left lateral position (Fig. 10.2), which usually means a three-quarter prone position. Alternatively, which side should to turn downwards can be decided according to the pathology. The head is anteflected and rotated towards the floor and fixed in the three-pin head-rest clamp to avoid any pressure to the head or motion during surgery.

10.1.3 Prone Position

Some surgeons prefer a prone position for the midline posterior fossa approach. We usually use the semisitting and three quarter lateral position to avoid venous congestion and bleeding. In rare cases in small children with infratentorial tumors the prone position may be an alternative when sharp head fixation is impossible (Fig. 10.3).

10.2 Surgical Approaches

10.2.1 Supracerebellar Infratentorial Approach

10.2.1.1 Indications

The supracerebellar infratentorial approach provides an excellent view to the pineal region, the posterior third ventricle, the posterior and posterolateral portion of the midbrain and the medial superior surface of the cerebellar hemispheres. Therefore, this approach might be chosen for tumors of the pineal region (pineocytoma, pineoblastoma, pineal cysts) or tumors of the posterior third ventricle or lesions deriving from the cerebellum and expanding upwards such as pilocytic astrocytomas (Fig. 10.4).

10.2.1.2 Technique

The skin incision is always individually adapted to the pathology but usually extends from about 2 cm above the inion to the level of the foramen magnum. A galea periost flap can be dissected as an autologous graft for dural repair after successful surgery. This is done by separating the soft tissue from the fascia around the inion. A Y-shaped incision of the muscles begins at the superior nuchal line lateral to the external occipital protuberance on both sides joining 1 to 2 cm below the

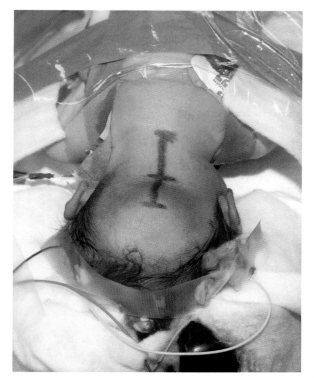

Fig. 10.3 The head of this infant is placed in a horseshoe head holder. IOM electrodes can be placed in small children

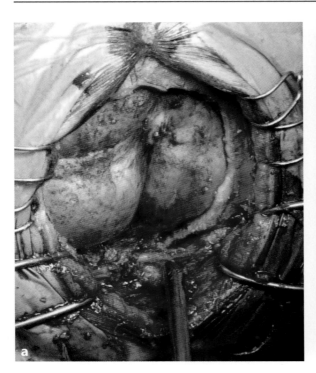
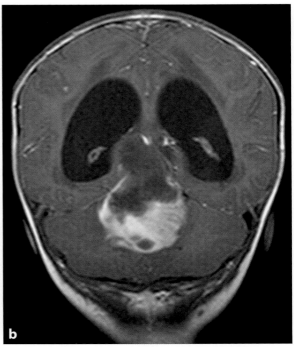

Fig. 10.4 Large polycystic astrocytoma. **a** Surgical exposure after midline dissection and craniotomy with bilateral exposure of the transverse sinus. **b** The preoperative T1-weighted contrast-enhanced coronal MRI image shows the large tumor with a cystic component growing towards the pineal region

inion. The muscles in the neck are dissected strictly in the midline and suboccipital bone is exposed. Complete dissection of the foramen magnum is not always necessary and can be avoided in patients with a lesion in the upper part of the posterior fossa. The burr hole is placed about 1–2 cm above the inion in the midline. The bone is sometimes very thick in the midline and has a wedge shape which can be drilled with a diamond to carefully expose the dura on both sides. The dura is dissected from the bone using a dissector and the craniotomy is performed beginning about 1 cm above the sinus on each side and turning down the craniotomy about 3–4 cm lateral to the midline. Care is taken not to injure the transverse sinus, which can cause bleeding. Craniotomy is extended downward to a level about 1 cm above the foramen magnum. After dissecting the dura from the bone the flap can be removed (Fig. 10.4). Especially in older patients, the dura can be very adherent and tear during craniotomy or dissection. The authors prefer a Y-shaped dura incision, which can be enlarged at the base laterally depending on the approached target. Microsurgical dissection above the

cerebellum is performed in the midline or laterally if large veins are present to approach the lesion. Preservation of veins draining in the vein of Galen is very important. In some cases the supracerebellar infratentorial approach can be combined with a supratentorial transtentorial approach.

10.2.2 Inferior Suboccipital Median Approach

10.2.2.1 Indications

Lesions of the vermis, the medial part of the cerebellar hemispheres and the tonsils (metastases), the fourth ventricle (ependymoma) or pontobulbar region (exophytic brainstem glioma, cavernoma) and around the foramen magnum (meningiomas in the upper spinal canal and posterior or posteriolaterally at the foramen magnum) can be approached via an inferior suboccipital median approach.

However, this approach is also appropriate for removing midline cerebellar arteriovenous malformations, to clip distal posterior inferior cerebellar artery (PICA) aneurysm or if combined with a laminectomy C1 to treat Chiari malformation.

10.2.2.2 Technique

A midline skin incision is performed from the inion down to C2/C3. A monopolar knife is used to split the superficial and deep muscles of the neck in the midline, which can be extended down to C1 or C2 depending on the size of the lesion and the extension of the approach. As described for the superior median approach the muscles are dissected bilaterally from the inion in a Y shape. During lateralization of the muscles in the craniocervical junction care is taken not to injure the vertebral artery in its course around the lateral part of the posterior arch of C1. For lesions extending to or below the foramen magnum the posterior arch of the lamina C1 and C2 can be drilled off to facilitate a larger dura opening, which enables the surgeon to have a better view from below into the fourth ventricle. Placement of the burr hole is directly on the external prominence (inion) and a lateral curved craniotomy is performed bilaterally including the foramen magnum at the lower end (Fig. 10.5). Alternatively, the rim of the foramen magnum can be dissected and the craniotomy started from below without placing a burr hole in the upper part of the planned craniotomy. However, there might be a risk of damage to the vertebral artery or the extracranial branching PICA. After craniotomy the dura is dissected from the bone flap and the flap is removed. The craniotomy can be enlarged laterally according the extension of the lesion and the space needed for dissection. The dura incision is usually in the midline in the lower part, but can be Y-shaped in the upper part and fixed with tack-up sutures. Sometimes a midline suboccipital sinus can be encountered during opening of the dura but bleeding can be controlled with bipolar coagulation and placement of hemoclips. After incision of the arachnoidea and opening the cisterns of the foramen magnum cerebrospinal fluid is released.

Further dissection can be done in the midline with extension upwards with splitting of the inferior two-thirds of the vermis cerebelli or via a velotonsillar approach.

For closure a pericranial or fascial graft or synthetic dura substitute can be used to achieve water tight closure if the patient's own dura is torn or constrict neural structures.

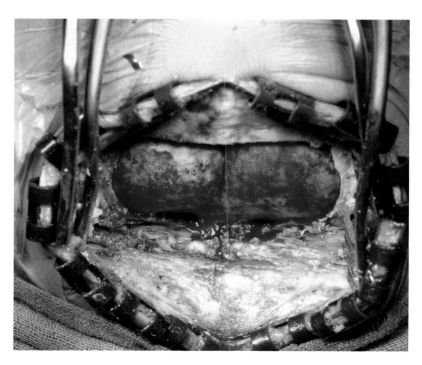

Fig. 10.5 Median inferior suboccipital approach

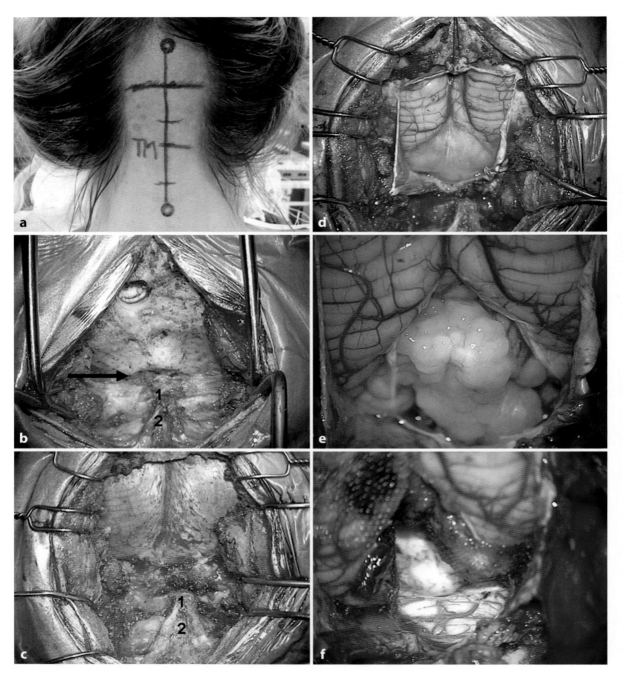

Fig. 10.6 Stepwise surgical technique for an inferior suboccipital approach in the case of a subependymoma of the fourth ventricle in a 20-year-old woman. **a** After the hair has been shaved the planned skin incision is marked with a pen. An important landmark is the tip of the mastoid which (TM). The transverse sinus is about two fingers above the tip of the mastoid (longer transverse line). The skin incision is planned from above the inion down to the spinous process of C3. **b** The muscles have been dissected in the midline with a monopolar knife and the posterior arch of C1 (*1*) and C2 (*2*) is exposed. A burr hole is place slightly lateral to the left below the level of the transverse sinus. The blue curved line (*black arrow*) marks the foramen magnum. **c** A craniotomy is performed and the foramen magnum is opened. **d** After removing the upper part of the posterior arch of C1 the dura is opened in the midline in a Y-shaped manner and retracted with stitches. **e** After opening the arachnoid membranes of the cisterna magna the large subependymoma is visible between the cerebellar hemispheres below the vermis. **f** View after complete tumor resection with a broad view to the floor of the fourth ventricle and the posterior part of the medulla

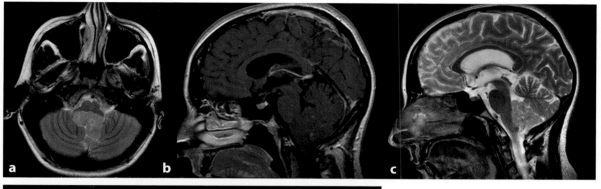

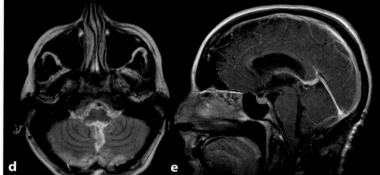

Fig. 10.7 MR images in the 20-year-old woman with a subependymoma of the fourth ventricle. *Top row* Preoperative images: T2-weighted axial (**a**), contrast-enhanced T1-weighted sagittal (**b**) and T2-weighted sagittal (**c**) images show a large hypointense lesion close to the floor of the fourth ventricle and medulla. *Bottom row* Postoperative images: T2-weighted axial (**d**) and T1-weighted contrast-enhanced sagittal (**e**) images show complete tumor removal

10.3 Illustrative Case

Figure 10.6 illustrates the stepwise surgical technique for an inferior suboccipital approach in the case of a subependymoma of the fourth ventricle.

Preoperative and postoperative MR images in the same patient are shown in Figure 10.7. The patient was operated in a semisitting position. Although the tumor was very adherent at the floor of the forth ventricle, the tumor could be completely removed as shown in Fig. 10.6f and was confirmed by postoperative MRI (Fig. 10.7d,e). There were no changes of the evoked potentials during resection and the patient had no postoperative deficit.

She was discharged home after an uneventful postoperative course a few days later.

References

1. Jadik S, Wissing H, Friedrich K et al (2009) A standardized protocol for the prevention of clinically relevant venous air embolism during neurosurgical interventions in the semisitting position. Neurosurgery 64(3):533–538; discussion 538–539

Middle Cranial Fossa Approach

Alessandro Ducati, Luciano Mastronardi, Luc De Waele
and Takanori Fukushima

11.1 Introduction

The middle fossa approach is an extradural subtemporal route consisting of an anterior petrosectomy. The most relevant indications for the middle cranial fossa approach are: intradural lesions medial to the trigeminal nerve and ventral to the internal auditory canal (IAC), including IAC pathology, mostly in patients with normal hearing [1–7].

Together with mastoidectomy, retrosigmoid, suboccipital, and supramastoid drilling, the middle fossa approach is a fundamental step of the combined petrosal approach useful for exposure of the petroclival area, the medial cerebellopontine angle, and the posterior cavernous sinus [2, 3, 6, 8]. The most common indications for the combined petrosal approach are: (1) sphenopetroclival tumors, (2) removal of transtentorial (supra- and infratentorial) extending neoplasms, and (3) vertebrobasilar aneurysms [1–10].

If this approach is extended anteriorly it becomes the so-called extended middle fossa approach which is indicated for: (1) intradural lesions of superior cerebellopontine angle and prepontine clivus (retroclival lesions, ventral brainstem tumors and cavernomas); (2) by-pass at the level of the C6 segment of the internal carotid artery (ICA) (Kawase's triangle of the cavernous sinus); (3) cavernous sinus (we use Fukushima's nomenclature for the carotid segments, illustrated in Fig. 11.4, because we think it is easier to remember

owing to the correspondence between the carotid segment and the cranial nervelesions) [5, 6].

With the aim of simplifying the recognition of all anatomical structures during this technically demanding approach, on the basis of cadaveric dissections we developed a simple learning method that we hope will be useful for young neurosurgeons during their first middle fossa approaches.

11.2 Description of Technique

The optimal surgical position for the middle fossa approach is Fukushima's lateral position, with the head positioned so that the sagittal plane is parallel to the floor (Fig. 11.1). Alternatively, the patient is placed supine, with the head rotated to the contralateral side, parallel to the floor. These two operative positions are described in detail in Chapter 8.

A preauricular linear o "lazy S" incision and a small square craniotomy (about 4×4 cm) with a temporal groove (Fig. 11.2) [6, 11] are carried out, providing a working plane parallel to the lateral skull base (Fig. 11.3). The epidural exposure of the middle fossa starts with identification and elevation of the "dura propria", the key step for dissection and exposure of all anatomical structures (Fig. 11.4). The "dura propria" is the dura mater of the temporal lobe, that during the procedure must be separated from a second layer of dura covering the trigeminal nerve and gasserian ganglion by a fatty inner reticular layer. For this reason this approach is also called the "interdural approach" [10].

In order to avoid severe injuries, at this stage of the dissection it is very important to locate all anatomical

L. Mastronardi (✉)
Dept of Neurosurgery, Sant'Andrea Hospital
"Sapienza" University of Rome, Italy

P. Cappabianca et al. (eds.), *Cranial, Craniofacial and Skull Base Surgery*.
© Springer-Verlag Italia 2010

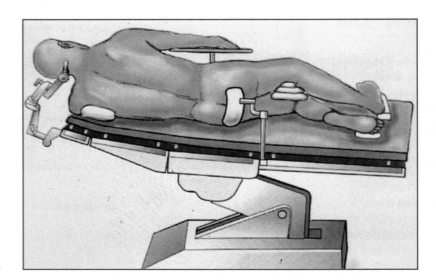

Fig. 11.1 Fukushima's lateral position

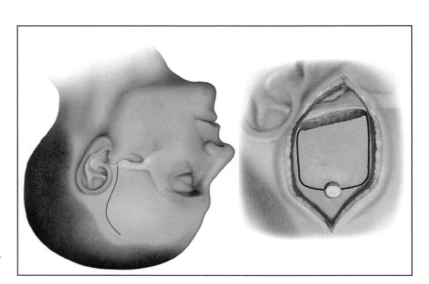

Fig. 11.2 Incision and small square craniotomy with temporal groove

structures, especially the C5–C6 tract of the ICA, according to Fukushima's classification (Fig. 11.4), and the IAC [6, 8, 11]. The middle meningeal artery at the level of foramen spinosum and the tensor tympani muscle are two important landmarks. Once the middle meningeal artery has been divided at the level of the foramen spinosum, it is possible to elevate the dura propria from the layer close to the bone, both in cadavers and in patients. At this point it is necessary to identify the greater superficial petrosal nerve (GSPN), covering the C6 segment of the ICA. The GSPN arises from the geniculate ganglion (GG) and runs anteriorly under V3.

At this level it joins with the deep petrosal nerve in the vidian nerve, which supplies ganglionic fibers to the lacrimal gland.

At this stage of the dissection, attention and know-how is required concerning frequent and relevant anatomical variations. In fact, the GG, the GSPN, and the C6 segment of the ICA are not always covered by bone [6, 11]. Absence of bone over the GG occurs in 15–17% of patients and the length of the bony canal covering the GSPN from the GG ranges from 0 to 7.6 mm (mean 3.8 mm) [11]. In 20% of patients, the petrous ICA is exposed along the carotid canal because of the absence of bone in the roof of the canal [6, 11]. In order to safely localize the GSPN, it usually has to be searched for just deeper to the posterior border of V3, half way between the foramen ovale (mean distance 7.3 mm) and the gasserian ganglion [6, 11]. Iden-

tification of the GSPN at this level is a "key point" that allows the nerve to be followed posteriorly, toward the GG and the hiatus fallopii, and over the C6 segment of the ICA.

Elevation of the dura propria continues to identify the arcuate eminence (AE) that overlies (although not always [11, 12]) the superior semicircular canal, the V3 from the foramen ovale to the gasserian ganglion, the porus trigeminus, V2, and V1. In order to mobilize V2 and V3 safely, decompression of the foramen rotundum and foramen ovale with the drill is advisable.

The next step of the dissection is the identification of the so-called "rhomboid fossa" and the location of the possible position of the IAC. The rhomboid fossa is a rhomboid-shaped construct of middle fossa landmarks, and serves as a guide to maximally removing the petrous apex. It is a bony area delimited by: (a) the petrous ridge and the superior petrosal sinus (from the porus trigeminus to the AE), (b) the AE (from the petrous ridge to the GG), (c) the GSPN (from the intersection with the GG and AE to V3), and (d) the posterior border of V3 (from the intersection with the GSPN to the porus trigeminus) (Fig. 11.5).

Rules for location of the possible position of the IAC inside the rhomboid fossa have been suggested by several authors [3, 4, 6, 8, 13] (Fig. 11.6). In our opinion, the method suggested by Cokkeser et al. seems to be the safest (Sanna's method) [13]. In their study on 20 temporal bones, the authors evaluated and measured the medial and lateral ends of the IAC. Measure-

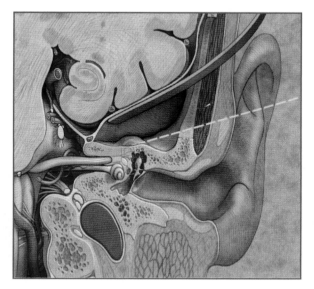

Fig. 11.3 Middle fossa approach: working plane parallel to the lateral skull base

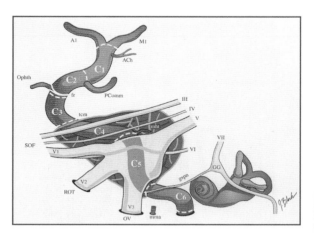

Fig. 11.4 Fukushima's ICA segments and nomenclature [6]. *ACh* anterior choroidal artery, *fr* fibrous ring, *GG* geniculate ganglion, *gspn* greater superficial petrosal nerve, *mma* middle meningeal artery, *mht* main hypophyseal trunk, *Ophth* ophthalmic artery, *OV* foramen ovale, *PComm* posterior communicating artery, *ROT* foramen rotundum, *SOF* superior orbital fissure, *tcm* tentorial cavernous membrane, *III* oculomotor nerve, *IV* trochlear nerve, *V* trigeminal nerve end branches, *VI* abducens nerve, *VII* facial nerve

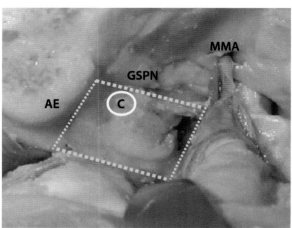

Fig. 11.5 Rhomboid fossa construct [6]. *AE* arcuate eminence, *C* cochlea, *GSPN* greater superficial petrosal nerve, *MMA* middle meningeal artery

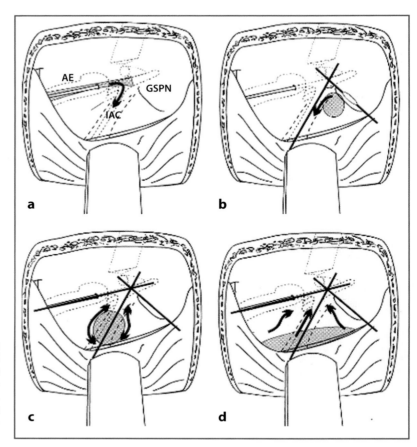

Fig. 11.6 Methods of identification of the internal auditory canal in the rhomboid fossa [6]. **a** House's method: *AE* arcuate eminence, *GSPN* greater superficial petrosal nerve, *IAC* internal auditory canal. **b** Fisch's method. **c** Garcia-Ibañez's method. **d** Sanna's method (medial-to-lateral direction)

ments were obtained at three levels: (1) the width of the IAC at the fundus, (2) the width of the IAC at the porus, and (3) a safe distance around the IAC at the meatal level. The mean width of the IAC at the porus level is more than three times that at the level of Bill's bar (between GG and AE). The width of the medial safe area around the IAC is more than seven times the width of the IAC at the lateral end. Therefore, in order to obtain quick direct exposure of the IAC without handling the facial nerve and the inner ear structures, the authors suggest that the drilling of the roof of the IAC should be started from the medial safe area (petrous ridge), continuing the unroofing in the lateral direction (toward the GG) [13].

With the IAC unroofed, the drilling is continued in the premeatal (limited anteriorly by V3) and postmeatal (limited posteriorly by the AE) triangles of the cavernous sinus (Fig. 11.7) until the posterior fossa dura is reached, taking care to spare the cochlea. A geometric construct assists in locating the cochlea: it is positioned

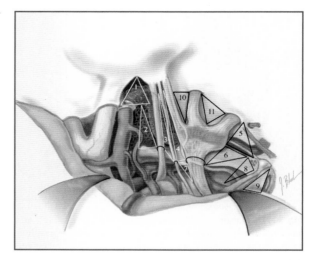

Fig. 11.7 Triangles of the cavernous sinus [6]. *1* anteromedial, *2* medial, *3* superior, *4* lateral, *5* posterolateral, *6* posteromedial, *7* posteroinferior, *8* premeatal, *9* postmeatal, *10* anterolateral, *11* farlateral

in the corner between the GG, GSPN and IAC, about 4–5 mm under and anterior to the GG, and medial and posterior to the C6 segment of the ICA, at about 1 mm from the carotid genu between C6 and C7 (vertical intrapetrous ICA) [6].

At this point, maximal bone removal is extended inferiorly, beyond the inferior petrosal sinus to reach the clivus, and anteriorly under the gasserian ganglion, following the ICA as far as the petrous apex (extended middle fossa approach) [6]. The dissection inside the cavernous sinus triangles and in proximity to the superior orbital fissure allows visualization of V1, III and IV cranial nerves and, close to the C4 segment of the ICA, the VI cranial nerve.

Both in cadaver dissection and in patients without an intracavernous tumor, it is possible to follow the abducens nerve that runs close to the inferior petrosal sinus inside Dorello's canal, from the posterior petrosphenoidal and Gruber's ligaments to the superior orbital fissure [2, 3, 5, 6, 9–11].

11.3 Cadaver Head Study and Technical "Tricks"

The study was performed in the Skull Base Microdissection Laboratory of Anspach Company in West Palm Beach (FL), in the Carolina Neuroscience Institute for Skull Base Surgery Temporal Bone Laboratory (Raleigh, NC), in the University of Morgantown Skull Base Microdissection Laboratory (WV), and in the II

Faculty of Medicine of the University of Roma "La Sapienza" Temporal Bone Laboratory (Sant'Andrea Hospital, Rome, Italy), during single dissections and skull-base courses.

Dissections of 15 fixed human cadaver heads and 20 isolated temporal bones were performed to yield 50 sides studied. As described in a previous article [8], in order to identify and scheletonize all nervous, vascular, fibrous, and osseous structures contained in this lateral skull-base approach, two fans bordering each other at an angle of 90° can be schematically identified (Fig. 11.8) [8]. The base of posterior fan can be considered the GG, and the base of anterior fan the gasserian ganglion. Proceeding in posterior–anterior and medial–lateral directions, the rays of the posterior fan are: the AE, the IAC, the cochlear line (an ideal line passing through the cochlea), and the GSPN. It is very important to remark that cochlea lies in a plane deeper than the IAC and GSPN, in front of the "genu" (loop) between the C6 and C7 segments of the ICA [6]. Proceeding in posterior–anterior and lateral–medial directions, the rays of the anterior fan are: third (V3), second (V2), and first (V1) branches of the trigeminal nerve, and the petrous ridge. The two fans border the rhomboid fossa in the following way: (1) GSPN–V3 junction; (2) lateral edge of the porus trigeminus; (3) intersection of the petrous ridge and the AE; and (4) intersection of the GSPN and the AE [3, 4, 6, 8].

In order to remember the different segments of the ICA, according to Fukushima's classification [6], the C6 segment of the ICA lies under the GSPN, C5 under the fifth cranial nerve (V2–V3), and C3–C4 under the

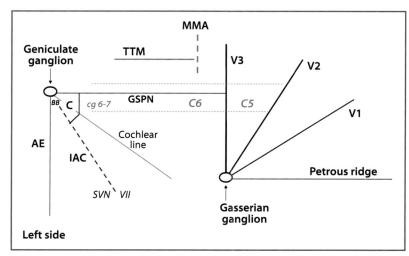

Fig. 11.8 Schematic drawing of the "rule of two fans". Vascular, nervous, fibrous, and osseous structures are localized within two bordering fans (posterior and anterior) positioned at an angle of 90°. Posterior fan: the GG is the base. The rays of the fan are: the arcuate eminence (*AE*), the IAC, the cochlear line (an ideal line passing through the cochlea), and the greater superficial petrosal nerve (*GSPN*). Anterior fan: the gasserian ganglion is the base. The rays of the fan are: V3, V2, V1, and the petrous ridge. *MMA* middle meningeal artery, *SVN* superior vestibular nerve, *TTM* tensor tympani muscle

oculomotor (third) and trochlear (fourth) nerves (close to the superior orbital fissure).

11.4 Conclusions

When performed properly, this technique provides a solid adjunct to treating complex skull-base lesions. Although the anatomical landmarks of the lateral skull base are well known, the simple rule and tricks that we propose aim to simplify the recognition of vascular, nervous, osseous, and fibrous structures during the middle fossa dissection and approach.

The cochlea, labyrinth, ICA, and cranial nerves five through eight are all at risk during drilling and dissection [3, 6–8]. Therefore, practicing this technique in the cadaver laboratory is a mandatory prerequisite to its clinical performance in patients for all neurosurgeons, especially those unfamiliar with this approach.

References

1. Al-Mefty O, Ayoubi S, Gaber E (2002) Trigeminal schwannomas: removal of dumbbell-shaped tumors through the expanded Meckel cave and outcomes of cranial nerve function. J Neurosurg 96:453–463
2. Day JD, Fukushima T, Giannotta SL (1994) Microanatomical study of the extradural middle fossa approach to the petroclival and posterior cavernous sinus region: description of the rhomboid construct. Neurosurgery 34:1009–1016
3. Day JD, Fukushima T, Giannotta SL (1996) Innovations in surgical approach: lateral cranial base approaches. Clin Neurosurg 43:72–90
4. Day JD, Fukushima T (1998) The surgical management of trigeminal neuromas. Neurosurgery 42:233–240
5. Inoue T, Rhoton AL Jr, Theele D, Barry ME (1990) Surgical approaches to the cavernous sinus: a microsurgical study. Neurosurgery 32:903–932
6. Sameshima T, Mastronardi L, Friedman A, Fukushima T (eds) (2007) Middle fossa dissection for extended middle fossa and anterior petrosectomy approach. Fukushima's microanatomy and dissection of the temporal bone for surgery of acoustic neuroma, and petroclival meningioma, 2nd edn. AF Neurovideo, Raleigh, pp 51–83
7. Samii M, Migliori MM, Tatagiba M, Babu R (1995) Surgical treatment of trigeminal schwannomas. J Neurosurg 82:711–718
8. Mastronardi L, Sameshima T, Ducati A et al (2006) Extradural middle fossa approach. Proposal of a learning method: the "rule of two fans." Technical note. Skull Base 16:181–184
9. Day JD, Kellogg JX, Tschabitscher M, Fukushima T (1996) Surface and superficial surgical anatomy of the posterolateral cranial base: significance for surgical planning and approach. Neurosurgery 38:1079–1083
10. Kawase T, van Loveren H, Keller JT, Tew JM (1996) Meningeal architecture of the cavernous sinus: clinical and surgical implications. Neurosurgery 39:527–534
11. Maina R, Ducati A, Lanzino G (2007) The middle cranial fossa: morphometric study and surgical considerations. Skull Base 17:395–404
12. Kartush JM, Kemink JL, Graham MD (1985) The arcuate eminence: topographic orientation in middle cranial fossa surgery. Ann Otol Rhinol Laryngol 94:25–28
13. Cokkeser Y, Aristegui M, Naguib MB et al (2001) Identification of internal acoustic canal in the middle cranial fossa approach: a safe technique. Otolaryngol Head Neck Surg 124:94–98

Translabyrinthine and Transcochlear Petrosal Approaches

12

Antonio Bernardo and Philip E. Stieg

12.1 Introduction

The objective of transtemporal surgery is wide skull-base exposure obtained by precise anatomic management of the temporal bone. These techniques involving the collaboration of neurotologists and neurosurgeons provide ample surgical exposure and minimize brain retraction during access to posterior and lateral skull-base lesions. The transpetrosal surgical routes can be classified broadly into anterior and posterior. The posterior transpetrosal approaches include the retro-labyrinthine, translabyrinthine and transcochlear, whereas the anterior approaches are extensions of the basic middle fossa approach. The posterior approaches are based on the standard mastoidectomy, and involve resection of the otic capsule to various degrees which provides the most direct route to the internal auditory canal (IAC) and the cerebellopontine angle (CPA) without the need for brain retraction.

12.2 Translabyrinthine Approach

The translabyrinthine approach provides wide and direct access to CPA tumors with minimal cerebellar retraction. The versatility of this approach for both large and small tumors makes it very popular for resection of acoustic neuromas [1-6]. A significant advantage of the translabyrinthine approach is that it permits positive

identification of the facial nerve, lateral at the fundus, and medial at the brainstem. Additional advantages of this exposure include complete lateral exposure of the IAC, including the vestibule. The disadvantage of this approach is that hearing cannot be preserved. Realistically, however, preservation of useful hearing in tumors greater than 2.0 cm in the CPA is unlikely.

The translabyrinthine approach is applicable to CPA and IAC lesions of all sizes, especially in patients with poor hearing. While the approach was popularized for acoustic neuromas [1-6], it is suitable for any neoplasms requiring exposure of the CPA, including meningiomas [5, 7-9], nonacoustic neuromas, gliomas, and skull-base chondrosarcomas. It can be used to access lesions localized more medially, towards the clivus, beyond the VII/VIII nerve complex. It can also be combined in varying degrees with other skull-base approaches such as subtemporal transtentorial routes for lesions involving the entire length of the clivus [10, 11] or with transcervical dissection for jugular foramen lesions with superior and inferior extension. In patients without functional hearing, the translabyrinthine approach is also useful for facial nerve decompression, facial nerve tumors, and vestibular neurectomy.

12.2.1 Surgical Technique

12.2.1.1 Anatomical Landmarks

Knowledge of temporal bone anatomy is essential to identify external features during surgical exposure and also in gaining three-dimensional orientation [12-13].

At our institution we currently use virtual reality technology to teach neurosurgeons the visuospatial

A. Bernardo (✉)
Dept of Neurological Surgery, Weill Medical College
Cornell University, New York, NY, USA

P. Cappabianca et al. (eds.), *Cranial, Craniofacial and Skull Base Surgery*.
© Springer-Verlag Italia 2010

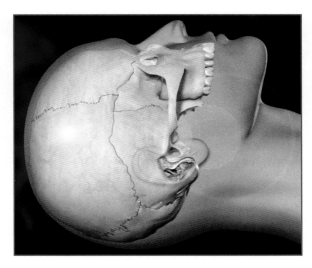

Fig. 12.1 Position of the patient for a translabyrinthine approach in the virtual reality module at the Cornell University Microneurosurgery Skull Base Laboratory

skills required to navigate through a transpetrosal approach (Fig. 12.1). This technology now permits the computed 3-D images obtained from cadaveric dissections and diagnostic imaging to be manipulated with an intuitive immediacy similar to that of real objects, and by engaging other senses, such as touch and hearing, to enrich the simulation [15] (Fig. 12.2).

Temporal bone surgery is based upon landmarks. Landmarks should always be identified before cutting and should always be preserved until other landmarks are located at deeper levels.

There are several bony landmarks, readily palpable through the skin overlying the occipital and mastoid areas, which are helpful to the surgeon in planning the approach.

Externally, the *external auditory meatus*, the *mastoid tip*, the *root of the zygoma*, and the *external occipital protuberance* must be identified first. The *transverse sinus* lies deep to the *superior nuchal line*, between the inion and the asterion. The *asterion*, defined by the convergence of the lambdoid, occipitomastoid, and parietomastoid sutures typically overlies the transverse sinus–sigmoid sinus junction. The *suprameatal spine*, or *Henle's spine*, is a small bony prominence that is located at the posterosuperior rim of the external auditory meatus and is useful as a guide in exposing the incus.

In the inferior portion of the mastoid, the *digastric ridge* constitutes an important landmark in locating the facial nerve at the stylomastoid foramen. The ridge is formed by the impression of the digastric groove, which houses the origin of the posterior belly of the digastric muscle. This ridge leads directly to the stylomastoid foramen.

The internal anatomy of the mastoid bone is largely composed of air cells. These air cells communicate with the middle ear cavity via the mastoid *antrum*. Opening the mastoid antrum exposes deeper anatomical structures. The *sinodural angle* begins at the convergence of the middle fossa plate dura and the sigmoid sinus. It continues forward to the antrum. In this angle the superior

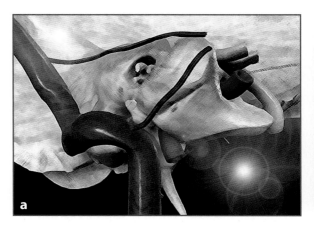
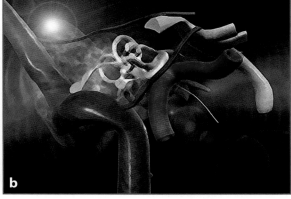

Fig. 12.2 Computed 3-D images obtained from cadaveric dissections and diagnostic imaging are imported into computer simulation modules to be manipulated with an intuitive immediacy similar to that of real objects. **a** 3-D reconstruction of the intracranial view of the temporal bone. **b** Subtraction of bone reveals the intrapetrosal anatomical structures from the same perspective

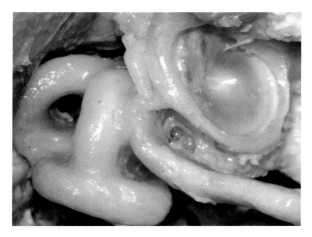

Fig. 12.3 Anatomical view of the semicircular canals and their relationships with the tympanic membrane, the incus, and the tympanic portion of the facial nerve

petrosal sinus joins the transverse sinus–sigmoid sinus junction. The *fallopian canal* houses the *facial nerve*. It runs on the anterior wall of the petrous bone, approximately 12 to 15 mm deep to the auditory meatus. The canal runs parallel to, and below, the lateral semicircular canal for a short distance before turning downward. The *corda tympani* exits the nerve in the fallopian canal at the level of the external auditory canal and travels at an acute angle to the nerve into the tympanic cavity.

The nerve is surrounded by a nerve sheath in its course inside the fallopian canal. The sheath merges with the periosteum of the *stylomastoid foramen* at its exit for the mastoid tip at the level of the digastric groove. The *retrofacial air cells* comprise part of the petrous bone between the fallopian canal and the presigmoid dura. This space houses the *jugular bulb*. The *labyrinth* lies in denser, harder bone, medial to the tympanic cavity posterior to the cochlea and to the *internal acoustic meatus*, anterior to the mastoid air cells, and immediately underneath the superior surface of the petrous bone.

The axes of the *anterior* and *posterior canals* are at right angles to each other (Fig. 12.3). The *horizontal semicircular canal* is plainly seen in the open antrum, oriented in the axial plane. The ascending limb of the posterior semicircular canal joins the posterior limb of the superior semicircular canal to form the *common crus*. The vestibule is the middle part of the bony labyrinth and lies medial to the tympanic cavity, posterior to the cochlea and anterior to the semicircular canal. It contains the *utriculus* and *sacculus* of the

membranous labyrinth and it is an important surgical landmark as its anterior wall is the last bone structure in the process of exposing the posterior wall of the internal acoustic meatus.

The *cochlea* is the most anterior part of the labyrinth, lying anterior to the vestibule, anterior to the tympanic portion of the facial nerve, and medial to the genu of the intrapetrous carotid artery.

12.2.1.2 Patient Positioning

The patient is placed supine with the ipsilateral shoulder elevated and the head turned to the opposite side in order to position the mastoid surface at the highest point (Fig. 12.4). Electromyographic intraoperative facial nerve monitoring is necessary in every transpetrosal approach. Perioperative antibiotics are continued for 48 hours, and steroids are used if there is evidence of brainstem compression. Hyperventilation is usually sufficient for brain relaxation.

12.2.1.3 Incision

A C-shaped scalp incision is started above the pinna of the ear. It curves posteriorly and inferiorly behind the body of the mastoid and ends below the mastoid tip. The incision is carried directly down the bone. The scalp flap is elevated and retracted anteriorly. During flap elevation, emissary veins are divided and bleeding controlled with bone wax.

12.2.1.4 Superficial Bone Removal

Using a large, high-speed cutting burr and continuous suction/irrigation the cortex over the mastoid bone is removed in a systematic, progressive fashion with the deepest portion of penetration in the triangle of Macewen, which is the area of mastoid behind the spine of Henle and which actually overlies the mastoid antrum. The cortical dissection proceeds from the posterior aspect of the external auditory canal to a line 1–2 cm behind the sigmoid sinus. The superior limit of the dissection corresponds to a line extending from the zygomatic root to the asterion.

12.2.1.5 Sigmoid Sinus Skeletonization

As the cortical bone is removed, air cells will be opened. Posteriorly the sigmoid sinus is uncovered. The

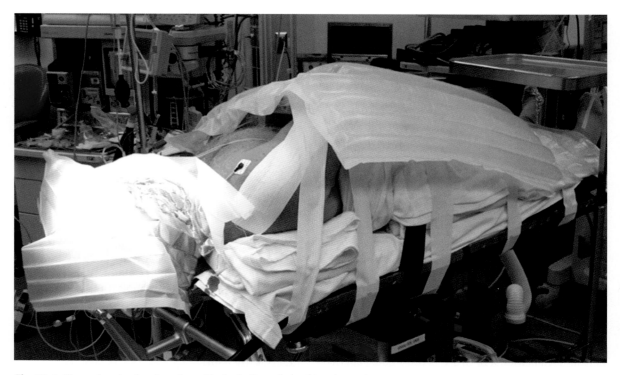

Fig. 12.4 The patient is placed supine with the ipsilateral shoulder elevated and the head turned to the opposite side so that the mastoid surface is at the highest point

sigmoid sinus generally appears in the posterior portion of the dissection as a blue discoloration of smooth dural bony plate. Thinned dural plate can usually be identified by a change in the sound of the burr vibrating on it. Once the sigmoid sinus has been located, the area between the sigmoid and the middle fossa plate, or the sinodural angle, can be fully evacuated of air cells. It is always advisable to leave a thin depressible shell of bone over the sinus to protect the sinus from inadvertent injury while continuing the dissection towards deeper targets (Fig. 12.5).

12.2.1.6 Middle Fossa Dura Exposure

Once skeletonizing of the sigmoid sinus is completed, mastoid air cells are removed anteriorly and superiorly to expose the middle fossa dura (Fig. 12.5). Exposing the middle dura is critical for best possible access into the antrum and epitympanic areas. Once the heavier bone is removed, thinning can be performed with a diamond tip, which results in less bleeding and less risk of lacerating the dura. Subsequently, the air cells surrounding the inferior segment of the sigmoid sinus and the digastric ridge are removed. When adequate cortical removal has been accomplished, a kidney bean-shaped cavity will result extending from the mastoid tip inferiorly to the sinodural angle superiorly, to the posterior bony canal anteriorly (Fig. 12.5). The next most important landmark is the posterior wall of the external canal and the mastoid antrum.

12.2.1.7 Opening the Antrum

The next step is opening the mastoid antrum in the superior portion of the exposure. The antrum lies immediately below the deepest point of penetration into the temporal bone posterior to the spine of Henle and the zygomatic root. By keeping the external canal wall bone thin and avoiding the nearby middle fossa dura, progressively deeper penetration will reveal the antrum. Normally the antrum can be identified as a larger air-containing space, at the bottom of which lies the basic landmark of the hard labyrinthine bone of the horizontal semicircular canal (Fig. 12.5).

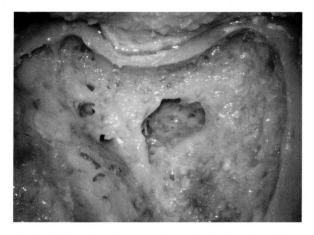

Fig. 12.5 The sigmoid sinus and the middle fossa dural plate have been skeletonized; the antrum is identified as a larger air-containing space

12.2.1.8 Labyrinth Exposure and Isolation

Exposure should be carried anteriorly until the entire length of the lateral semicircular canal is visible in the medial wall of the antrum, thus revealing the short process of the incus. Identification of the horizontal semicircular canal allows exposure of the fossa incudis, the epytimpanum anteriorly and superiorly, and the external genu of the facial nerve medially and inferiorly

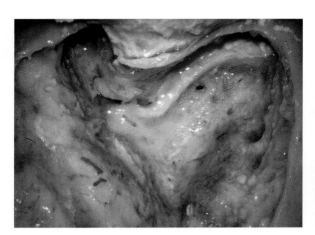

Fig. 12.6 The facial nerve is skeletonized distally along its descending portion in the mastoid to the stylomastoid foramen. The posterior bony wall of the external acoustic canal has been thinned, and the sinodural angle completely skeletonized. Note that the vertical segment of the facial nerve, the incus, and the lateral semicircular canal all lie in the same surgical plane

(Fig. 12.6). By removing cells between the horizontal canal and the sinodural angle, the hardest bone of the body, the so-called "hard angle", which is part of the otic capsule, may be encountered.

At this stage, the posterior fossa dura between the sigmoid sinus and the labyrinth is uncovered, and the tegmen mastoideum and tympani are removed. Inferior to the posterior canal, the posterior fossa dural plate overlies the endolymphatic sac. The sac is located in a thickened portion of the posterior fossa dura, medial to the sigmoid sinus and inferior to the posterior canal. The exact location of the sac, which varies, is usually identified by the presence of thickened white dura (Fig. 12.7). The middle fossa dura is skeletonized and the bone in the sinodural angle is completely removed (Fig. 12.6).

12.2.1.9 Identification of the Incus

The fossa incudis is most easily identified by removing bone in the zygomatic root overlying the antrum (Fig. 12.6). The superficial landmark for the incus is the spine of Henle. By drilling deeper, to thin the posterior bony wall of the external canal at the level of the spine of Henle, the incus is exposed.

12.2.1.10 Facial Nerve Dissection

In large tumors, or for targets located toward the clivus, the vertical segment of the facial nerve is also skeletonized to facilitate exposure of the anterior CPA. The

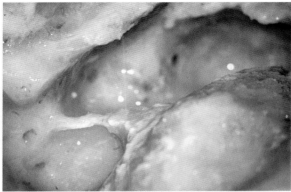

Fig. 12.7 The endolymphatic sac is located in a thickened portion of the posterior fossa dura, medial to the sigmoid sinus, and inferior to the posterior semicircular canal

facial nerve is normally localized inferior and slightly medial to the horizontal semicircular canal by thinning the posterior canal wall bone and carefully removing bone in the facial recess area. The facial recess area is delineated by the fossa incudis, the chorda tympani, and the facial nerve. Dissection of the facial recess begins by identifying the external genu, or the descending portion of the facial nerve in the mastoid cavity. Generally, this dissection is accomplished with a cutting burr until a change in bone character is identified. Further dissection is performed with a diamond burr, and profuse irrigation is used to prevent frictional heating of the nerve. A thin shell of bone is left on the facial nerve. Identification of a facial recess cell tract is often possible by thinning the posterior wall of the external canal (Fig. 12.6). Care must be taken not to perforate the canal wall, disrupt the chorda tympani, or transect the annulus.

Once the facial sheath is safely identified, the nerve is skeletonized distally along its descending portion in the mastoid to the stylomastoid foramen (Fig. 12.6). As the stylomastoid foramen is approached, the periosteum of the digastric muscle will blend with the sheath of the facial nerve. Inferiorly the chorda tympani nerve is detected as it leaves the facial nerve. The chorda tympani nerve joins with the tympanic membrane anteriorly and laterally at the annular edge. The nerve is further exposed medial to its external genu into the facial recess. This exposure allows visualization of the horizontal portion of the nerve (Fig. 12.3). The incus, already exposed, can be disarticulated from the stapes in order to better visualize this portion of the nerve (Fig. 12.8). With the fallopian canal defined, the remaining (retrofacial) air cells between the facial nerve and the jugular bulb are

removed. Removal of these air cells extending from the mastoid into the middle ear will result in skeletonization of the lateral portion of the jugular bulb (Fig. 12.7).

12.2.1.11 Labyrinth Dissection

At this point, the sinodural angle must be completely drilled out to provide adequate exposure of the area of the vestibule later. The middle fossa plate has to be thinned completely to provide access to the superior semicircular canal. These maneuvers will result in complete isolation of the labyrinthine complex.

The first portions of the labyrinth to be removed are the upper part of the posterior semicircular canal and the superior aspect of the lateral canal. The labyrinthectomy is then deepened to open, and then remove, the superior semicircular canal. The subarcuate artery usually penetrates the hard labyrinthine bone in the center of the circle inscribed by the superior canal. The dissection further advances into the horizontal semicircular canal and care must be exercised when working on the anterior edge of the lateral canal not to injure the exposed tympanic segment of the facial nerve. The anterior wall of the horizontal canal is preserved to protect the horizontal portion of the facial nerve until further thinning over the facial nerve becomes necessary to expose more of the vestibule. All three semicircular canals must be opened and the common crus exposed. Subsequently, the common crus is followed until it enters the

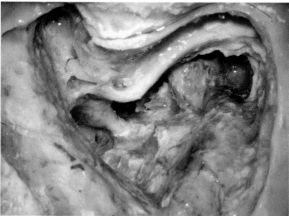

Fig. 12.9 Translabyrinthine approach, final dural exposure. The internal auditory canal is exposed through 270° of its circumference, the middle and posterior fossa dural plates have been completely skeletonized, and the sigmoid sinus and the jugular bulb have been fully exposed

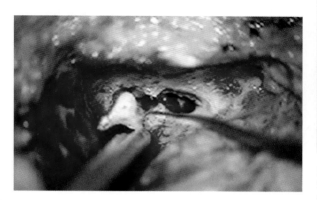

Fig. 12.8 The incus can be disarticulated from the stapes in order to better visualize the horizontal portion of the facial nerve

vestibule. The endolymphatic aqueduct is severed at its operculum, and the vestibule is opened widely. In approaching the internal auditory canal, it must be kept in mind that the anterior wall of the vestibule represents the posterior wall of the canal. Drilling at this level will expose the internal auditory canal fundus, where the nerve enters the inner ear structures. The internal auditory canal lies in the bone deep to the labyrinth. The canal is initially identified in its midsection and towards the porus acusticus. The internal auditory canal must be exposed through 270° of its circumference to achieve proper dural exposure. Troughs are drilled above and below the canal, parallel to its long axis. Bone is removed along the posterior petrous face medial to the porus acusticus and inferiorly between the IAC and the jugular bulb revealing the dura overlying the ninth nerve (Fig. 12.9). The final step to complete the exposure of the internal auditory canal is excavation of the fundus until the transverse crest separating the superior and inferior vestibular nerves is exposed.

12.2.1.12 Dural Incision

The internal auditory canal is so exposed through 270° of its circumference and the surrounding dura completely uncovered (Fig. 12.9). The presigmoid dura is incised at the lateral sinodural angle towards the porus acusticus. A second limb of the incision is made in a perpendicular fashion, crossing the first limb near the porus acusticus. The arachnoid space is sharply opened using microscissors. If cerebrospinal fluid has to be released, the cisterna magna should be entered at this point by dissecting between the lower pole of the tumor and the nerves of the jugular foramen. The size of the dural opening may be tailored to meet the amount of opening necessary to adequately expose the tumor.

This standard translabyrinthine exposure can be extended by removing bone above and below the internal auditory canal until the lateral aspect of the clivus is reached, thus improving the surgical view anteriorly into the prepontine cistern. The superior vestibular nerve is transected by placing an angled instrument adjacent to Bill's Bar and reflecting the superior vestibular nerve inferiorly. Sharp and blunt dissection can proceed with scissors and angled hooks without placing traction on the facial nerve. In large tumors CPA exposure is necessary. The dural opening at the completion of the translabyrinthine approach reveals the contents of the internal auditory canal and the CPA (Fig. 12.10). Posterior fossa exposure extends from the tentorium

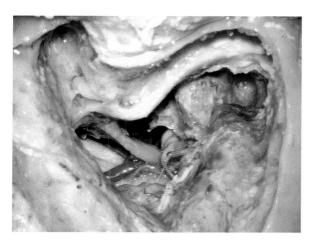

Fig. 12.10 After opening the dura, the posterior fossa exposure extends from the tentorium above to the lower cranial nerve inferiorly, affording exposure to the lateral aspect of the pons and the upper medulla. Anterior exposure toward the clivus is somewhat limited by the presence of the VII–VIII cranial nerve complex

above to the IX–X cranial nerve complex inferiorly, affording exposure to the lateral aspect of the pons and upper medulla. The translabyrinthine approach also affords good visualization of lesions extending toward the clivus and the midline, although exposure is somewhat limited by the presence of the VII–VIII cranial nerve complex (Fig. 12.10).

12.2.1.13 Closure

At the end of the approach (the incus has already been removed, and the facial recess opened), after transecting the tensor tympani tendon, the eustachian tube and antrum are filled with small pieces of Surgicel and temporalis muscle. Strips of fat, previously harvested from the abdomen or hip are then laid into the craniotomy defect to obliterate the dead space. The wound is closed in layers, and a compression dressing is kept in place for four postoperative days.

12.3 Transcochlear Approach

While the translabyrinthine approach offers wide exposure of the CPA, the cochlea, the petrous apex and the VII–VIII nerve complex, access to the anterior aspects of the CPA and the ventral brainstem is blocked. Modifications for improved anterior exposure, especially for petroclival lesions, and for vascular lesions of the mid-portion of the basilar artery, are the transcochlear modifications of the translabyrinthine approach. These approaches have been modified from their original description, and now represent a spectrum of transcochlear approaches to the ventral brainstem, beginning with the transotic and extending to the true transcochlear, with the widest exposure being the total petrosectomy [16-21]. All of these approaches, by definition, remove the cochlea following a translabyrinthine approach to extend the exposure anteriorly. The distinction between the transotic and the transcochlear dissections is that the facial nerve remains in situ (although skeletonized) in the transotic approach, while the nerve is transposed posteriorly in the transcochlear approach [22]. The transcochlear approach combines the translabyrinthine dissection with removal of the cochlea; however, wide access to the anterior CPA is provided by posterior transposition of the facial nerve. Thus, the exposure extends from the sigmoid sinus posteriorly to the petrous carotid artery anteriorly. By rerouting the facial nerve and exenterating the entire otic capsule, petrous apex, and lateral aspect of the clivus, an unobstructed view of the ventral aspect of the pons is obtained (Fig. 12.16). The principal indications for this approach are large petroclival meningiomas, epidermoids, extensive glomus jugulare tumors, temporal bone malignancies, and aneurysms of the mid-portion of the basilar artery [19, 22, 24-26].

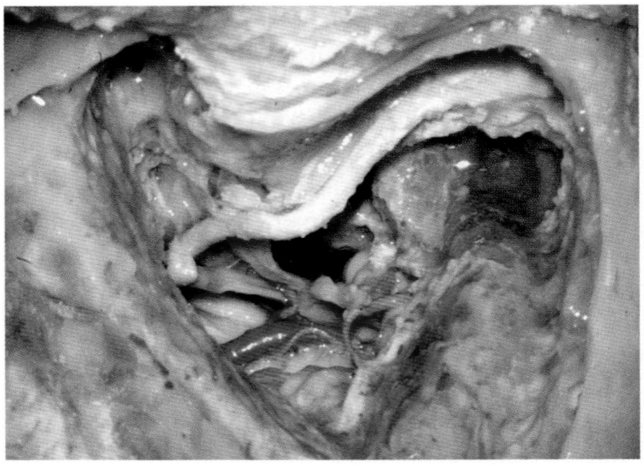

Fig. 12.11 Transcochlear approach. The tympanic portion of the facial nerve is skeletonized to the geniculate ganglion; the greater superficial petrosal nerve is sectioned at its origin from the ganglion, permitting posterior displacement of the nerve

12.3.1 Surgical Technique

The initial mastoidectomy and facial nerve dissection are performed in the same fashion as in the translabyrinthine approach (Figs. 12.1 to 12.10). The internal auditory canal is also skeletonized as in the translabyrinthine approach. With a medium cutting burr, the posterior wall of the external auditory canal is removed, opening the middle ear cavity. The ossicles and tympanic membrane are removed. The descending portion of the facial nerve is decompressed. An essential element of the transcochlear approach is to open the fallopian canal without injuring the facial nerve. The same surgical techniques as in the translabyrinthine approach are used to localize and expose the facial nerve in its tympanic and fallopian segments. During the initial stages of the dissection, a cutting burr rapidly locates the nerve, leaving a thin bony covering in place. A diamond burr is then used to partially remove the last

eggshell-thin bone from the epineurium. Once the entire horizontal and descending portions of the nerve have been exposed, the remaining egg-shell-thin bone is gently peeled off the sheath of the facial nerve using any thin, sharp pick tool. Elevation of the facial nerve from its bony channels proceeds from inferior to superior. The chorda tympani is transected sharply. With a small diamond burr, the tympanic portion of the facial nerve is skeletonized to the geniculate ganglion.

The anterior aspect of the ganglion is exposed to visualize the greater superficial petrosal nerve which

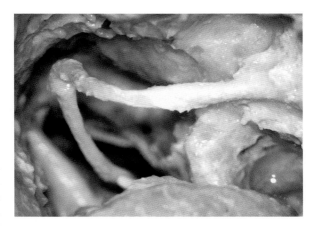

Fig. 12.12 Transcochlear approach. Anatomosurgical view of the entire intrapetrosal course of the facial nerve completely skeletonized. Note the relationship of the nerve to the jugular bulb and to the intrapetrous carotid artery

is sectioned at its origin from the ganglion, permitting posterior displacement of the nerve (Fig. 12.11). Elevation of the tympanic segment requires transection of the facial nerve to the stapedius muscle. The dura of the internal auditory canal is opened and the facial nerve is separated from the vestibulocochlear complex. The eighth nerve (cochlear and both vestibular branches) is transected. After the necessary amount of sharp arachnoid dissection the facial nerve is reflected out of its position in the internal auditory canal and fallopian canal (Figs. 12.11 and 12.12) and transposed posteriorly (Fig. 12.13). For the remainder of the procedure the nerve is kept out of the surgical field covered with a moistened Telfa strip and a nerve retractor. With the facial nerve out of the field, using a medium diamond burr, the basal turn of the cochlea is opened. The cochlea is located directly below the geniculate ganglion, surrounded by compact bone, and is removed by drilling anteriorly (Fig. 12.14).

Anteriorly, a thin wall of bone separates the cochlea from the intrapetrous carotid artery (jugulocarotid spine). Removal of this thin wall of bone exposes the genu of the intrapetrous carotid artery (Fig. 12.13). Once the intrapetrous carotid artery is localized and partially exposed, the petrous apex is removed. The superior limit of the exposure will be the dural-periosteal lining of Meckel's cave. Inferiorly, the jugular bulb will form the bottom portion of the exposure. Bone removal progresses medially to the clivus, working in a surgical corridor defined by the two petrosal sinuses, inferior and superior (Fig. 12.15). Typically, diffuse venous oozing is encountered from the clival bone marrow and can be controlled with bone wax and Surgicel packing.

Dural incision is superficially similar to that in the translabyrinthine approach. Medial to the porus acusticus, a Y-shaped incision opens the dura over the apical petrous bone (Fig. 12.16).

The advantage of this approach as compared to the translabyrinthine approach is that the exposure includes, in addition to the contents of the CPA, an unobstructed view to the lateral and anterior faces of the

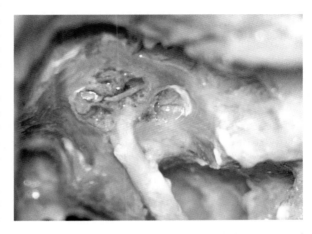

Fig. 12.14 Transcochlear approach. With the facial nerve out of the field, using a medium diamond burr, the basal turn of the cochlea is opened

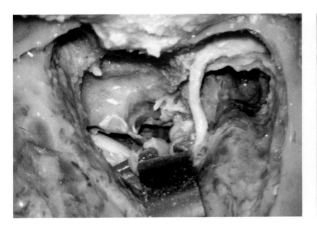

Fig. 12.13 Transcochlear approach. The facial nerve has been transposed posteriorly and the cochlea removed, thus exposing the genu of the carotid artery. Once the intrapetrous carotid artery is localized and partially exposed, the petrous apex is removed

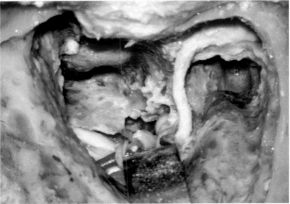

Fig. 12.15 Transcochlear approach. Bone removal progresses medially to the clivus. The petrous apex is removed working in a surgical corridor defined by the two petrosal sinuses, inferior and superior

pons, to the basilar artery and both the sixth nerves (Fig. 12.16). The cost of such wide exposure, however, is that posterior transposition of the facial nerve results inevitably in temporary facial paralysis that produces some degree of aberrant regeneration (usually House-Brackmann grade 3).

Closure is similar to that in the translabyrinthine approach, except that the external auditory canal must be sutured closed and the eustachian tube obliterated.

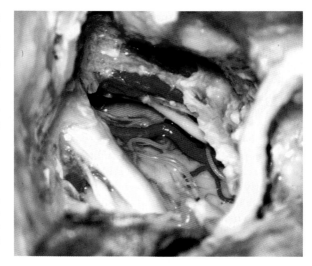

Fig. 12.16 Transcochlear approach. The final dural incision offers the same exposure of the CPA as in the translabyrinthine approach with the advantage of the added unobstructed view of the lateral and anterior faces of the pons, the basilar artery, and both sixth nerves

References

1. Mamikoglu B, Wiet RJ, Esquivel CR (2002) Translabyrinthine approach for the management of large and giant vestibular schwannomas. Otol Neurotol 23(2):224–227
2. Chen JM, Fisch U (1993) The transotic approach in acoustic neuroma surgery. J Otolaryngol 22(5):331–336
3. Hitselberger WE (1993) Translabyrinthine approach to acoustic tumors. Am J Otol. 14(1):7–8
4. Brackmann DE, Green JD (1992) Translabyrinthine approach for acoustic tumor removal. Otolaryngol Clin North Am 25(2):311–329
5. Giannotta SL (1992) Translabyrinthine approach for removal of medium and large tumors of the cerebellopontine angle. Clin Neurosurg 38:589–602
6. Maddox HE 3rd (1977) The lateral approach to acoustic tumors. Laryngoscope 87(9 Pt 1):1572–1578
7. Kirazli T, Oner K, Ovul L et al (2001) Petrosal presigmoid approach to the petro-clival and anterior cerebellopontine region (extended retrolabyrinthine, transtentorial approach) Rev Laryngol Otol Rhinol (Bord) 122(3):187–190
8. Hirsch BE, Cass SP, Sekhar LN, Wright DC (1993) Translabyrinthine approach to skull base tumors with hearing preservation. Am J Otol 14(6):533–543
9. Giannotta SL, Pulec JL, Goodkin R (1985) Translabyrinthine removal of cerebellopontine angle meningiomas. Neurosurgery 17(4):620–625
10. Sanna M, Taibah A, Falcioni M (2001) Translabyrinthine-transtentorial approach. J Neurosurg 95(1):168–170
11. Tedeschi H, Rhoton AL Jr (1994) Lateral approaches to the petroclival region. Surg Neurol 41(3):180–216
12. Sanna M, Saleh E, Russo A, Falcioni M (2001) Identification of the facial nerve in the translabyrinthine approach: an alternative technique Otolaryngol Head Neck Surg 124(1):105–106
13. Aslan A, Tekdemir I, Elhan A, Tuccar E (1999) Surgical exposure in translabyrinthine approaches – an anatomical study. Auris Nasus Larynx 26(3):237–243
14. Miller CG, van Loveren HR, Keller JT et al (1993) Transpetrosal approach: surgical anatomy and technique. Neurosurgery. 33(3):461–469; discussion 469
15. Bernardo A, Preul MC, Zabramski JM, Spetzler RF (2003) A three-dimensional interactive virtual dissection model to simulate transpetrous surgical avenues Neurosurgery 52(3):499–505; discussion 504–505
16. Angeli SI, De la Cruz A, Hitselberger W (2001) The transcochlear approach revisited. Otol Neurotol 22(5):690–695
17. Sanna M, Mazzoni A, Saleh E et al (1998) The system of the modified transcochlear approach: a lateral avenue to the central skull base. Am J Otol. 19(1):88–97; discussion 97–98
18. Arriaga MA, Gorum M (1996) Indications and variations of transcochlear exposure of the ventral brainstem. Laryngoscope 106(5 Pt 1):639–644
19. Sanna M, Mazzoni A, Saleh EA et al (1994) Lateral approaches to the median skull base through the petrous bone: the system of the modified transcochlear approach. J Laryngol Otol 108(12):1036–1044
20. Tedeschi H, Rhoton AL Jr (1994) Lateral approaches to the petroclival region. Surg Neurol 41(3):180-216<21
21. Horn KL, Hankinson HL, Erasmus MD, Beauparalant PA (1991) The modified transcochlear approach to the cerebellopontine angle. Otolaryngol Head Neck Surg 104(1):37–41
22. Selesnick SH, Abraham MT, Carew JF (1996) Rerouting of the intratemporal facial nerve: an analysis of the literature. Am J Otol 17(5):793-805; discussion 806–809
23. Thedinger BA, Glasscock ME 3rd, Cueva RA (1992) Transcochlear transtentorial approach for removal of large cerebellopontine angle meningiomas. Am J Otol 13(5):408–415
24. De la Cruz A (1981) Transcochlear approach to lesions of the cerebellopontine angle and clivus. Rev Laryngol Otol Rhinol (Bord) 102(1-2):33–36
25. House WF, De la Cruz A, Hitselberger WE (1978) Surgery of the skull base: transcochlear approach to the petrous apex and clivus. Otolaryngology 86(5):ORL-770–779
26. House WF, Hitselberger WE (1976) The transcochlear approach to the skull base. Arch Otolaryngol 102(6):334–342

Dorsolateral Approach to the Craniocervical Junction

13

Helmut Bertalanffy, Oliver Bozinov, Oguzkan Sürücü, Ulrich Sure, Ludwig Benes, Christoph Kappus and Niklaus Krayenbühl

13.1 Introduction

The region of the craniocervical junction is the site of various pathological lesions. Due to the complex topographical anatomy, performing surgery within this area requires great experience and knowledge in both spinal and skull-base anatomy. The most frequent tumors located within the craniocervical junction area are meningiomas. These lesions may occur in a great variety of appearances in terms of histological type, size, extension, insertion, vascularity, invasiveness, involvement of the vertebral artery, and growth pattern. Accordingly, the surgical removal of such tumors must be adequately adapted to all these variations. Apart from meningiomas, we have also treated a number of other lesions within this area such as neurinomas, ependymomas, hemangioblastomas, etc.

Generally, when discussing surgery of the craniocervical junction area, mainly those pathological lesions that originate between the lower third of the clivus and the superior rim of the C2 vertebral arch are considered. However, many lesions, including extradural pathology (tumors, granulomas, etc.), may extend beyond these boundaries, requiring a more extensive procedure. The majority of craniocervical lesions are located predominantly posterior or posterolateral to the lower brainstem and upper cervical cord; nevertheless, quite a number of tumors and vascular lesions are found anterior or anterolateral to the neuraxis. The former lesions may easily be accessed by the traditional posterior approach comprising a median suboccipital craniotomy that includes opening of the posterior foramen magnum and, depending upon the size and extent of the lesion, sometimes also including a C1 or even a C2 laminectomy. The latter lesions cannot adequately be accessed by this standard posterior approach without the risk of injuring the neuraxis or the rootlets of the lower cranial nerves. These lesions can best be approached via the dorsolateral access route that includes a special design and is the topic of the present chapter.

13.2 Review of the Literature

Seeger was the first to describe a dorsolateral approach to the vertebrobasilar junction and to use the term "transcondylar" in the present context [1]. Traditionally, the midline posterior approach was used to expose most intradural lesions located lateral or posterior to the neuraxis at the cervicomedullary junction. Being associated with significant disadvantages, the direct transoral approach to intradural pathology of the foramen magnum region has not gained wide acceptance. Instead, multiple variations of the suboccipital approach were elaborated and published in the 1980s and early 1990s [2–10]. George and Laurian advocated the lateral enlargement of the usual posterior opening [4]. This exposure requires control of the vertebral artery and sigmoid sinus. For further enlargement, medial transposition of the vertebral artery and transection of the sigmoid sinus with inferior petrosal resection are necessary.

Heros described in 1986 a modification of the unilateral suboccipital approach with extended bone

H. Bertalanffy (✉)
Dept of Neurosurgery
University Hospital of Zurich, Switzerland

P. Cappabianca et al. (eds.), *Cranial, Craniofacial and Skull Base Surgery.*
© Springer-Verlag Italia 2010

drilling [6]. His technique entails an extreme lateral removal of the rim of the foramen magnum towards the condylar fossa and the posterolateral removal of the atlantal arch towards the exposed vertebral artery. This approach was recommended for aneurysms of the vertebral artery and as an access route to the ventral surface of the brainstem with an inferolateral view. The exposure requires gentle upward and medial retraction of the tonsil, but no retraction of the medulla. In 1990 and 1991, Sen and Sekhar added the so-called "extreme" to the lateral approach by partially drilling the condyle to yield a wider angle [8, 9]. A similar technique with condylar drilling was almost simultaneously reported by Bertalanffy and Seeger [2], Menezes [7] and Spetzler and Grahm [10].

In the following years technical improvements and refinements were obtained by systematic anatomical dissections and from increased clinical input, and the results were published by several skull-base groups [11–21]. Morphometric and comparative studies of various bone resections as well as stability studies have increased our understanding of these access routes [10, 13, 14, 19]. The necessity for partial condylar resection has been widely discussed, leading to the conclusion that the final individual decision should be mainly based on the origin of the lesion. Thus, cadaveric dissections and clinical publications have encouraged a number of skull-base centers to adopt this extended transcondylar approach for lesions of the anterior or anterolateral cervicomedullary junction [22–24, 26–36].

Instability through partial condylar resection has only rarely been mentioned (for example, in 2 out of 23 series of foramen magnum meningioma [26]). Both series were small (comprising a total of 13 patients) and gave only few technical details. None of the 330 patients from the remaining 21 published series showed instability that would have required stabilization. In addition to the well-established indication for foramen magnum meningiomas [4, 23, 26, 29, 30, 34] including pediatric cases [31], the transcondylar approach has also been found advantageous for extradural lesions [22, 36], vascular lesions [24, 35], upper cervical spine tumors [6, 22], and various other tumors [4, 26, 30, 31, 33]. Recently, Bruneau and George have reported a classification system that helps anticipate the lateral extent of drilling in relation to the lower cranial nerves when operating on foramen magnum meningiomas. Their paper summarizes the knowledge gained over three decades by a very experienced skull-base group, and provides a valuable review of the literature [26].

13.3 Microsurgical Anatomy

At first glance, the anatomy of the craniocervical junction appears quite complicated (Fig. 13.1). This area comprises muscles, vascular and bony structures of the skull base and the first two cervical vertebrae, the atlantooccipital and atlantoaxial joints, the dura mater, the neuraxis, the rootlets of the caudal cranial nerves and superior cervical nerve roots, and a number of arachnoid membranes. Detailed descriptions of the craniocervical anatomy are available and may serve as valuable references to those working in this area [3, 18, 21]. However, the best knowledge concerning the craniocervical anatomy is obtained from anatomical dissections performed in the neuroanatomical laboratory. This is strongly recommended to all those who wish to learn the surgical techniques described in the present chapter.

The muscles of the craniocervical junction are organized anatomically in three different layers (Fig. 13.2). The external layer attached to the superior nuchal line is formed by the trapezius and sternocleidomastoid muscles. The posterior belly of the digastric muscle is located in the digastric groove between the mastoid and the jugular process and serves as an important landmark. The middle layer is composed of the semispinalis and splenius capitis muscles. In the deep layer the most important muscles are the rectus capitis posterior major and minor muscles and the superior and inferior oblique muscles. The rectus capitis lateralis muscle inserts on the transverse process of the atlas and on the jugular process of the occipital bone and covers the jugular vein below the jugular foramen.

Bony structures that may serve as important landmarks include: the occipital protuberance, the asterion, the mastoid process, the digastric groove, the jugular process and the supracondylar fossa, the condylar emissary canal, the posterior rim of the foramen magnum, the occipital condyle, the C1 arch, the transverse process and the lateral mass of the atlas, and the C2 arch with the atlantoaxial joint located between the first two vertebrae (Fig. 13.3). At the level of the foramen magnum region, the vertebral artery comprises the vertical V3 segment below the transverse foramen of the atlas, and the horizontal V3 segment lying in the sulcus of the atlantal arch and surrounding the lateral mass of the atlas. The arterial course is C-shaped and runs from medial to lateral in its distal extradural portion to enter the dura mater just medial to the lateral portion of the occipital condyle where it continues as the V4 intradural portion. Among the extradural branches of the vertebral artery are small muscular and dural suppliers

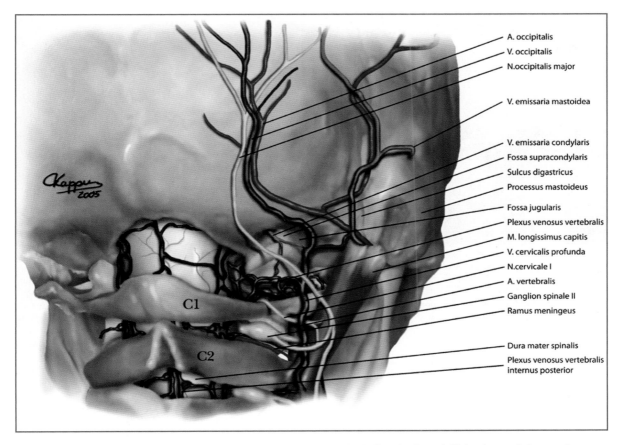

A. occipitalis
V. occipitalis
N.occipitalis major

V. emissaria mastoidea

V. emissaria condylaris
Fossa supracondylaris
Sulcus digastricus
Processus mastoideus

Fossa jugularis
Plexus venosus vertebralis
M. longissimus capitis
V. cervicalis profunda
N.cervicale I
A. vertebralis
Ganglion spinale II
Ramus meningeus

Dura mater spinalis
Plexus venosus vertebralis
internus posterior

Fig. 13.1 Illustration of the craniocervical region viewed dorsolaterally including the C1 and C2 laminae and the prominent extracranial neurovascular structures

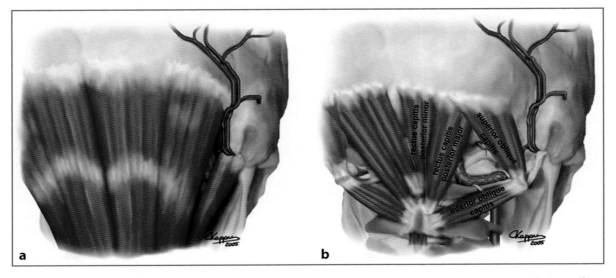

Fig. 13.2 Illustration of the dorsal craniocervical region showing the superficial muscular layers (**a**) and deep muscular layers (**b**)

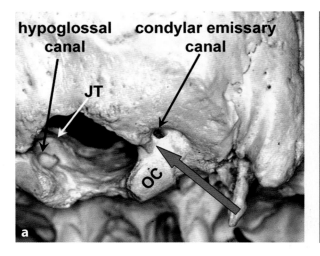

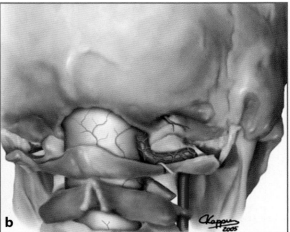

Fig. 13.3 Dry skull without cervical spine viewed from a right dorsolateral and inferior angle (**a**) and illustration of the right dorsolateral craniovertebral region (**b**). As indicated by the *large arrow*, a straight-line view to the anterior rim of the foramen magnum and to the anterior surface of the neuraxis is obstructed by the lateral rim of the foramen magnum, the posterior condylar emissary canal and the medial portion of the atlantooccipital joint. By partially drilling these structures located immediately lateral to the dural entrance of the vertebral artery, the viewing angle can be sufficiently enlarged to allow safe manipulation anterolateral to the neuraxis. *OC* occipital condyle, *JT* jugular tubercle

that can be coagulated and divided during dissection. In rare instances, the posterior inferior cerebellar artery has an extradural origin while the intradural origin shows a variable location from very proximal up to the distal portion of the intradural vertebral artery.

The most important venous structure in this area is the jugular bulb. However, this part of the venous drainage system can be exposed only after drilling the jugular process. A number of extracranial muscular and epidural veins, the plexus venosus vertebralis surrounding the vertebral artery and the condylar emissary vein draining into the jugular bulb are other important venous structures encountered in this area (Fig. 13.1). They should be well known to the surgeon who should also master several techniques of avoiding venous congestion and severe venous bleeding in this area.

The dura mater encountered in the craniocervical region consists of the suboccipital dura covering the cerebellum and the spinal dura covering the spinal cord. At the entrance point of the vertebral artery, the dura mater forms a ring similar to the dural ring of the carotid artery. The dura is continuous with the nerve sheath of the hypoglossal nerve running through the hypoglossal canal, and in a similar fashion also forms the proximal part of the C2 root up to the spinal ganglion. The marginal sinus is located between the suboccipital and spinal dura.

13.4 Clinical Application

The cervical approach described in this chapter can be used for access to a variety of intradural and extradural lesions. Intradural lesions may be totally intraaxial, partially exophytic or entirely extraaxial. Some lesions such as meningiomas or neurinomas may sometimes be located in both areas, intradural and extradural. Other lesions are exclusively located extradurally and may involve not only the foramen magnum region in the strict sense (from the lower third of the clivus to the upper rim of the C2 arch) but may sometimes extend into the petrous bone and the superior clivus as well as below the C2 level and into the odontoid process.

13.4.1 General Considerations

In view of the complex anatomy of the craniocervical junction, both the initial extracranial approach and the specific exposure of the dura mater following craniotomy, partial condylectomy, drilling of the jugular tubercle and perhaps C1 hemilaminectomy, are time-consuming surgical steps that may not always be necessary to the same extent. This is the reason why we do not advocate a rigid standard approach to the posterolateral craniocervical junction. Instead, we design and perform the procedure in an individually tailored fashion paying great attention to the principle of minimal invasiveness. For us, minimal invasiveness as applied to skull-base surgery means obtaining maximum microsurgical exposure (as required by the underlying lesion) with the least possible amount of surgical trauma.

13.4.2 Radiological Considerations

Obviously, the more the information that can be obtained before surgery, the better the design of the surgical approach. Therefore, apart from three-planar MRI, angiography may be helpful in the evaluation of vascular lesions, complemented by CT angiography with three-dimensional reconstruction, and also thin-slice CT scans with or without three-dimensional reconstruction. These investigations also provide sufficient information about local anatomical variations and bony destruction or pertinent distortions caused by the pathological lesion. We consider it advisable to focus on two other specific aspects: (1) the loop of the horizontal portion of the vertebral artery in relation to the atlas, and (2) the size of the posterior condylar canal containing the condylar emissary vein. In some instances the horizontal portion of the vertebral artery may form a prominent posterior loop extending 10 mm or more beyond the level of the lateral atlantal arch, an anatomical variation of which the surgeon must be aware in order to avoid injuring the artery. Similarly, incising a large condylar emissary vein may cause severe venous bleeding. This can be avoided by separating the vein from the surrounding bone within the emissary canal and then by coagulating the dissected vein.

13.4.3 Goals of Surgery and Preoperative Planning

The goal of surgery may vary according to the pathological lesion that is to be treated. Particularly in nonaggressive benign tumors, total tumor resection may be a practical goal of surgery, but this may be a goal that cannot be accomplished in certain cases except at the price of significant morbidity. Therefore, the surgeon must anticipate the specific risks of morbidity in order to better define the prognosis and thus the goal of sur-

gery. For instance, in the treatment of vascular lesions such as aneurysms, the surgeon must be prepared not only to exclude the malformation from the circulation by clipping but also be able to apply revascularization methods if necessary. In practically all intradural lesions, an important secondary goal of surgery should be preserving the function of the atlantooccipital joint. As occasionally encountered in our series, extensive extradural lesions such as plasmacytomas or tuberculomas may infiltrate the atlantooccipital joint so that fusion may be necessary at the end of the procedure. A lesion that extends into the lower petrous bone may similarly require a special design and additional bony drilling that must be anticipated by the surgeon.

Thus, preoperative planning should be based on high-quality preoperative imaging, knowledge of local anatomical structures and variations, and upon the patient's clinical condition before surgery. This planning is an important part of the entire surgical procedure that should receive the highest priority and concentration; it should always be undertaken individually in a case-by-case manner. With such a strategy and proper patient selection, satisfactory surgical results can be achieved and morbidity can be kept to a minimum.

13.5 Surgical Technique

The following is a detailed step-by-step description of our preferred technique. We also try to consider variations of this technique. However, all possible variations encountered in a great variety of lesions over the years cannot be entirely included in a chapter. We emphasize that although this description may suggest a standard approach, some individual variation is practically always present. We also estimate the expected benefit for the patient obtained by an extensive and time-consuming exposure in close relationship with the associated risks. Thus, we always try to find an optimal compromise between these two extremes.

13.5.1 Anesthesia, Monitoring, Neuronavigation and Endoscopy

The goal and type of surgery must be discussed with the anesthesiologist before commencing the procedure, including the issue of venous pressure that should generally be kept as low as possible. Without doubt, good cooperation between surgeon and anesthesiologist is an important prerequisite for avoiding venous congestion and profuse venous bleeding while performing the extracranial dissection and craniotomy. In practically all procedures involving the neuraxis, electrophysiological long-tract monitoring is performed (somatosensory, auditory and motor evoked potentials), and in many instances cranial nerve EMG is indicated and helpful. Most of the peripheral and scalp electrodes can be placed outside the operating room before starting positioning the patient. Neuronavigation and endoscopy can be prepared for intraoperative guidance and for endoscopically assisted microsurgery. Neither is mandatory but both are helpful tools.

13.5.2 Patient Positioning

Generally, we prefer the sitting position for patients under the age of approximately 60 years and if there is no other contraindication such as an open foramen ovale that should be excluded preoperatively with cardiac sonography. When the sitting position is used, continuous cardiac sonographic monitoring is mandatory to detect possible air embolism. In recent years we have regularly used transesophageal cardiac sonography which is far more sensitive than precordial Doppler monitoring for detecting even extremely small amounts of air bubbles within the atrium. If the sitting position is not considered appropriate, the lateral park-bench position is most suitable. In either case the patient's head is turned and oriented in three different planes: (1) anteflexion to extend the dorsal anatomical structures and expose the posterior aspect of the occipital condyle, (2) ipsilateral rotation of the head to avoid obstruction by the patient's shoulder, and (3) slight contralateral tilting of the head to better expose the lateral suboccipital region. The patient's head is always fixed in a Mayfield holder that is placed so as not to interfere with the surgical field.

13.5.3 Skin Incision and Exposure of the Deep Suboccipital Region

While some surgeons prefer a so-called hockey-stick skin incision, we have always used a slight curvilinear or straight skin incision between the mastoid and midline in the retroauricular area except in a few patients in whom dorsal craniocervical fusion has been planned

preoperatively (Fig. 13.4). Before incision, the scalp is infiltrated with local anesthetic and adrenaline (1:200,000). After exposing the fascia of the outer muscle layer, pieces of fascia are harvested for eventual use as a graft for watertight dural closure. To adequately place the skin incision, the course of the transverse and sigmoid sinuses, the tip of the mastoid process and the inferior nuchal line are clearly marked on the patient's shaved skin. Skin incision is followed by detaching the muscle insertions on the superior nuchal line and mastoid, with the sternocleidomastoid and splenius capitis muscles laterally and trapezius and semispinal capitis muscles medially. The muscles are partially divided as much as possible in the direction of their fibers, and the occipital artery deep to the splenius capitis muscle is coagulated and divided. In clinical practice we usually do not obtain an anatomical exposure of the deep muscle triangle that is formed by the rectus capitis posterior major, and the superior and inferior oblique capitis muscles (Fig. 13.2). The posterior lateral part of the atlantal arch and the horizontal portion of the vertebral artery lie within this triangle. To identify the artery at an early stage of this exposure, palpating the sharp dorsal lateral rim of the atlantal arch is the best procedure. Once the periosteal sheath of the atlantal arch is dissected sharply, the exact location of the vertebral loop is confirmed. It now becomes easy to detach the rectus capitis posterior major and minor and the superior oblique muscles from the inferior nuchal line and to gradually expose the supracondylar fossa and the posterior rim of the foramen magnum. In meningiomas it is useful to also expose the atlantal arch beyond the midline by detaching the muscle insertions.

Laterally, the exposure extends toward the jugular process and digastric groove. Dissection within the deep suboccipital area is facilitated not only by detaching the small deep muscles but also by partially or completely excising these muscles. These muscle pieces are harvested and used to obliterate the mastoid cells at the end of the procedure if necessary. To keep the area centered on the vertebral artery open, one or two self-retaining retractors can be placed, taking care not to interfere with the vertebral artery by excessive traction (Fig. 13.4). For this reason, it is helpful to expose the artery and muscle branches that may be distorted by the muscle retractor. The craniocaudal extension of the exposure depends upon the underlying lesion. Usually, exposure of the atlantal arch is sufficient. In some instances, however, complete exposure of the C2 arch may also be necessary. In a similar fashion, the transverse process of the atlas is not routinely completely

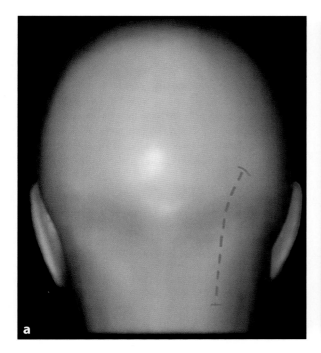
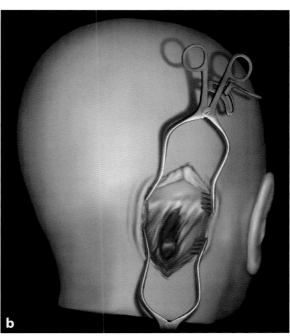

Fig. 13.4 Illustration showing the slightly curved skin incision (**a**) and the surgical exposure in the initial stage using two self-retaining retractors (**b**)

exposed but this may be necessary in lesions that extend towards the jugular foramen.

During this exposure, as mentioned above, identifying and coagulating the posterior condylar emissary vein is important, particularly when this vein is of large caliber. It has proven helpful to use a diamond drill to remove the remaining muscle insertions within the supracondylar fossa to better identify and recognize the local bony surface. The capsule of the atlantooccipital joint is opened in the lateral portion and is partially excised together with portions of the atlantooccipital membrane. During this step, avoiding venous bleeding or, if venous hemorrhage has occurred, obtaining quick hemostasis is most important. If obvious venous congestion occurs despite positioning or measures taken by the anesthesiologist, local injection of fibrin glue into the epidural and periarterial venous plexus may be very effective. Sometimes, local packing with Surgicel are additionally needed, and bipolar coagulation within the periarterial region or around the dural entrance of the vertebral artery may be required as well. If possible, the C1 root that exits the dura below the vertebral artery is preserved. Dividing this root, however, does not cause clinically detectable neurological or functional deficits.

13.5.4 Craniotomy and Extradural Exposure

Most neurosurgeons perform a routine retrosigmoid craniotomy that is gradually extended medially and caudally to include the foramen magnum. However, the key points of our preferred approach are the partial resection of the occipital condyle and jugular tubercle. Depending upon necessity, drilling the medial part of the lateral atlantal mass enlarges the approach caudally, and removing the jugular process exposes the jugular bulb laterally.

This exposure may be rendered difficult by the proximity of the vertebral artery, and the presence of the periarterial venous plexus, the condylar emissary vein and the jugular bulb.

On the other hand, for an experienced surgeon these anatomical structures do not pose serious problems. To improve understanding of the microsurgical anatomy of this region and to render this exposure less difficult than it may appear, we have elaborated a concept for those who wish to learn our technique of safely performing the transcondylar approach.

13.5.5 The "C-Zero" (C0) Concept

The first step is exposure of the lateral suboccipital craniocervical region as shown in Fig. 13.5. Following this, a suboccipital lateral craniectomy of sufficient size is carried out so as to leave the posterior rim of the foramen magnum in place as shown in Fig. 13.6. By carefully inspecting the exposed area and gently detaching the dura mater laterally and inferiorly to separate the posterior rim of the foramen magnum from the dura, one can identify the distal sigmoid sinus and proximal jugular bulb (Fig. 13.7). It is helpful to expose the medial portion of the distal sigmoid sinus because this structure is a good landmark that indicates the lateral limit of this exposure.

The dorsal rim of the foramen magnum contains more cancellous bone and is thicker than the squama, thus resembling the atlantal arch. Regarding the occipital bone as a modified vertebra facilitates our understanding of the craniocervical anatomy. Indeed, embryologically, portions of the occipital bone stem from the proatlas, the fourth occipital sclerotome [37]. Thus, the remaining posterior rim of the foramen magnum may be regarded as a modified vertebral arch that, in analogy to the C1 arch, can be termed the "C0" ("C-zero") arch. In this concept, the atlantooccipital joint is just a slightly modified intervertebral joint, similar to those below this level, except for the presence of the vertebral artery and,

perhaps, the condylar emissary vein. When dealt with properly, however, these two vascular structures do not pose serious problems during exposure. For instance, after detachment from the surrounding bone that forms the condylar emissary canal, the vein can be easily coagulated and shrunk. Using a diamond drill, the emissary canal is gradually opened and exposed up to the jugular bulb. Concomitantly, the posterior rim of the foramen magnum is removed and, if necessary, the atlantal arch can be resected too, as shown in Fig. 13.8.

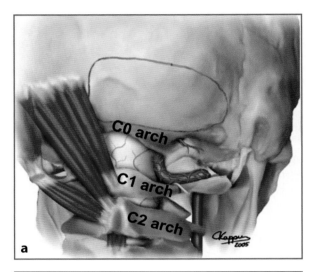

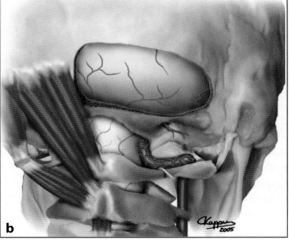

Fig. 13.6 a Illustration showing the outline of the planned craniotomy on the squama of the occipital bone. b The suboccipital craniectomy exposes the cerebellar dura while the dorsolateral rim of the foramen magnum (the so-called "C0" arch) has been left in place. In practice, the craniectomy does not necessarily extend as far as the midline as shown in this illustration

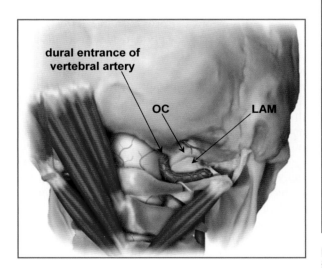

Fig. 13.5 The surgical exposure for the transcondylar approach is centered over the dorsal rim of the foramen magnum, the dural entrance of the vertebral artery and the atlantooccipital joint. *OC* occipital condyle, *LAM* lateral atlantal mass

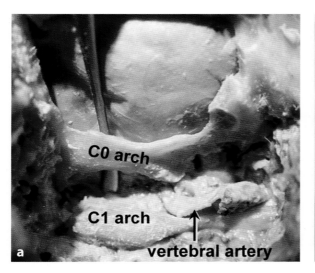

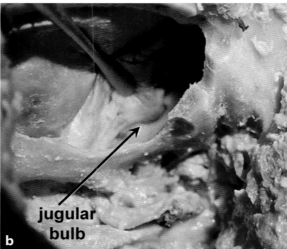

Fig. 13.7 Photograph of a cadaveric dissection showing an exposure similar to that illustrated in Fig. 13.6 a. The dorsal rim of the foramen magnum (the "C0" arch) is left in place and a dissector separates the dura mater from this rim (**a**). The remaining lateral squama of the occipital bone, the lateral rim of the foramen magnum, the jugular process, and the medial portion of the atlantooccipital joint correspond to the area of subsequent resection, the key point of the transcondylar approach (**b**)

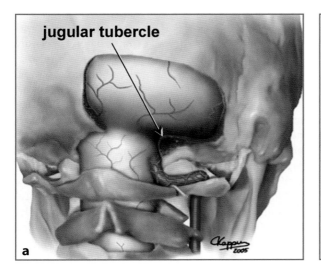

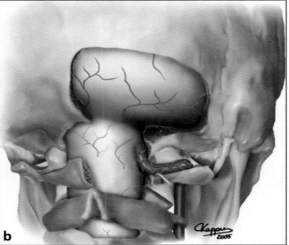

Fig. 13.8 Illustration showing the typical exposure after having removed the dorsal rim of the foramen magnum (the so-called "C0" hemilaminectomy) and after having partially drilled the occipital condyle and jugular tubercle; this exposure can be carried out either without (**a**) or including (**b**) a C1 hemilaminectomy

In routine practice these hemilaminectomies "C0" and C1 provide optimal exposure of the dorsolateral craniocervical junction (Fig. 13.9). Nevertheless, a straight-line view to the anterolateral surface of the neuraxis may still be obstructed by the lateral rim of the foramen magnum that is continuous with the jugular tubercle (Fig. 13.10). The shape of the tubercle can be quite variable as can be seen on preoperative CT scans. It may sometimes be flat and in other instances rather high. Just below the jugular tubercle,

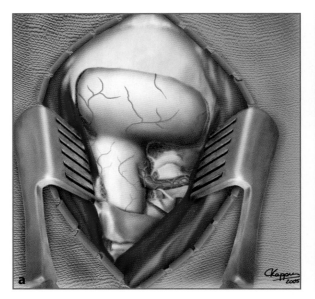
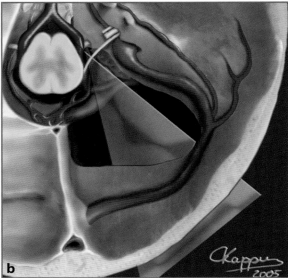

Fig. 13.9 Ideally, a single self-retaining retractor is sufficient for an adequate dorsolateral craniocervical exposure with the dural entrance of the vertebral artery forming more or less the center of this approach (*left*). The additional removal of the lateral rim of the foramen magnum close to the jugular bulb enlarges the viewing angle and offers a straight-line view to the anterolateral aspect of the neuraxis (*right*)

the hypoglossal canal passes through the occipital condyle in a medial-to-lateral and superior-to-inferior direction (Fig. 13.11). Drilling within the occipital

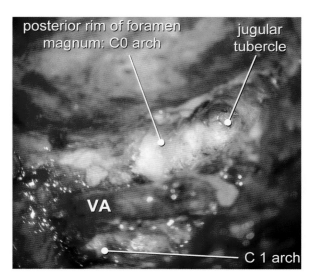

Fig. 13.10 Intraoperative photograph showing the V3 horizontal segment of the vertebral artery (*VA*) surrounding the lateral atlantal mass and the posterolateral rim of the foramen magnum forming the lateral portion of the so-called "C0" arch

condyle allows more or less extensive bony exposure along the dura mater in a posterior-to-anterior direction, and the hypoglossal canal can be exposed to a variable degree.

The jugular tubercle is a bony prominence that separates the jugular bulb laterally from the foramen magnum medially. Drilling is performed stepwise with diamond burrs after gently detaching the dura mater and jugular bulb from the bone (Fig. 13.12). The amount of drilling of the jugular tubercle depends upon the size and location of the underlying lesion and upon the local anatomical situation. The more anteriorly the jugular tubercle is removed, the better becomes the intradural view. Drilling within the occipital condyle sparing the articular facet guarantees that the function of the atlantooccipital joint remains intact, even if large portions of the medial condyle and lateral atlantal mass are drilled away to better expose the dural entrance of the vertebral artery. This latter step is particularly important in meningiomas that encase the artery. In such instances, the dural ring of the vertebral artery can be opened and the artery can be sufficiently mobilized to allow complete tumor resection in this area as we have done in several cases.

Drilling 6 or 7 mm of the medial occipital condyle and lateral atlantal mass can be regarded as partial face-

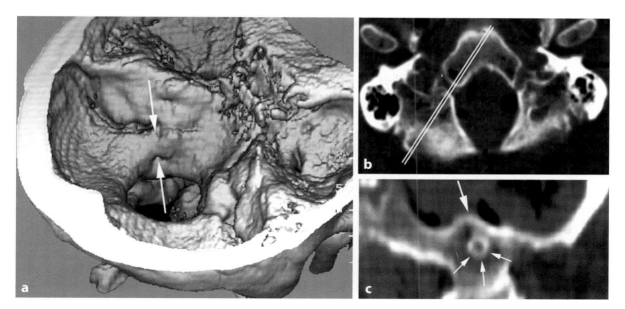

Fig. 13.11 a Three-dimensional CT reconstruction of the middle and posterior fossa; the jugular tubercle is located between the *two white arrows*. **b** Thin-slice CT scan at the level of the hypoglossal canal; the *white lines* indicate the plane of vertical reconstruction taken in a direction perpendicular to the direction of the hypoglossal canal. **c** On the CT reconstruction the jugular tubercle is visible (*large arrow*); the *small arrows* indicate the hypoglossal canal located directly below the jugular tubercle

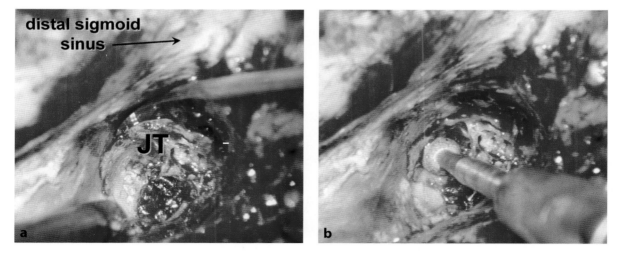

Fig. 13.12 Intraoperative photographs centered over the jugular tubercle (*JT*) as exposed with the transcondylar approach. The dura mater and the wall of the jugular bulb are gently separated with a dissector (**a**). The residual jugular tubercle is gradually resected with a diamond drill (**b**).

tectomy in analogy to spinal surgery where such a partial facetectomy is useful, for instance, to expose a neurinoma that extends into the intervertebral foramen. At this juncture, we have never destabilized the atlantooccipital joint with such an exposure when treating intradural lesions; neither did instability occur in a large series published for foramen magnum meningioma resections [26]. In certain instances, depending upon the local situation, opening of the transverse foramen of the atlas to completely mobilize the vertebral artery may also be necessary. However, to save time this is not done routinely.

13.5.6 Intradural Stage

We prefer to open the dura mater in a longitudinal or Y-shaped fashion, the lower part of the incision being placed medial to the vertebral artery (Fig. 13.13). In meningiomas that encase the intradural portion of the vertebral artery, we usually open the dural ring. In the remaining procedures this step is avoided to facilitate rapid and watertight dural closure. In tumors such as meningiomas, neurinomas or certain gliomas, the brainstem may be considerably distorted and displaced. Sufficient working space is gradually obtained by reducing the tumor volume in a piecemeal fashion. In other lesions that do not distort or displace the brainstem, for example aneurysms or intraaxial lesions, the exposure described above provides the optimal straight-line view to the anterolateral aspect of the lower brainstem and upper cervical cord without the need to retract the neuraxis or damage the rootlets of the lower cranial nerves. As a general principle, performing surgery in the intradural area within a bloodless surgical field is advised for clear visualization of all anatomical structures. However, to maintain a bloodless surgical field

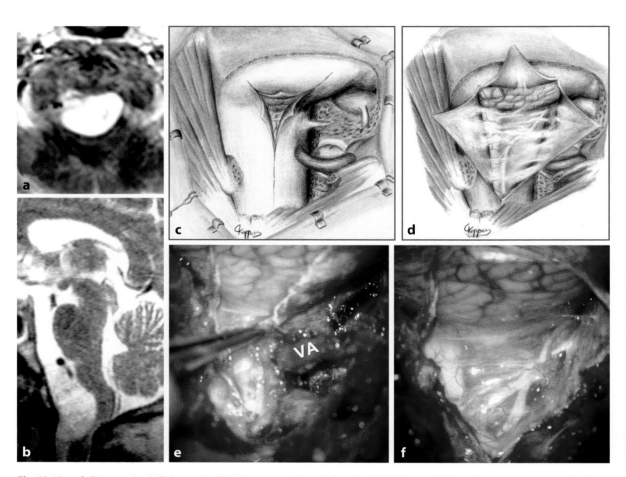

Fig. 13.13 a, b Preoperative MR images (**a** T1-W contrast-enhanced, **b** sagittal T2-W) reveal a large foramen magnum meningioma that displaces the medulla dorsally and severely compresses the cervical cord at level C1. **c, d** Illustrations show the dural incision and exposure of the dorsolateral and ventral tumor portion by reflecting the dura mater laterally together with the distal V3 portion of the vertebral artery. **e, f** Corresponding intraoperative photographs demonstrate the direct access to the dural attachment of the tumor by reflecting the dura mater laterally

even in vascular tumors, a special microsurgical technique is necessary. Accordingly, we undertake immediate hemostasis of new hemorrhage and try to avoid causing further bleeding.

13.5.7 Dural Closure, Cranioplasty and Wound Closure

At the end of the intradural stage we direct our attention towards avoiding postoperative complications such as cerebrospinal fluid (CSF) leakage or local hemorrhage. To avoid CSF leakage, the dura mater is sutured watertight, and the sutured area is covered with portions of muscle fascia that was harvested at the beginning of the procedure. These grafts are fixed with fibrin glue. When the dural ring of the vertebral artery has been opened, dural suture in this area includes pieces of muscle to facilitate watertight closure. Additionally, any opened mastoid cell is covered with muscle pieces. We avoid applying bone wax in this area to prevent postoperative local infection. Meticulous hemostasis in the epidural area is obtained by packing with collagen sponge or Surgicel fixed with fibrin glue. If available, a bone flap is fixed with osteosynthetic material. If the craniectomy is quite small, the area is filled merely with bone dust obtained from the initial trepanation. If there is insufficient bone available, cranioplasty is performed using polymethyl methacrylate. If the mastoid process has been largely resected, a titanium mesh is inserted. This helps the cosmetic reconstruction of the outer contour of the mastoid process. We avoid leaving the craniectomy area without any cranioplasty, as this may lead to an unsatisfactory cosmetic result due to significant retroauricular excavation. Usually, we place a wound drain for 48 hours, and the wound is closed in several muscle layers. During this last step of the surgical procedure, attention is paid to obtaining meticulous local hemostasis.

13.6 Specific Considerations

In light of the great variety of pathological entities encountered in the craniocervical junction, we use a wide range of surgical techniques to deal with these lesions in a specific manner. The following is a discussion of the most frequently encountered tumors and vascular lesions and a brief description of the microsurgical technique used in the intradural stage.

13.6.1 Meningiomas

Typically, meningiomas have a dural insertion which is the site of their vascular supply (Fig. 13.13). Some meningiomas show an en-plaque growth pattern; in others the dural attachment area is limited and smaller than the diameter of the tumor. In our clinical routine, these are two different situations. Devascularizing a meningioma with a small insertion area is easily performed while en-plaque meningiomas have a higher tendency to bleed and require more bipolar coagulation. Moreover, the latter tumors also tend to encase the rootlets of cranial nerves IX–XII and to invade the hypoglossal canal and pars nervosa of the jugular foramen rendering resection more difficult. In either case, our general principle is to incise the first dentate ligament and to devascularize the meningioma by coagulating its dural insertion (Fig. 13.13). In the next step, the tumor portions closest to the ventral dura mater are sharply resected to create a working space that allows stepwise mobilization of the remaining dorsal tumor portions in a direction from the lower brainstem towards the ventral dura (Fig. 13.14). During this maneuver, every effort should be made to avoid compression of the neuraxis. The level of the dorsal atlantal arch is frequently the site of maximum compression of the neuraxis (Fig. 13.14). In such cases, instead of C1 hemilaminectomy, it can be helpful to perform a C1 laminectomy before opening the dura to avoid any additional compression of the neuraxis during intradural manipulation.

Most meningiomas are very fibrous and not easily resectable with the aid of an ultrasonic aspirator. Pieces of such tumors are sharply cut with microscissors, while the arachnoid surrounding the tumor is gently incised to separate nerve rootlets and branches of the PICA and draining veins from the tumor. In many instances, the meningioma extends far beyond the midline and also involves the contralateral vertebral artery. This must be taken into account when removing such distal tumor portions in order to avoid damaging small distal vessels. In a similar fashion, the contralateral hypoglossal nerve may also be involved by the tumor. These rootlets are also preserved by sharp arachnoid dissection.

After total macroscopic removal, the area of tumor attachment is generously coagulated for two reasons: 1) to obtain sufficient local hemostasis and 2) to avoid tumor recurrence when it is not possible to completely resect the infiltrated dura mater as within the hypoglossal canal.

While most of the meningiomas consist of an intracranial and intraspinal portion, other tumors may be confined to the C1 level as shown in Fig. 13.15. In such

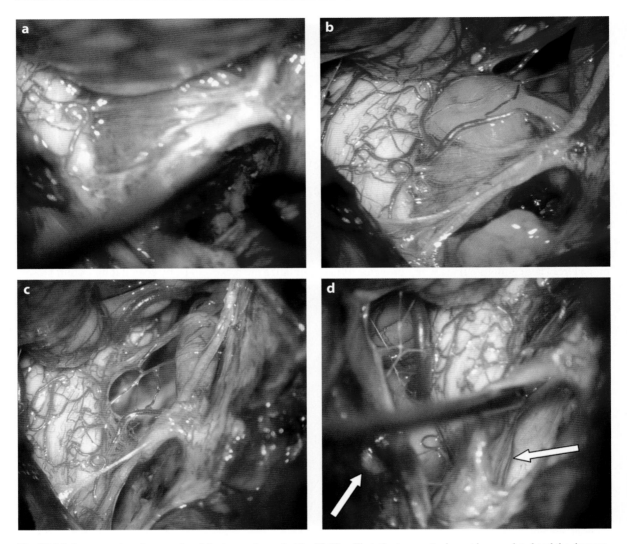

Fig. 13.14 Intraoperative photographs of the tumor shown in Fig. 13.13. **a** First, the tumor attachment is coagulated and the devascularized portions of the tumor are sharply excised. **b** This technique of devascularization is continued in a craniocaudal contralateral direction until the entire tumor is separated from its vascular supply. The remaining avascular tumor portions can now be gently separated from the neuraxis and rootlets of the lower cranial nerves and are excised in a piecemeal fashion. **c** After complete tumor removal, the neuraxis is still distorted, but the proximal V4 portion of the vertebral artery and the cranial nerves are completely free of tumor. **d** The C1 level is the site of maximal compression of the upper cervical cord where the tumor had pressed the neuraxis against the atlantal arch

cases a limited extradural exposure centered to the dural entrance of the vertebral artery is sufficient (Fig. 13.15).

13.6.2 Neurinomas

Neurinomas (schwannomas) of the foramen magnum may originate from the first two cervical roots or from the hypoglossal nerve. While the tumor may compress the neuraxis in a similar fashion to a meningioma, schwannomas usually lack a dural attachment and their growth pattern is different from that of meningiomas. Tumors arising from the C2 root typically extend between the atlas and axis and may be composed of an intraspinal and an extraspinal portion. Similarly, tumors arising from the C1 root or from the hypoglossal nerve

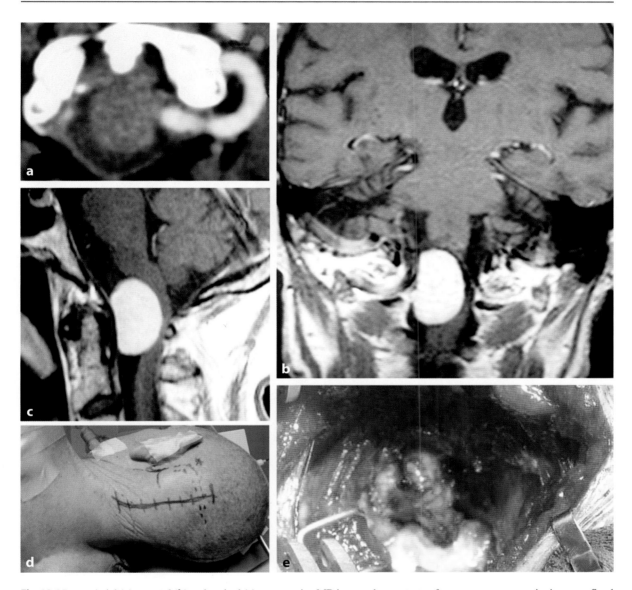

Fig. 13.15 a–c Axial (**a**), coronal (**b**) and sagittal (**c**) preoperative MR images demonstrate a foramen magnum meningioma confined to the C1 level in a 69-year-old patient. **d** The tumor was excised with the patient placed in the right lateral park bench position. **e** The surgical exposure was minimal and centered on the dural entrance of the vertebral artery

may show a dumbbell shape (Fig. 13.16). The goal of surgery is the same as in meningiomas: complete excision with decompression of the neuraxis. Tumor exposure may require a C1 and perhaps a C2 hemilaminectomy combined with a small suboccipital craniectomy that includes the foramen magnum. In hypoglossal neurinomas the hypoglossal canal is opened by drilling within the occipital condyle sparing the articular facet (Fig. 13.16). To start with, the tumor mass is gradually reduced. This is best accomplished with an ultrasonic aspirator. After sufficient tumor volume reduction, the origin of the tumor, usually one of the sensory rootlets of C1 or C2, or one of the hypoglossal rootlets, must be sharply divided. The remaining nerve root is gradually separated from the residual tumor and preserved. The intracisternal or intraspinal tumor portion is gently

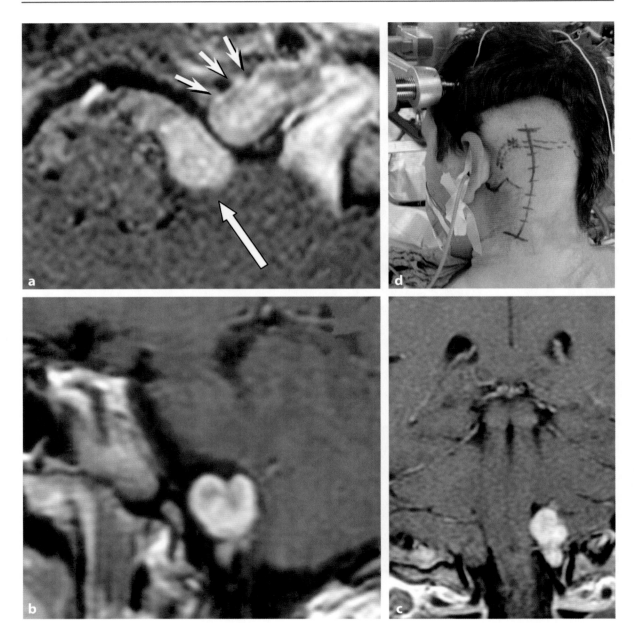

Fig. 13.16 a–c Preoperative axial (**a**), sagittal (**b**) and coronal (**c**) contrast-enhanced T1-W MR images in a 31-year-old man reveal a dumb-bell shaped neurinoma. The patient presented with hypoglossal palsy. The tumor is composed of an intradural cisternal portion (*large arrow*) and a second extradural portion that fills the enlarged hypoglossal canal (*small arrows*). **d** The patient was operated on in the sitting position, and the postoperative course was uneventful

separated from the neuraxis, nerve rootlets and surrounding vessels, paying attention to small tumor-supplying arteries that must be coagulated and cut. The distal extracranial/extraspinal tumor portion is continuous with the affected rootlet that must be divided as well.

In many instances, the proximal portion of the dura forming the dural sleeve of the affected nerve root is adherent to the tumor capsule. This part must be excised to a certain degree in order to achieve total tumor removal, leaving a dural defect of variable size. At the end of tumor resection, this dural defect is closed with the aid of a dural graft. We prefer to use a piece of muscle fascia; however, other graft material can be used as well to obtain a watertight dural closure.

13.6.3 Gliomas

Most gliotic tumors of the foramen magnum region can be accessed by a dorsal midline exposure. However, among the various gliomas we have encountered in this region (from pilocytic astrocytomas to WHO grade IV glioblastomas), some were exophytic and extended predominantly anterolateral to the neuraxis (Fig. 13.17). In such tumors, a standard posterior exposure is not sufficient. Instead, we prefer the transcondylar approach because it allows good visualization of the anterior tumor portions and because the structures involved by the tumor (rootlets of the caudal cranial nerves, vertebral artery and PICA) can be adequately dissected and preserved.

The goal of surgery in intraaxial gliomas is to remove as much as possible of the tumor avoiding any damage to the neuraxis and its normal vascular supply. While most parts of an exophytic glioma can be resected in a straightforward fashion with an ultrasonic aspirator, the deep intraaxial tumor portions do not have a clear-cut boundary that would allow precise radical resection. Therefore, the extent of tumor removal depends upon the macroscopic aspect of the tumor, its consistency and vascularity, and also upon the surgeon's experience.

Electrophysiological monitoring is mandatory in such procedures. Sudden changes in somatosensory and motor evoked potentials provide important feedback that influences the decision to continue or to stop the intraaxial tumor resection.

13.6.4 Aneurysms

Although endovascular techniques play an increasing role in the management of aneurysms of the VA-PICA complex, there are still indications for microsurgical treatment, either aneurysm clipping or revascularization procedures [24, 25].

The transcondylar approach is an excellent access route to expose this group of difficult aneurysms of the posterior circulation. It not only offers good control of the vertebral artery proximal to the aneurysm but also gives good access to the distal portion of the artery up to the vertebrobasilar junction. Moreover, this approach offers a better overview of the complex anatomical relationships between aneurysm and caudal cranial nerves (Fig. 13.18). This is important particularly in small aneurysms where the brainstem is not distorted or displaced, and where the space for microsurgical dissection is limited.

13.6.5 Cavernous Malformations

Intraaxial cavernous malformations that reach the surface of the brainstem or upper cervical cord dorsally can be exposed via a standard posterior approach. In our series, more than 20 lesions were located in the anterolateral portion of the neuraxis, within the lower pons, the pontomedullary junction, the medulla or the spinal cord. All these lesions were exposed via the transcondylar approach, modified according to the exact location. With this approach we obtained an optimal trajectory to the anterior and anterolateral surface of the neuraxis that allowed entering the brainstem or spinal cord at the point where the lesion was closest to the surface. Moreover, with this approach unnecessary and hazardous retraction of the brainstem is avoided (Fig. 13.19).

13.6.6 Extradural Lesions

In a series of more than 40 patients treated surgically for foramen magnum meningioma, in only two did the meningioma extend from intradurally to the extradural region along the course of the vertebral artery. Other lesions such as the hypoglossal neurinoma seen in Fig. 13.16 may also show both an intradural and extradural extension.

Apart from these tumors, we have treated a number of plasmacytomas, chordomas, glomus tumors, metastatic tumors, tuberculomas and arteriovenous fistulas of the jugular bulb with transosseous arterial feeders [23, 35]. All of these extradural lesions involved the craniocervical junction including the atlantooccipital joint; some of them also invaded the lower petrous bone and jugular foramen. These complex lesions require a modified transcondylar approach that extends laterally and into the petrous bone and exposes not only the jugular foramen but also the intrapetrous carotid artery and fallopian canal [23].

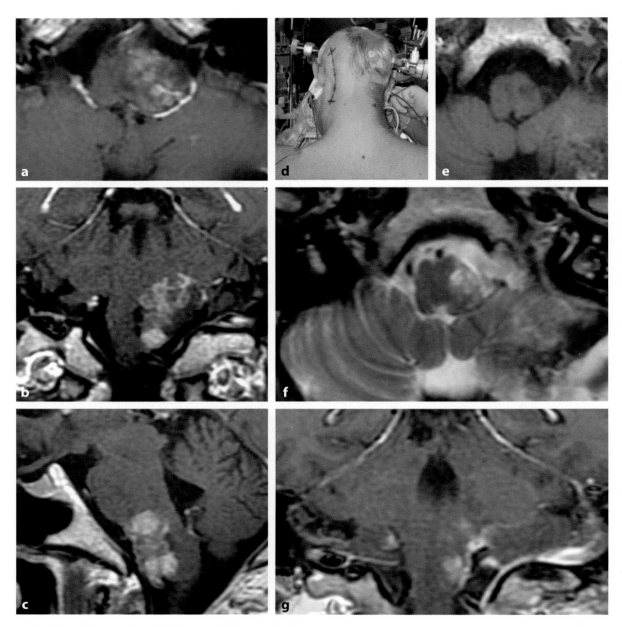

Fig. 13.17 a–c Preoperative axial (**a**), coronal (**b**) and sagittal (**c**) contrast-enhanced T1-W MR images in a 66-year-old man suffering from dysphagia and gait ataxia show an exophytic intraaxial glioma that involves the left anterolateral region of the medulla and upper cervical cord. **d** The patient was operated on in the sitting position via a left transcondylar approach. **e–g** Postoperative MR images show that approximately 80% of the tumor volume has been resected. Histological examination revealed pilocytic astrocytoma. The patient experienced no additional neurological deficits

The transcondylar exposure is most appropriate in osteodestructive lesions such as tuberculomas of the axis body and odontoid process (Fig. 13.20). To treat such a lesion, the initial exposure is identical to that described in this chapter. At an early stage of the procedure, the upper spinal cord is relieved from the compression caused by the atlantal arch by performing a complete C1 laminectomy. After completely

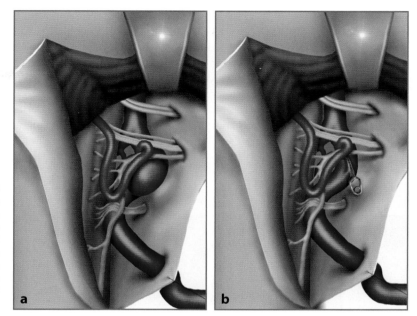

Fig. 13.18 Illustration shows the right V4 intradural vertebral artery and an aneurysm that arises at the origin of the posterior inferior cerebellar artery located below the rootlets of cranial nerves IX, X and XI (a). With this exposure, all neurovascular structures anterolateral to the neuraxis are clearly visualized, and aneurysm clipping is readily achievable (b)

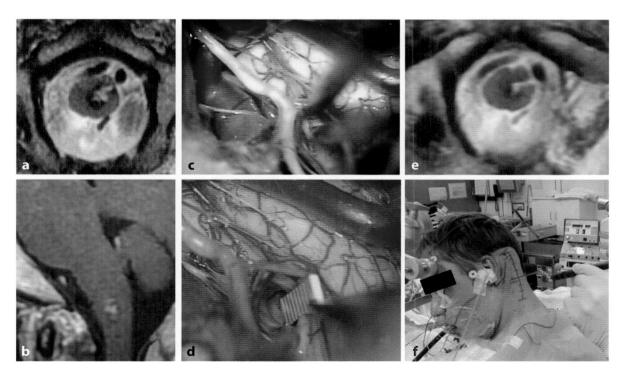

Fig. 13.19 a, b Preoperative axial (a) and sagittal (b) MR images in a 33-year-old patient demonstrates an intraaxial cavernous malformation. The patient suffered two episodes of intralesional bleeding. c, d A left-sided transcondylar approach was used to obtain a lateral-to-medial viewing angle that allowed entry to the neuraxis anterolaterally (c) and total excision of the malformation (d). e Postoperative MR image confirms total excision. f The patient underwent surgery in the sitting position

freeing the horizontal portion of the V3 segment of the vertebral artery, drilling is carried out in the medial portion of the lateral atlantal mass and continued in an anterior direction lateral to and in close proximity to the dura mater until the invaded odontoid process is reached. By also drilling the lateral part, a lateral-to-medial viewing trajectory is obtained that allows removal of the entire destroyed odontoid process and even of the superior portion of the body of the axis (Fig. 13.20d).

Planning the surgical procedure included the final occipitocervical stabilization. For this purpose the patient was placed in the sitting position with the head fixed in the Mayfield holder in a neutral position that was chosen to be the final position of the head in relation to the cervical spine. It is important to use SEP monitoring during the positioning in order to detect any additional compression of the upper cervical cord during this maneuver involving a highly unstable atlantooccipital segment.

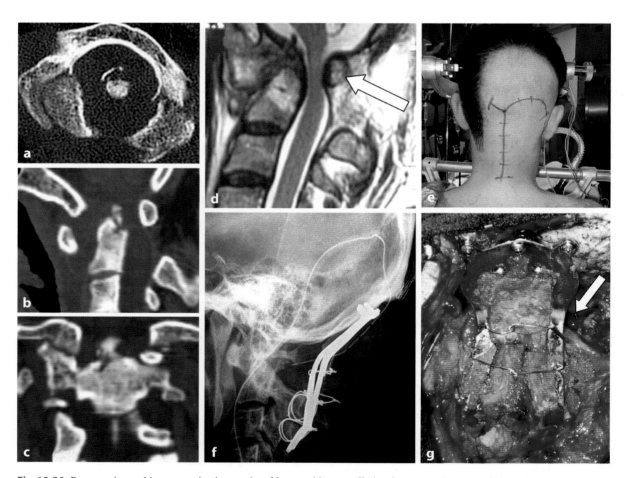

Fig. 13.20 Preoperative and intraoperative images in a 30-year-old man suffering from osteodestructive tuberculoma that involved the odontoid process and the body of the axis. The patient presented with severe neck pain. **a–c** The axial CT scan (**a**) with sagittal (**b**) and coronal reconstruction (**c**) demonstrate both the destruction of the superior odontoid and superior articular facets of the axis and the atlantoaxial dislocation. **d** Preoperative sagittal MR shows that the atlantoaxial dislocation has led to significant anterior displacement of the posterior atlantal arch (*arrow*) that compresses the upper cervical cord. **e** The patient was operated on in the sitting position, and a modified "hockey-stick" skin incision was used. **f** At the end of surgery, occipitocervical fusion was performed with the head fixed in a neutral position as seen on the lateral plain radiograph. **g** A horseshoe-shaped osteosynthetic plate was fixed with screws to the occipital squama and with wires to the C2 and C3 vertebral arches on both sides; for osseous fusion, an iliac crest graft was inserted between occipital bone and C2 spinous process. The odontoid process was partially resected by drilling through the lateral atlantal mass from the right posterolateral region below the vertebral artery (*arrow*).

In the same fashion, other osteodestructive lesions such as plasmacytomas, chordomas and metastatic tumors have been completely removed, in most instances, however, without the necessity of additional atlantooccipital fusion. Arteriovenous fistulas of the jugular bulb are a special pathological entity where transosseous arterial feeders have direct connection to the jugular bulb. As many of these lesions could not be obliterated endovascularly, a microsurgical procedure was carried out that exposed the jugular bulb and interrupted these transosseous arterial feeders by extensively drilling within the occipital condyle [35].

13.7 Outcome and Complications

The transcondylar approach always provides sufficient exposure of the dorsolateral craniospinal region with excellent visualization of the neuraxis, vertebral artery and branches, and of the caudal cranial nerves and upper cervical roots. Owing to this wide exposure, all extraaxial and intraaxial lesions can be well treated without the need to retract the lower brainstem and upper cervical cord, and damage to other neurovascular structures of this area can be avoided. With the exception of a few patients with CSF leakage or wound infection, there have been no serious approach-related complications. In particular, no craniocervical or atlantoaxial instability has been created in any of the patients harboring an intradural lesion, even after extensive drilling within the condyle and jugular tubercle. The reason why we are able to continuously maintain stability lies in our technique of preserving the main portion of the articular facet of the condyle and lateral atlantal mass.

13.8 Lessons Learned

Over the past two decades we have used the transcondylar approach in more than 200 patients and have continuously optimized our technique. The following are important lessons learned from these demanding procedures:

- The patient should be positioned with the head rotated ipsilaterally and flexed so that the posterior portion of the occipital condyle articular facet becomes visible during surgery. Care is taken to avoid compression of the jugular vein during positioning, par-

ticularly when the patient is placed in the lateral parkbench position.

- Avoiding venous congestion during the extradural stage and injection of fibrin glue into the periarterial or epidural venous plexus are helpful measures to maintain a bloodless surgical field.
- At an early stage of the exposure, the exact location of the vertebral artery should be identified by palpating the posterior sharp edge of the atlantal arch. Once the vertebral artery has been localized, all muscles superior to the artery can readily be divided or partially excised so that the extradural exposure can be performed within less than one hour. The incision of the dorsolateral muscles of the craniocervical junction must be carried out so as to provide an intraoperative viewing trajectory that is not obstructed by the retracted muscle mass. When a significant lateral-to-medial viewing trajectory is necessary, the muscle incision is carried out more laterally; conversely, if the trajectory needs to be oriented more laterally towards the jugular bulb, the muscle incision is carried out more medially.
- In many cases, a muscular branch of the vertebral artery emerges from its lateral horizontal loop. By coagulating and dividing this branch, excessive retraction of the vertebral artery can be avoided when the self-retaining retractor is inserted.
- An early exposure of the supracondylar fossa, incising the capsule of the atlantooccipital joint dorsally and drilling the muscular and capsular insertion from the bone clearly facilitate anatomical orientation. Extensive condylar drilling without resecting a significant portion of the articular facet of both condyle and lateral and atlantal mass is crucial for preserving the function of the atlantooccipital joint.
- Opening the dura mater lateral to the dural entrance of the vertebral artery is sufficient in the majority of cases. This facilitates watertight dural closure at the end of the intradural procedure. However, the dural ring of the vertebral artery should be opened if the tumor has encased the proximal portion of the intradural vertebral artery. This allows free mobilization of the artery and better tumor dissection.
- The transcondylar approach can easily be combined with an additional jugular foramen exposure by extending the dissection laterally as previously described [23].
- The surgeon should be prepared to perform cranioverrtebral stabilization in extensive extradural osteodestructive lesions of the occipital condyle, atlas or axis.

References

1. Seeger W (1978) Atlas of topographical anatomy of the brain and surrounding structures. Springer, Vienna, pp 486–489

2. Bertalanffy H, Seeger W (1991) The dorsolateral, suboccipital, transcondylar approach to the lower clivus and anterior portion of the craniocervical junction. Neurosurgery 29:815–821

3. de Oliveira EP, Rhoton AL Jr, Peace D (1985) Microsurgical anatomy of the region of the foramen magnum. Surg Neurol 24:293–352

4. George B, Laurian C (1980) Surgical approach to the whole length of the vertebral artery with special reference to the third portion. Acta Neurochir (Wien) 51:259–272

5. George B, Dematons C, Cophignon J (1988) Lateral approach to the anterior portion of the foramen magnum: application to surgical removal of 14 benign tumors – technical note. Surg Neurol 29:484–490

6. Heros RC (1986) Lateral suboccipital approach for vertebral and vertebrobasilar artery lesions. J Neurosurg 64:559–562

7. Menezes AH (1991) Surgical approaches to the craniocervical junction. In: Frymoyer JW (ed) The adult spine: principles and practice. Raven, New York, pp 967–985

8. Sen CN, Sekhar LN (1990) An extreme lateral approach to intradural lesions of the cervical spine and foramen magnum. Neurosurgery 27:197–204

9. Sen CN, Sekhar LN (1991) Surgical management of anteriorly placed lesions at the craniocervical junction: an alternative approach. Acta Neurochir (Wien) 108:70–77

10. Spetzler RF, Grahm TW (1990) The far-lateral approach to the inferior clivus and the upper cervical region: technical note. Barrow Q 6:35–38

11. Babu RP, Sekhar LN, Wright DC (1994) Extreme lateral transcondylar approach: technical improvements and lessons learned. J Neurosurg 81:49–59

12. Baldwin HZ, Miller CG, van Loveren HR et al (1994) The far lateral/combined supra- and infratentorial approach. A human cadaveric prosection model for routes of access to the petroclival region and ventral brain stem. J Neurosurg 81:60–68

13. Dowd GC, Zeiller S, Awasthi D (1999) Far lateral transcondylar approach: dimensional anatomy. Neurosurgery 45(1):95–99

14. Kawashima M, Tanriover N, Rhoton AL Jr et al (2003) Comparison of the far lateral and extreme lateral variants of the atlanto-occipital transarticular approach to anterior extradural lesions of the craniovertebral junction. Neurosurgery 53:662–674

15. Lanzino G, Paolini S, Spetzler RF (2005) Far-lateral approach to the craniocervical junction. Neurosurgery 57(4 Suppl):367–371

16. Nanda A, Vincent DA, Vannemreddy PS et al (2002) Far-lateral approach to intradural lesions of the foramen magnum without resection of the occipital condyle. J Neurosurg 96:302–309

17. Rhoton AL Jr (2000) The far-lateral approach and its transcondylar, supracondylar, and paracondylar extensions. Neurosurgery 47 [Suppl 1]:S195–S209

18. Rhoton AL Jr (2000) The foramen magnum. Neurosurgery 47 [Suppl 1]:S155–S193

19. Spektor S, Anderson GJ, McMenomey SO et al (2000) Quantitative description of the far-lateral transcondylar transtubercular approach to the foramen magnum and clivus. J Neurosurg 92(5):824–831

20. Vishteh AG, Crawford NR, Melton MS et al (1999) Stability of the craniovertebral junction after unilateral occipital condyle resection: a biomechanical study. J Neurosurg Spine 90:91–98

21. Wen HT, Rhoton AL Jr, Katsuta T, de Oliveira EP (1997) Microsurgical anatomy of the transcondylar, supracondylar, and paracondylar extensions of the far-lateral approach. J Neurosurg 87:555–585

22. Al-Mefty O, Borba LA, Aoki N et al (1996) The transcondylar approach to extradural nonneoplastic lesions of the craniovertebral junction. J Neurosurg 84:1–6

23. Bertalanffy H, Sure U (2000) Surgical approaches to the jugular foramen. In: Robertson JT, Coakham HB, Robertson JH (eds) Cranial base surgery. Churchill Livingstone, London, pp 237–258

24. Bertalanffy H, Sure U, Petermeyer M et al (1998) Management of aneurysms of the vertebral artery-posterior inferior cerebellar artery complex. Neurol Med Chir (Tokyo) 38 Suppl:93–103

25. Bertalanffy H, Tirakotai W, Bozinov O et al (2005) Surgical management of aneurysms of the vertebral and posterior inferior cerebellar artery complex. In: Schmidek HH, Roberts DW (eds) Schmidek and Sweet's operative neurosurgical techniques, 5th edn. Elsevier, Philadelphia, pp 1209–1223

26. Bruneau M, George B (2008) Foramen magnum meningiomas: detailed surgical approaches and technical aspects at Lariboisière Hospital and review of the literature. Neurosurg Rev 31:19–32

27. George B, Lot G (1995) Anterolateral and posterolateral approaches to the foramen magnum: technical description and experience from 97 cases. Skull Base Surg 5:9–19

28. George B, Lot G, Tran Ba HP (1995) The juxtacondylar approach to the jugular foramen (without petrous bone drilling). Surg Neurol 44:279–284

29. George B, Lot G, Boissonnet H (1997) Meningioma of the foramen magnum: a series of 40 cases. Surg Neurol 47:371–379

30. Kratimenos GP, Crockard HA (1993) The far lateral approach for ventrally placed foramen magnum and upper cervical spine tumors. Br J Neurosurg 7(2):129–140

31. Menezes AH (2008) Surgical approaches: postoperative care and complications "posterolateral-far lateral transcondylar approach to the ventral foramen magnum and upper cervical spinal canal". Childs Nerv Syst 24(10):1203–1207

32. Lot G, George B (1999) The extent of drilling in lateral approaches to the cranio-cervical junction area from a series of 125 cases. Acta Neurochir (Wien) 141:111–118

33. Salas E, Sekhar LN, Ziyal IM et al (1999) Variations of the extreme-lateral craniocervical approach: anatomical study and clinical analysis of 69 patients. J Neurosurg 90 [Suppl 4]:206–219

34. Samii M, Klekamp J, Carvalho G (1996) Surgical results for meningiomas of the craniocervical junction. Neurosurgery 39:1086–1095

35. Tirakotai W, Benes L, Kappus C et al (2007) Surgical management of dural arteriovenous fistulas with transosseous arterial feeders involving the jugular bulb. Neurosurg Rev 30(1):40–48

36. Ture U, Pamir MN (2002) Extreme lateral-transatlas approach for resection of the dens of the axis. J Neurosurg 96 [Suppl 1]:73–82

37. Garber JN (1964) Abnormalities of the atlas and axis vertebrae – congenital and traumatic. J Bone Joint Surg Am 46:1782–1791

14

Transsphenoidal Approaches: Endoscopic

Paolo Cappabianca, Luigi M. Cavallo, Isabella Esposito, and Manfred Tschabitscher

14.1 Introduction

The endonasal transsphenoidal route has become a mainstay of contemporary neurosurgical practice for pituitary lesions and is used for more than 95% of surgical indications in the sellar area. Lesions located in this area represent nearly 20% of surgically treated primary brain tumors; benign tumors of the pituitary constitute the majority of sellar lesions. Advances in surgical technology, and the use of the endoscope above all, have played a central role in the recent evolution of transsphenoidal surgery [1–4].

The endoscope was initially used to highlight dark and deep corners during microscopic transphenoidal surgery, but thanks to the increasing use of the endoscope by ENT surgeons in functional endoscopic sinus surgery, it has gradually become possible for the endoscope to be the only optical device used during the whole surgical procedure [5–7].

The advantages of this technique are listed in Table 14.1. Its use requires an in-depth knowledge of endonasal skull-base anatomy and specific endoscopic skills (Table 14.2) [8–13].

Several endonasal landmarks improve orientation during the approach, and the neurosurgeon needs to become familiar with them through anatomic studies and check their configuration preoperatively by means of a high-resolution CT scan with sagittal and coronal reconstructions.

The main features of the endonasal corridor are:

- The nasal mucosa is highly vascularized and should be preserved to prevent postoperative adhesions and discomfort. The tip of the instruments should always be under direct view, including during their insertion through the endonasal corridor.
- The surgical trajectory is in a posterior upward direction. However, the floor of the nose and the free-hanging portions of the turbinates run nearly parallel to the skull base. Inserting the instruments parallel to these structures reduces the risk of damaging the skull base.
- The keystone to a successful endoscopic approach is the quality of vision which depends on the lens cleaning system employed (i.e. a continuous irrigation system) and the ability to manage intraoperative bleeding.

Table 14.1 Advantages of the endoscopic transsphenoidal approach

	Advantages
Patient	Less nasal trauma
	No nasal packing
	Less postoperative pain
	Lower incidence of complications
	Quick recovery
Surgeon	Wider and orientable view of the surgical field
	Closer look "inside" the anatomy (better definition of tumor/gland/arachnoid interfaces)
	Easier treatment of recurrences
	Increase in scientific and research activity
	Promotion of interdisciplinary cooperation
Institution	Shorter postoperative hospital stay
	Increase in case load

P. Cappabianca (✉)
Dept of Neurological Science, Division of Neurosurgery
Università degli Studi di Napoli Federico II, Naples, Italy

Table 14.2 Principles of training in endoscopic endonasal transsphenoidal surgery

Specific requirements	Learning strategies
Basic knowledge of each component of the endoscopic equipment	Self-learning and collaboration with industry
Hand–eye coordination and dexterity	Endoscopic anatomic dissections
	Video games
Confidence with the bidimensional view of the anatomic structures	In-depth anatomic training (structured training sessions)
	Review of surgical videos
	Identify surgical landmarks during surgery and gain a sense of depth with in and out movements
Endoscopic bleeding management	Master hemostatic materials and techniques
	Practice the use of the bipolar forceps in training models
	Practice the use of the bipolar forceps in the surgical environment
Endoscopic skull base reconstruction	Master state-of-the-art materials and techniques
	Practice and compare the techniques in anatomic models

14.2 Surgical Anatomy

14.2.1 Endonasal Corridor

The surgical anatomy of the endonasal corridor (Fig. 14.1) is variable and it is important to know the surgical significance of these variations.

The *middle turbinate* has a characteristic three-dimensional orientation. Anteriorly, it is directly attached to the cribriform plate (sagittal portion). It then has a coronal course and is attached to the lamina papyracea (coronal portion or basal lamella) while, posteriorly, it attaches to the medial wall of the maxillary sinus (axial portion). During the nasal step of the procedure, the middle turbinate should be luxated laterally by pushing at the level of its head, thus reducing the risk of fracturing the cribriform plate and of postoperative maxillary sinusitis due to its destabilization. The head of the middle turbinate may be pneumatized ("concha bullosa") so narrowing the surgical corridor; in such cases its resection is required. The *bulla ethmoidalis* is an anterior ethmoid air cell with variable degrees of pneumatization. If it fills the whole middle meatus, it can be opened medially and anteriorly, preserving its lateral part, which is contiguous with the lamina papyracea.

The *posterior ethmoid* may have critical relationships with the sphenoid. It may extend laterally or superiorly to the anterior wall of the sphenoid and impinge on the optic nerve ("Onodi-Grünwald cell"). The relationships between the roof of the ethmoid and the ethmoidal arteries are critical since their damage during the approach can lead to vascular complications. The anterior ethmoidal artery runs in a lateral to medial and

posteroanterior direction and in a well-pneumatized bulla ethmoidalis its bone canal can be separated from the ethmoid roof by a thin bony mesentery. This artery can be damaged while removing the anterosuperior component of the bulla ethmoidalis and its bone canal can be dehiscent. The posterior ethmoidal artery, which is inconstant, has a horizontal course and runs in the ethmoidal roof, where the lamella of the superior turbinate inserts in the lamina papyracea, about 3–8 mm anteriorly to the anterior wall of the sphenoid sinus and runs about 7 mm away from the optic nerve, thus representing a valuable landmark during further extension of the anterior sphenoidotomy upward.

The sphenoid and ethmoid sinuses share a common wall in the lateral two-thirds while the medial one-third of the anterior sphenoid sinus wall is a free surface called the *sphenoethmoidal recess* where the ostium of the sphenoid sinus is identified, less or more laterally, depending on the pneumatization of the sphenoid prow.

The sphenopalatine artery is the terminal branch of the internal maxillary artery; it comes out from the homonymous foramen, behind the tail of the middle turbinate, and divides into two main branches: the nasopalatine artery and the posterior nasal artery. The former runs above the upper border of the choana, and the latter sends branches to the inferior and middle turbinates.

The *sphenoid sinus* is located in a central position in the skull base and represents the keyhole to unlock the whole midline skull base and the middle cranial fossa. The anatomical landmarks on its posterior wall provide a precise map for the safe and precise use of the transsphenoidal route (Fig. 14.2). The degree of pneumatization of the sphenoid sinus and the configuration of its septa present the surgeon with different dif-

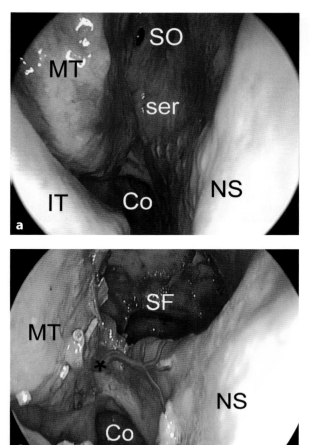

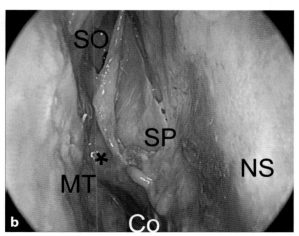

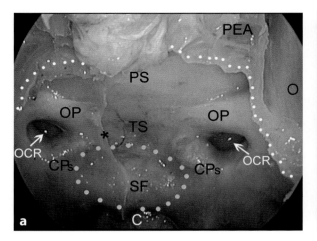

Fig. 14.1 Anatomic view; nasal stage; right nostril approach. **a, b** Identification of the landmarks inside the nostril. **c** The superimposed diagram shows the whole course of the septal branch of the sphenopalatine artery above the choana. It should be respected during the anterior sphenoidotomy. ✱ septal branch of the sphenopalatine artery, *Co* choana, *IT* inferior turbinate, *MT* middle turbinate, *NS* nasal septum, *ser* sphenoethmoid recess, *SF* sellar floor, *SO* sphenoid ostium, *SP* sphenoid prow

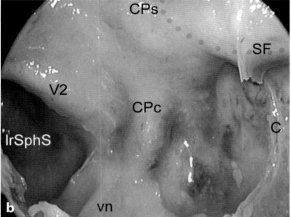

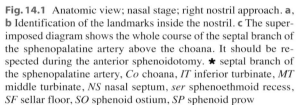

Fig. 14.2 Anatomic view. Exposure of the bony protuberances and depressions on the posterior wall of a well-pneumatized sphenoid sinus (**a**) with a wide lateral recess (**b**). ✱ flattened sphenoidal septum, *C* clivus, *CPc* paraclival segment of the carotid protuberance, *CPs* parasellar segment of the carotid protuberance, *dotted line* sellar bone window, *lrSphS* lateral recess of the sphenoid sinus, *O* orbit, *OCR* lateral opto-carotid recess, *OP* optic protuberance, *PEA* posterior ethmoidal artery, *PS* planum sphenoidale, *SF* sellar floor, *TS* tuberculum sellae, *V2* maxillary nerve, *vn* vidian nerve

ficulties. The bony landmarks on the posterior wall of the sphenoid sinus can be easily identified in a sellar-type sphenoid sinus while a presellar or conchal-type sphenoid sinus make orientation more difficult. A pre-operative CT or MRI scan provides the definition of the size and shape of the sphenoid septa, which often lead to the optical canal or the parasellar carotid artery. They should be carefully removed, avoiding twisting and fracturing them. Furthermore, a high degree of sphenoid sinus pneumatization may be associated with dehiscence of the bone covering the optic nerve, the carotid artery, the pterygoid canal and/or the groove of the maxillary nerve. Care should be taken when pinching off the sphenoid mucosa since such dehiscence may result in direct contact between the sinus mucosa and the overlying dura. The landmarks on the posterior wall of the sphenoid guide the approach to the sella which is defined laterally by the carotid prominences, superiorly by the tuberculum sellae and inferiorly by the clivus.

14.2.2 Sellar Region

The *sellar dura*, which is formed by a dense junction of the periosteal and meningeal dural layers, can host the *intercavernous sinuses* whose configuration is highly variable and which should be avoided or coagulated before dura opening. During periost and dura opening the surgeon should not go too deep into the gland since it is surrounded by a thin capsule which should be preserved. The color of the *pituitary gland* (Fig. 14.3a) is butter orange which reflects its microvascular organization. It is surrounded by a connective tissue capsule which serves as the route for blood vessels and from which spreads the connective tissue framework for the pituitary cells. The arteries of the pituitary gland arise from the internal carotid arteries as the superior and inferior hypophyseal arteries (Fig. 14.3b, c). The superior hypophyseal arteries supply the optic chiasm, the floor of the hypothalamus and the median eminence. They distribute vertical branches to the hypophyseal stalk and give off a vertical branch, the artery of the trabecula, which represents an anastomosis between the superior and inferior hypophyseal artery branches. Each inferior hypophyseal artery divides into a medial and a lateral branch which anastomose with the corresponding vessels of the opposite side, forming an arterial ring around the hypophysis.

Above the sella, the opening of the *diaphragma sellae* can be wide thus allowing descent of the suprasellar cistern into the sellar cavity. Such intrasellar arachnoid

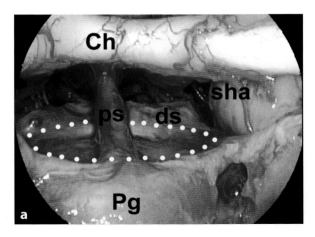

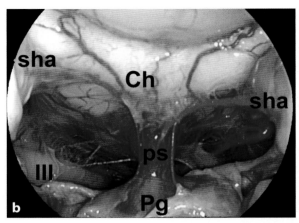

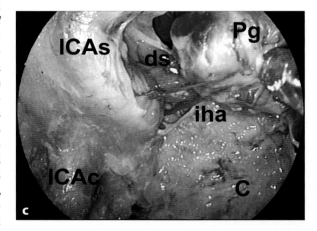

Fig. 14.3 Sellar area. Vascularization of the pituitary gland. *C* clivus, *Ch* chiasm, *ds* dorsum sellae, *dotted line* opening of the diaphragma sellae, *ICAc* paraclival segment of the internal carotid artery, *ICAs* parasellar segment of the internal carotid artery, *iha* inferior hypophyseal artery, *III* oculomotor nerve, *Pg* pituitary gland, *ps* pituitary stalk, *sha* superior hypophyseal artery

diverticula can be identified before dural opening as blue areas. However, a wide superior intercavernous sinus can have the same effect, although it will change in color when probed with a sharp instrument ("refilling effect").

14.2.3 Parasellar Area

In a widely pneumatized sphenoid sinus, the *vidian* and the *maxillary nerves* can be visualized as well, under the thin bony covering. These two nerves cross through the lateral recess of the sphenoid sinus, which extends out-

ward from the main sinus cavity into the greater wing of the sphenoid bone and is highly variable. This recess can be involved by sellar lesions and represents a gate to unlock the cavernous sinus, the middle skull base and the infratemporal fossa. To highlight the lateral recess of the sphenoid sinus an endonasal transmaxillary transpterygoid route can be followed (Fig. 14.4).

By removing the bone that covers the parasellar carotid artery both the medial and lateral compartments of the cavernous sinus are exposed. After dura opening, by lateralizing the intracavernous carotid artery, the inferior hypophyseal artery is highlighted

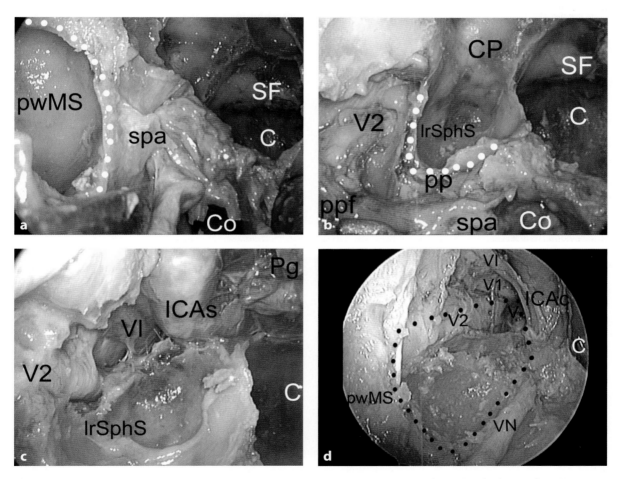

Fig. 14.4 Right nostril approach. Transantrum transpterygoid approach to the lateral recess of the sphenoid sinus (**a, b**) and exposure of the lateral compartment of the cavernous sinus (**c**) through the quadrangular area enclosed between the maxillary and the vidian nerves (**d**). The *dotted lines* indicate the medial antrostomy in **a**, the removal of the pterygoid process in **b**, and the boundaries of the quadrangular area in **d**. *C* clivus, *Co* choana, *CP* carotid protuberance, *ICAc* paraclival segment of the internal carotid artery, *ICAs* parasellar segment of the internal carotid artery, *lrSphS* lateral recess of the sphenoid sinus, *pwMS* posterior wall of the maxillary sinus, *Pg* pituitary gland, *pp* pterygoid process, *ppf* pterygopalatine fossa, *SF* sellar floor, *spa* sphenopalatine artery, *V1* ophthalmic nerve, *V2* maxillary nerve, *V* gasserian ganglion, *VI* abducens nerve, *VN* vidian nerve

(Fig. 14.5a, b). Passing laterally to the internal carotid artery, the oculomotor, trochlear, abducens and maxillary nerves are visualized along the lateral compartment of the cavernous sinus. The ophthalmic nerve can be identified behind the abducens nerve, while slight medialization of the internal carotid artery allows identification of the trochlear nerve and of the inferolateral trunk (Fig. 14.5c, d). The inferolateral trunk usually crosses over the middle segment of the abducens nerve and its branches provide blood supply to the cranial nerves [14].

14.3 Procedure

14.3.1 Preoperative Workup

MRI and CT scans with coronal reconstruction should be reviewed; attention should be paid to the following items [15]:
- Nasal anatomy: septal deviations, presence of concha bullosa or turbinate hypertrophy.
- Configuration of the floor of the anterior skull base, presence of Onodi-Grünwald cells.

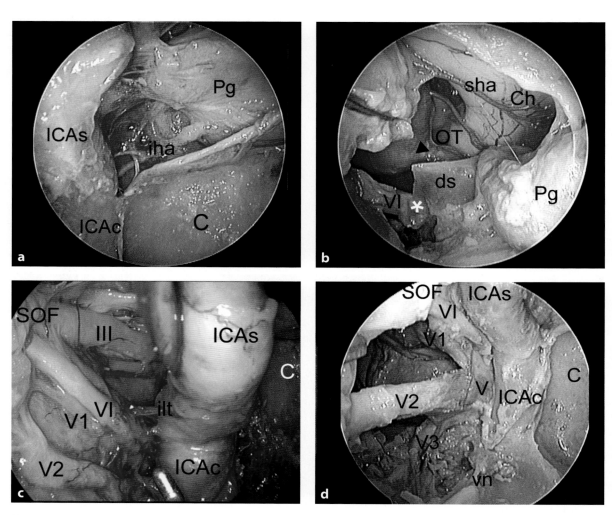

Fig. 14.5 Intradural exploration of the medial (**a, b**) and lateral (**c, d**) compartments of the right cavernous sinus. The abducens nerve can be followed running through the Dorello's canal (**b**) and into the cavernous sinus (**c**), toward the superior orbital fissure (**c, d**). ▲ right posterior communicating artery, ✱ Dorello's point, *C* clivus, *Ch* optic chiasms, *ds* dorsum sellae, *ICAc* paraclival segment of the internal carotid artery, *ICAs* parasellar segment of the internal carotid artery, iha inferior hypophyseal artery, *III* oculomotor nerve, *ilt* infero-lateral trunk, *OT* optic tract, *Pg* pituitary gland, *sha* superior hypophyseal artery, *SOF* superior orbital fissure, *V* Gasserian ganglion, *VI* ophthalmic nerve, *V2* maxillary nerve, *V3* mandibular nerve, *VI* abducens nerve, *vn* vidian nerve

- Pneumatization of the sphenoid sinus, distribution of its septa and their relationship with the optic canal and the internal carotid artery.
- Intercarotid distance at the level of the sella (so-called kissing carotids, when very close to each other).
- At level of the sella, beside the lesion, partial empty sella or arachnoid diverticula should be noted preoperatively.

We advise the use of preoperative neuronavigation in the following cases [16]:
- Presellar or conchal-type sphenoid sinus
- Recurrences previously operated upon transsphenoidally
- Huge lesions with wide suprasellar and parasellar extension

14.3.2 Operating Room Set-up and Patient Positioning

In the operating room, the endoscopic surgery equipment (monitor, video camera, cold light source, and video recording system) is placed behind the head of the patient in such a way that both the operating surgeon and the second surgeon can comfortably look at the monitor. Each component of the equipment should be checked before the start of the procedure. The operating surgeon is usually on the right side of the patient and the second surgeon on the left. The anesthesiologist and the anesthesiologist's equipment are positioned to the left and the scrub nurse next to the patient's legs. The image guidance system, when used, is put beside the main endoscopic monitor.

The patient is placed supine on the operating table, under general anesthesia and orotracheal intubation. The back is elevated by about 10°, and the head, in neutral position, is rotated 10° towards the operating surgeon and secured in a horseshoe headrest. His/her eyes should be protected with antibiotic eye ointment and a wet pad should be inserted in his/her throat to plug the oropharynx and prevent fluid collection in the airway. A Foley urinary catheter should be used if it is possible that the surgery will last more that 3 hours. Preoperative antibiotics are routinely administered whereas intraoperative corticosteroid is reserved for patients with hypopituitarism. The nose is prepped with pledgets soaked in 50% povidone-iodine gently inserted through a small Killian-type nasal speculum and avoiding scarring the nasal mucosa.

Before scrubbing up the surgeons should adjust the operating table to a comfortable working height [17].

14.3.3 Surgical Technique

The procedure is performed with a rigid endoscope inserted into one nostril, usually the right one. We currently use a rigid 0° endoscope, 18 cm in length and 4 mm in diameter, (Karl Storz, Tuttlingen, Germany) as the visualizing instrument, without any working channel and inserted in an irrigation shaft to keep the lens clean. It is held in the surgeon's nondominant hand until the anterior sphenoidotomy is completed and then it can be either fixed to an adjustable table-mounted holder or better if held by a second surgeon [18].

The operation is usually performed through a single nostril up to the anterior sphenoidotomy. Then the endoscope plus the nondominant instrument is usually inserted through one nostril, while the main instrument is inserted through the other nostril. The procedure consists of three main steps: nasal, sphenoidal and sellar.

14.3.3.1 Nasal Step

The endoscope is inserted into the chosen nostril, usually the right, parallel to the nasal floor, and the nasal septum is visualized medially. The inferior turbinate is identified laterally and its tail is followed until the choana, which is limited by the vomer medially and the floor of the sphenoid sinus superiorly. The vomer and the sphenoid keel provide good guidance to the midline. Essential aspects of this stage include: tailored widening of the nasal corridor and access to sphenoid sinus.

Tailored Widening of the Nasal Corridor

Soft cotton pledgets, soaked in diluted adrenaline (1/10,000, 1:20 dilution) are slid between the middle turbinate and the nasal septum and a sharp instrument is used to gently luxate it laterally. The instrument should be parallel to the nasal floor thus reducing the risk of entering the ethmoid and the anterior skull base. Nasal crests can be fractured or septal deviations corrected, if necessary.

Access to Sphenoid Sinus

Once the choana is identified, the endoscope is angled upward, along the sphenoethmoid recess for approximately 1–1.5 cm above the roof of the choana and the sphenoid sinus can be unlocked either through its natural ostium or through the sphenoid prow.

14.3.3.2 Sphenoidal Step

Essential aspects of this stage include: anterior sphenoidotomy, removal of the sphenoidal septa, and identification of the anatomical landmarks on the posterior wall of the sphenoid sinus.

Anterior Sphenoidotomy

The mucosa of the spheno-ethmoid recess is coagulated bilaterally and the posterior part of the nasal septum is removed for about 1 cm allowing a binostril access. The nasal septum is detached from the anterior wall of the sphenoid sinus with a high-speed microdrill using a diamond burr of 5 mm diameter. The bone opening on the anterior wall of the sphenoid septum is enlarged circumferentially with a microdrill and/or bone punches. Inferolateral extension of the bone opening is usually not necessary but, if required, the mucosa is carefully detached from the bone and the major trunks of the sphenopalatine artery are coagulated with the bipolar forceps to avoid their bleeding.

Removal of the Sphenoidal Septa

After the anterior sphenoidotomy has been performed, the distribution of the sphenoid septa as shown by the preoperative neuroradiological studies is compared with the endoscopic view. They are removed carefully and not fractured, preserving the mucosa if not infiltrated by the tumor. Their insertion along the posterior wall of the sphenoid sinus may be a useful landmark for identification of the edges of the sella.

Identification of the Anatomical Landmarks on the Posterior Wall of the Sphenoid Sinus

After all the sphenoidal septa have been flattened, the posterior and lateral walls of the sphenoid sinus are visible with the sellar floor at the center, the planum sphenoidale above it, and the clival indentation below. Lateral to the sellar floor, the bony prominences of the intracavernous carotid artery, the optic nerve and, between them, the optocarotid recess can be observed. In the presence of a presellar or a conchal sphenoid sinus, there will be a paucity of anatomic landmarks and the identification of the lateral boundaries of the sella is mandatory. In these cases the use of a neuronavigation system and the microDoppler probe provide accurate information with regard to the midline and position of the parasellar internal carotid artery.

14.3.3.3 Sellar Step

From this step onwards the surgeon has absolutely to operate bimanually, i.e. with two instruments, usually one through each nostril, while the endoscope is held dynamically by a second surgeon (three-/four-hand technique). If necessary, but non recommendable, the endoscope can be fixed to an adjustable holder, either mechanical or pneumatic. Prior to opening the sellar floor, it is essential to check if the endoscope has the proper orientation to ensure that all anatomical landmarks inside the sphenoid cavity are displayed in their appropriate position. The correct orientation is crucial with respect to the midline and to the approach.

Essential aspects of this stage include: opening of the sellar floor, opening of the sellar dura, and tumor removal.

Opening of the Sellar Floor

The surgical window should be extended between the medial aspect of both cavernous sinuses. Depending on the bone thickness and/or tumor infiltration, the sellar floor is opened using a microdrill, a Kerrison rongeur, a Stammberger circular cutting punch or a blunt dissector. The bone opening is enlarged until the carotid prominences laterally and from the tuberculum to the clival indentation (Fig. 14.6).

Particularly in cases of macroadenoma, if intraoperative CSF leakage is foreseen, the sellar floor should not be flattened to the clivus since it could be useful to buttress further reconstruction of the osteodural defect. The sellar dura should be widely exposed from one cavernous sinus to the other and from the tuberculum sellae down to the junction of the sellar floor to the clivus.

Opening of the Sellar Dura

The superior intercavernous sinus should be identified and avoided or coagulated. Several strategies can be used to identify carotid arteries behind the dura such as the use of the ultrasound Doppler probe and intraoperative neuronavigation. The dura is incised sharply using a scalpel with a telescopic blade, in a linear or cruciate fashion. The direction of the dural opening should be

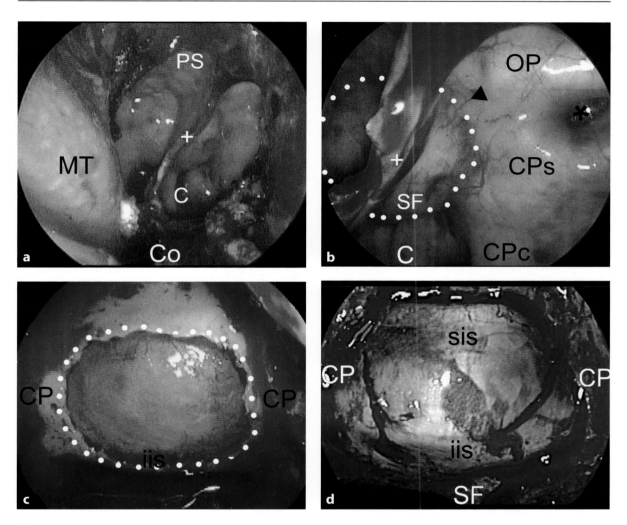

Fig. 14.6 Exposure and opening of the sellar floor. **+** flattened sphenoid septum, **▲** medial opto-carotid recess, **✱** lateral opto-carotid recess, *C* clivus, *Co* choana, *CP* carotid protuberance, *CPc* paraclival segment of the carotid protuberance, *CPs* parasellar segment of the carotid protuberance, *dotted line* sellar bone window, *iis* inferior intercavernous sinus, *MT* middle turbinate, *OP* optic protuberance, *PS* planum sphenoidale, *SF* sellar floor, *sis* superior intercavernous sinus

from lateral to medial and superior to inferior; further enlargement can be performed with scissors. During dura opening the pituitary gland should not be entered and both sellar dural layers should be incised, since interdural dissection will cause venous bleeding from the intercavernous sinuses.

Tumor Removal

There are different strategies for removal of a micro- or a macroadenoma which are discussed separately.

When a *microadenoma* is enclosed in the sella, it is critical to find a surgical plane at the margin of the adenoma and identify and preserve the normal gland. Providing one-third of the normal pituitary remains in the sella, there is no risk of producing panhypopituitarism, whereas manipulation of the pituitary stalk will cause an endocrinological deficit and diabetes insipidus. The development of a surgical plane at the margin of a microadenoma may be favored for the identification of a pseudocapsule which comprises compressed reticulin, and represents the scaffold of normal pituitary cells.

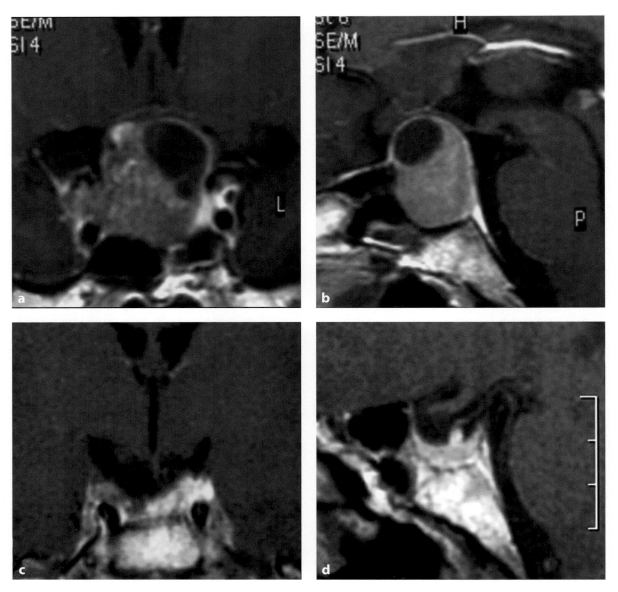

Fig. 14.7 Preoperative (**a**, **b**) and postoperative (**c**, **d**) MR imaging in a case of pituitary macroadenoma, The postoperative images (**c**, **d**) images show gross total removal of the tumor, decompression of the chiasm and residual pituitary gland

The adenoma enclosed in its pseudocapsule is dissected from the residual normal gland and removed en bloc, when possible, or piecemeal [19].

Identification of the adenoma is not always clear after opening of the dura, despite an accurate preoperative neuroimaging study. The endoscopic close-up view may improve the likelihood of identifying the pathological tissue, which differs in color and consistency from normal pituitary tissue. The normal pituitary is yellowish orange and not easily aspirated at low pressure, while adenomatous tissue is more yellow and soft than normal pituitary tissue.

In the case of a *macroadenoma*, the inferior and lateral components of the lesion should be loosened and removed before the superior part, to prevent redundant suprasellar cistern falling into the operative field, which

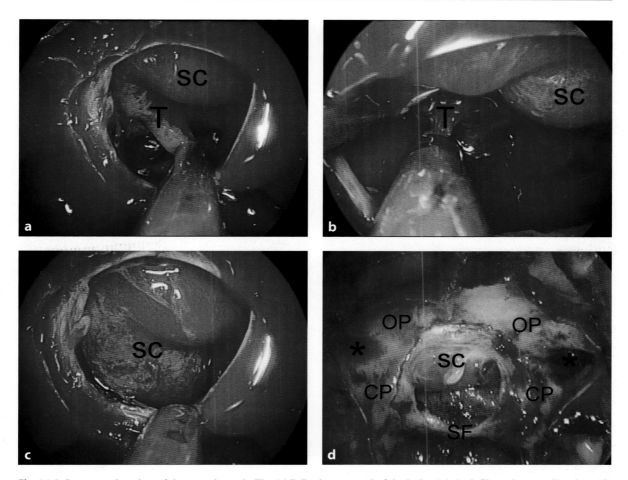

Fig. 14.8 Intraoperative view of the case shown in Fig. 14.7. During removal of the lesion (**a**) the infiltrated suprasellar cistern is highlighted. Painstaking peeling of its posterior part delivers some more tumor (**b**). The cistern drops into the sella (**c**), even down to the sellar floor (**d**). ★ lateral optocarotid recess, *CP* carotid protuberance, *OP* optic protuberance, *SC* suprasellar cistern, *SF* sellar floor, *T* tumor

would obstruct the view of the residual tumor (Figs. 14.7 and 14.8). The parasellar extension of the lesion should finally be removed under direct view and after identification of the carotid artery and management of venous bleeding.

The advantages of the endoscopic endonasal approach have led to the extension of its indications. The endoscopic approach extended to the planum can be used to manage fibrous adenomas or even giant adenomas, approached transcranially in the past [20–22]. Rare fibrous adenomas, because of their hard consistency, should be removed through an extracapsular dissection in which, after internal debulking, the tumor edge is gently pulled medially, allowing further visual-

ization of the outer surface of the lesion and its interface with the arachnoid. To allow such a view, the bone window is extended upward to the tuberculum sellae and sphenoid planum.

The endoscope also provides specific benefits during surgical management of lesions, mainly pituitary adenomas, extending to the cavernous sinus, along tongue-like projections of the pituitary gland itself or through weak points in the meningeal layer [23]. Different transsphenoidal corridors permit access either medially or laterally to the intracavernous internal carotid artery. The medial compartment is highlighted by inserting the endoscope through the nostril contralateral to the parasellar extension of the lesion. After identification of the intracav-

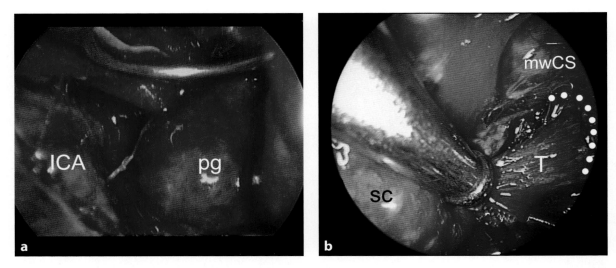

Fig. 14.9 Intrasellar exploration of an intact medial wall of the right cavernous sinus (**a**), and another case in which the medial wall of the left cavernous sinus has been violated by tumor extension (**b**). *Dotted line* opening in the medial wall of the cavernous sinus, *ICA* internal carotid artery, *mwCS* medial wall of the cavernous sinus, *pg* pituitary gland, *SC* suprasellar cistern, *T* tumor

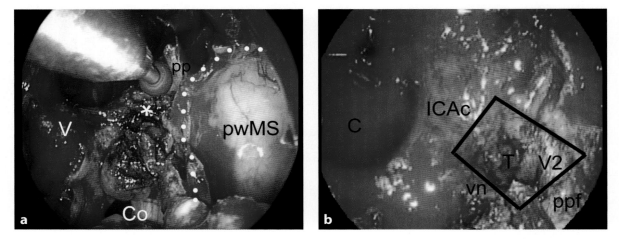

Fig. 14.10 Transantrum transpterygoid approach to the lateral compartment of the cavernous sinus through the quadrangular area. *∗* coagulated sphenopalatine artery, *C* clivus, *Co* choana, *ICAc* paraclival segment of the internal carotid artery, *MT* middle turbinate, *pp* pterygoid process, *ppf* pterygopalatine fossa, *pwMS* posterior wall of the maxillary sinus, *T* tumor, *V* vomer, *V2* maxillary nerve, *vn* vidian nerve

ernous carotid artery pulsation, atraumatic angled suctions cannulas and curettes can be inserted to remove tumor extensions through the enlarged C-shaped loop of the carotid artery (Fig. 14.9). Venous bleeding indicates complete tumor removal and is easily controlled. Lesions extending toward the lateral compartment of the cavernous sinus can be removed through the homolateral

transethmoid transpterygoid route directed to the lateral recess of the sphenoid sinus (Fig. 14.10). The transethmoid transpterygoid route provides a wide frontal exposure of the surgical target with the 0° endoscope and is indicated to treat lesions with a soft consistency, such as adenomas and chordomas. Resection of the middle turbinate, the ethmoid and the medial pterygoid process

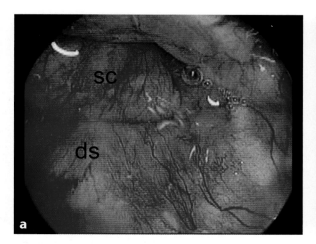
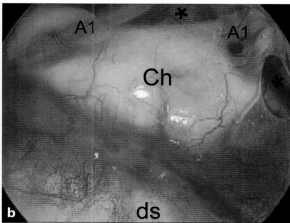

Fig. 14.11 Intrasellar exploration with zero (a) and 30° (b) endoscopes. Note how the angled view of the 30° endoscope improves the likelihood of finding tears in the cistern. * hole in the arachnoid space, *A1* precommunicating tract of the anterior cerebral artery, *Ch* chiasm, *ds* dorsum sellae, *sc* suprasellar cistern

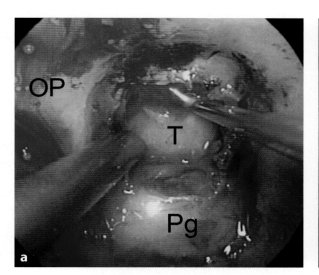
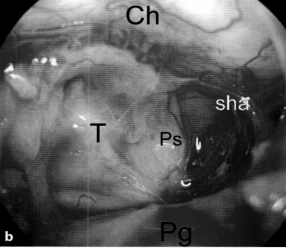

Fig. 14.12 Suprasellar Rathke's cleft cyst. a Before cyst evacuation, the thickened arachnoid of the chiasmatic cistern is carefully dissected. b After decompression, the cyst wall, tenaciously attached to the pituitary stalk, is left in place. *Ch* chiasm, *OP* optic protuberance, *Pg* pituitary gland, *Ps* pituitary stalk, *sha* superior hypophyseal artery, *T* tumor

highlights the lateral compartment of the sphenoid sinus, where a quadrangular area is bounded superiorly by V2, inferiorly by the vidian nerve and posteriorly by the parasellar and paraclival carotid artery.

The endoscopic transsphenoidal approach provides specific intraoperative advantages in the surgical management of sellar and intra- and suprasellar cystic lesions such as cystic pituitary adenomas and craniopharyngiomas, and arachnoid and Rathke's cleft cysts [24, 25]. During the sellar step of the procedure, the endoscopic view facilitates the dissection of the capsule from the suprasellar cistern and the identification of CSF leakage over the suprasellar cistern surface. The effectiveness of the endoscopic sellar exploration depends upon the width of the sella, the descent of the suprasellar cistern, which may obliterate the tumor cavity, and sellar and/or epidural venous bleeding.

For *arachnoid cysts*, after their evacuation, the sellar cavity is inspected with a 0° and/or an angled scope to evaluate the presence of communication with the subarachnoid space directly or indirectly, by identifying air bubbles over the cisternal surface. By maneuvering the endoscope within the sella, a greater area is exposed compared with the static anteroposterior perspective under the microscopic view. When the 30–45° endoscope is used, structures in the suprasellar and parasellar spaces come clearly into view (Fig. 14.11). For *intrasellar Rathke's cleft cysts*, a low midline vertical glandular incision is performed. Through this small corridor, the cyst contents are removed and the cyst wall is removed partially in order to preserve pituitary function. For suprasellar Rathke's cleft cyst, after evacuation, its wall is removed in fragments unless strictly adherent to the surrounding structures, specially to the pituitary stalk, where it is left in place to avoid post-op hypopituitarism (Fig. 14.12).

14.3.3.4 Sellar Reconstruction

Once the sellar lesion has been removed, the sella is repaired only in selected patients, mainly when intraoperative CSF leakage has occurred due to opening of the suprasellar cistern [26–28]. Autologous or heterologous materials, either resorbable or not, are used and the reconstruction technique is tailored to the leak entity, the size of the osteodural defect and the presence of "dead

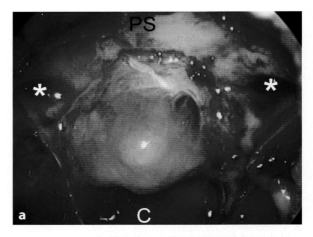
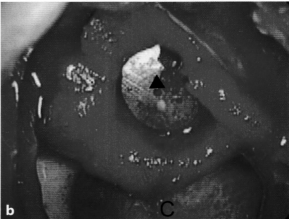
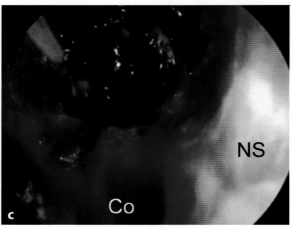

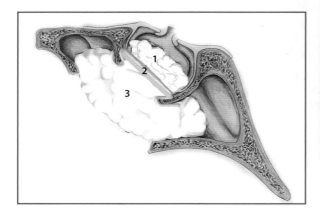

Fig. 14.13 Diagram showing the main steps of a multilayer reconstruction: *1* intrasellar dead space filled with fibrin glue (Tisseel), *2* osteodural defect plugged with bone and dural substitutes, *3* intrasphenoidal scaffold of the overhanging reconstruction

Fig. 14.14 Intraoperative images of the leading strategies in the multilayer reconstruction. **a** Intrasellar injection of fibrin glue (Tisseel). **b** Sealing the osteodural defect. **c** Buttressing the reconstruction by injection of DuraSeal. ▲ dural and bone substitutes jammed in the osteodural defect ("Granma's technique"), ✱ lateral optocarotid recess, *C* clivus, *Co* choana, *NS* nasal septum, *PS* planum sphenoidale

space" inside the sella. The aim of the repair is to guarantee a watertight closure, reduce the intrasellar dead space, and prevent the descent of the chiasm into the sellar cavity. Overpacking may lead to postoperative optic chiasm compression and should be avoided.

The key steps in the multilayer reconstruction (Figs. 14.13 and 14.14) are as follows:

1. Closure of the arachnoid defect, if identified, with fibrin glue (Tisseel; Baxter, Vienna, Austria). The suprasellar cistern can be reinforced with collagen sponge or Tissudura or another autologous dural substitute.
2. Reduction of the intrasellar dead space with fibrin glue (Tisseel).
3. Closure of the dura with a watertight seal using the granma's cup or gasket seal technique [28]. The dural substitute is positioned extradurally and the

bone substitute (LactoSorb, Walter Lorenz Surgical) is embedded in the extradural space dragging the dural substitute. Other layers of dural substitute or mucoperichondrium are overlapped.

4. Buttress the reconstruction by filling the sphenoid sinus with fibrin glue or DuraSeal (Confluent Surgical, Waltham, MA).

14.4 Pitfalls and Complication Avoidance

Each step of the procedure has different pitfalls which can lead to different complications (Tables 14.3 and 14.4) [29–32].

Table 14.3 Complication avoidance

Surgical step	Complication	Tricks
Nasal step	Anterior skull base CSF leakage Sphenopalatine artery branches bleeding	Gentle luxation of the middle turbinate Avoid inferolateral extension of the anterior sphenoidotomy Careful coagulation of the mucosal borders
Sphenoid step	Optic nerve/carotid artery injury	Check landmarks on the posterior wall of the sphenoid sinus and correct endoscope orientation Use microDoppler probe and neuronavigation system
Sellar step	CSF leakage	Avoid sharp dissection during tumor removal Remove the adenoma remaining in the extraarachnoid plane
	ICA injury	Remove the parasellar extension of the tumor under direct view and using dedicated curettes and atraumatic suction
	Hypopituitarism and diabetes insipidus	Debulk the macroadenomas sequentially Avoid traction on the stalk Prevent empty sella by filling the dead space
	Overpacking	Use low-swelling collagen sponges to fill a bloodless dead space

Table 14.4 Bleeding management

Source of bleeding	Control strategy
Nasal mucosa	Anticongestant-soaked pledget Analgesia Monopolar/bipolar electrocautery Radiofrequency coagulation
Septal artery	Bipolar electrocautery
Bone	Diamond burrs
Intercavernous sinuses	Bipolar electrocautery (to stick the two layers) Thrombin-gelatin matrix (Floseal) and pledget compression
Cavernous sinus	Continued irrigation Slight increase in arterial pressure Head elevation
Tumor bed	Irrigation Compression with pledgets Thrombin/gelatin matrix
Internal carotid artery	Tamponade with thrombin/gelatin matrix (Floseal) and cottonoids

References

1. Kennedy DW (2006) Technical innovations and the evolution of endoscopic sinus surgery. Ann Otol Rhinol Laryngol Suppl 196:27–34

2. Carrau RL, Jho HD, Ko Y (1996) Transnasal-transsphenoidal endoscopic surgery of the pituitary gland. Laryngoscope 106:914–918

3. Jho HD, Carrau RL, Ko Y (1996) Endoscopic pituitary surgery. In: Wilkins RH, Rengachary SS (eds) Neurosurgical operative atlas. American Association of Neurological Surgeons, Park Ridge, pp 1–12

4. Cappabianca P, Alfieri A, de Divitiis E (1998) Endoscopic endonasal transsphenoidal approach to the sella: towards functional endoscopic pituitary surgery (FEPS). Minim Invasive Neurosurg 41:66–73

5. Kennedy DW (1985) Functional endoscopic sinus surgery. Theory and diagnostic evaluation. Arch Otolaryngol 111:576–582

6. Kennedy DW (1985) Functional endoscopic sinus surgery. Technique. Arch Otolaryngol 111:643–649

7. Stammberger HR (1991) Functional endoscopic sinus surgery. The Messerklinger technique. Decker, Baltimore

8. Laws ER (1992) Pituitary tumours – therapeutic considerations: surgical. In: Barrow DL, Selman W (eds) Concepts in neurosurgery, vol 5. Williams and Wilkins, Baltimore, pp 395–400

9. Kassam AB, Carrau RL, Patel A, Herrera A (2000) Endoscopic intrasellar and parasellar anatomy: detailed anatomic dissections and nuisances to avoid complications. CNS Annual Meeting, San Antonio, Texas, Poster Program Book, p 137

10. de Divitiis E, Cappabianca P, Cavallo LM (2002) Endoscopic transsphenoidal approach: adaptability of the procedure to different sellar lesions. Neurosurgery 51:699–705; discussion 705–707

11. de Divitiis E, Cappabianca P, Cavallo LM (2003) Endoscopic endonasal transsphenoidal approach to the sellar region. In: de Divitiis E, Cappabianca P (eds) Endoscopic endonasal transsphenoidal surgery. Springer, Vienna New York, pp 91–130

12. Cappabianca P, Cavallo LM, de Divitiis E (2004) Endoscopic endonasal transsphenoidal surgery. Neurosurgery 55:933–940; discussion 940–931

13. Cappabianca P, Cavallo LM, Esposito F et al (2008) Extended endoscopic endonasal approach to the midline skull base: the evolving role of transsphenoidal surgery. Adv Tech Stand Neurosurg 33:151–199

14. Cappabianca P, Cavallo LM, Esposito F, de Divitiis E (2007) Endonasal approaches to the cavernous sinus. In: Anand VK, Schwartz TH (eds) Practical endoscopic skull base surgery, Plural Publishing, Oxford, pp 177–189

15. Zinreich SJ, Kennedy DW, Rosenbaum AE et al (1987) Paranasal sinuses: CT imaging requirements for endoscopic surgery. Radiology 163:769–775

16. Cappabianca P, de Divitiis E (2003) Image guided endoscopic transnasal removal of recurrent pituitary adenomas. Neurosurgery 52:483–484

17. Cavallo LM, Dal Fabbro M, Jalalod'din H et al (2007) Endoscopic endonasal transsphenoidal surgery. Before scrubbing in: tips and tricks. Surg Neurol 67:342–347

18. Castelnuovo P, Pistochini A, Locatelli D (2006) Different surgical approaches to the sellar region: focusing on the "two nostrils four hands technique". Rhinology 44:2–7

19. Oldfield EH, Vortmeyer AO (2006) Development of a histological pseudocapsule and its use as a surgical capsule in the excision of pituitary tumors. J Neurosurg 104:7–19

20. Laws ER (1997) Surgery for giant pituitary adenomas. In: Kobayashi S, Goel A, Hongo K (eds) Neurosurgery of complex tumors and vascular lesions, Churchill Livingstone, New York, pp 272–273

21. Kassam AB, Mintz AH, Snyderman CH et al (2007) Expanded endonasal approach to the sella and anterior skull base. In Badie B (ed) Neurosurgical operative atlas, 2nd edn. Thieme, New York, pp 21–30

22. Kaptain GJ, Vincent DA, Sheehan JP et al (2008) Transsphenoidal approaches for the extracapsular resection of midline suprasellar and anterior cranial base lesions. Neurosurgery 62 (6 Suppl 3):1264–1271

23. Frank G, Pasquini E (2002) Endoscopic endonasal approaches to the cavernous sinus: surgical approaches. Neurosurgery 50:675

24. Cavallo LM, Prevedello D, Esposito F et al (2008) The role of the endoscope in the transsphenoidal management of cystic lesions of the sellar region. Neurosurg Rev 31:55–64

25. Laws ER (2008) Endoscopic surgery for cystic lesions of the pituitary region. Nat Clin Pract Endocrinol Metab 4:662–663

26. Cavallo LM, Messina A, Esposito F et al (2007) Skull base reconstruction in the extended endoscopic transsphenoidal approach for suprasellar lesions. J Neurosurg 107:713–720

27. Esposito F, Dusick JR, Fatemi N et al (2007) Graded repair of cranial base defects and cerebrospinal fluid leaks in transsphenoidal surgery. Neurosurgery 60:ONS1–ONS9

28. Leng LZ, Brown S, Anand VK et al (2008) "Gasket-seal" watertight closure in minimal-access endoscopic cranial base surgery. Neurosurgery 62:ONSE342–ONSE343

29. Cappabianca P, Cavallo LM, Colao A, de Divitiis E (2002) Surgical complications associated with the endoscopic endonasal transsphenoidal approach for pituitary adenomas. J Neurosurg 97:293–298

30. Cavallo LM, Briganti F, Cappabianca P et al (2004) Hemorrhagic vascular complications of endoscopic transsphenoidal surgery. Minim Invasive Neurosurg 47:145–150

31. Kassam A, Snyderman CH, Carrau RL et al (2005) Endoneurosurgical hemostasis techniques: lessons learned from 400 cases. Neurosurg Focus 19(1):E7

32. Dusick JR, Esposito F, Malkasian D et al (2007) Avoidance of carotid artery injuries in transsphenoidal surgery with the Doppler probe and micro-hook blades. Neurosurgery 60 (4 Suppl 2):322–328

Endonasal Endoscope-Assisted Microscopic Approach

15

Daniel F. Kelly, Felice Esposito and Dennis R. Malkasian

15.1 Introduction

Transsphenoidal surgery was first described a century ago by, among others, Schloffer, Cushing and Hirsch [1]. In the 1950s and 1960s, Dott, Guiot and Hardy began using the sublabial transsphenoidal route for removal of pituitary adenomas. With the advent of the operating microscope and the technique of selective adenomectomy as described by Hardy in the early 1970s, transsphenoidal surgery emerged into the modern microsurgical era [2–4]. Additional experience in the 1970s and early 1980s by Wilson, Weiss, Laws, and others, further improved the safety and efficacy of transsphenoidal surgery [5–13]. Subsequent modifications were developed to minimize mucosal trauma and patient discomfort associated with the sublabial approach [14–20], most notable of which was the direct endonasal approach first described by Griffith and Veerapan in 1987 [17] and later by Cooke and Jones in 1994 [15]. This approach, which requires minimal posterior nasal mucosal dissection and no turbinate removal, is now commonly used with the operating microscope and often with endoscopic assistance [15, 17, 21–26]. Although it provides a somewhat more restricted exposure than the sublabial approach and a slightly off-midline trajectory, these factors can be addressed and used to one's surgical advantage for tumor removal.

The evolution of the technique over the last decade, resulting largely from better instrumentation, surgical navigation and, perhaps most importantly, endoscopy [27–32], has lead to the extension of the approach beyond treating pituitary adenomas to the management of a variety of parasellar tumors [33–38]. In this chapter we describe the operative technique, a summary of pathologies treated, potential pitfalls and surgical complications.

15.2 Surgical Technique

15.2.1 Instrumentation

Given the narrow working space and requirement for visualization from the operating microscope, all instruments are as low-profile as possible with angled or bayoneted handles to minimize visual obstruction and to maximize instrument maneuverability. Thus, Cottle dissectors, microdissectors, ring curettes and microblades are on bayoneted handles. Similarly, microscissors, tumor grasping forceps (both straight and up-angled) are used in a single-shaft pistol-grip construct to minimize visual obstruction. High-speed drills and ultrasonic aspirators also are of the lowest possible diameter with angled handpieces. Endoscopic equipment includes 4-mm rigid endoscopes (18 cm in length) with 0, 30 and 45° angled lenses (Karl Storz, Tuttlingen, Germany). A microDoppler probe is also used in all cases to localize the cavernous carotid arteries prior to dural opening.

15.2.1.1 Modified Endonasal Specula

Two new trapezoidal specula with a short length (60 or 70 mm) have been designed, one with a trapezoidal up-

D.F. Kelly (✉)
Brain Tumor Center and Neuroscience Institute
John Wayne Cancer Institute at Saint John's Health Center
Santa Monica, CA, USA

ward-angled distal end and one with a trapezoidal downward-angled distal end (Mizuho-America, Beverly, MA) [30].

In contrast to the longer (70–90 mm), oval-shaped endonasal specula, the new trapezoidal speculum blades have three segments. The first 20-mm segment is an oval shape similar to the traditional endonasal specula, to conform to the nostril and minimize mucosal trauma. The middle 20-mm segment is vertically oriented and the distal 20 to 30-mm segment transitions to a trapezoidal shape with either a 15° upward and outward orientation or a 15° downward and outward orientation for suprasellar and infrasellar access, respectively. Both the suprasellar and the infrasellar trapezoidal specula have a 5° outward flare at the distal end (Fig. 15.1a). Compared with the standard 70- and 80-mm endonasal oval-shaped specula in a transsphenoidal model, the 60-mm upward-angled trapezoidal speculum provides increased surface area exposure at the parasellar target and a wider angle of exposure, particularly in the superior parasellar area [30] (Fig. 15.1b). The trapezoidal design minimizes the problem of curved blade obstruction encountered with traditional oval specula. The combination of the distal trapezoidal construction and shorter length expands the working volume within the speculum, widens the degree of horizontal exposure in the parasellar space, and improves instrument maneuverability.

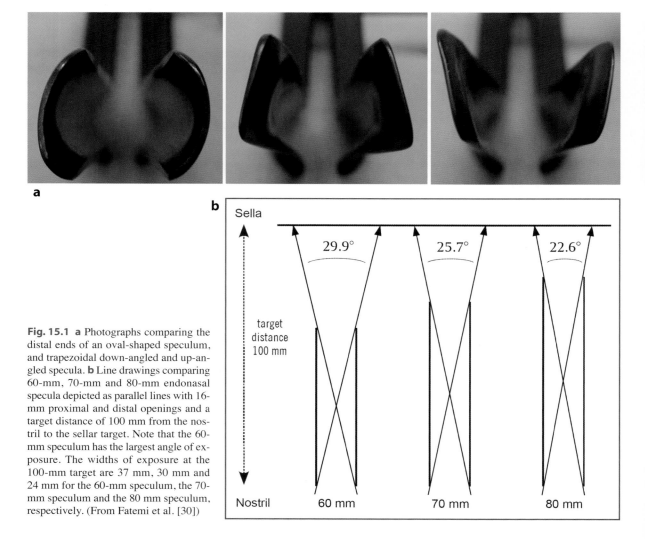

Fig. 15.1 a Photographs comparing the distal ends of an oval-shaped speculum, and trapezoidal down-angled and up-angled specula. **b** Line drawings comparing 60-mm, 70-mm and 80-mm endonasal specula depicted as parallel lines with 16-mm proximal and distal openings and a target distance of 100 mm from the nostril to the sellar target. Note that the 60-mm speculum has the largest angle of exposure. The widths of exposure at the 100-mm target are 37 mm, 30 mm and 24 mm for the 60-mm speculum, the 70-mm speculum and the 80 mm speculum, respectively. (From Fatemi et al. [30])

15.2.2 Patient Preparation, Positioning and Room Set-Up

Endonasal surgery is performed as originally described by Griffith and Veerapen with several modifications as described below [17, 33, 38]. Preoperative antibiotics (typically cefazolin) are given and continued for 24 hours. In patients with normal preoperative adrenal function or those with Cushing's disease, no perioperative glucocorticoids are administered [39]. Those with adrenal insufficiency or borderline adrenal function are given 100 mg of intravenous hydrocortisone.

Following induction of general anesthesia, the endotracheal tube emerges from the left corner of the mouth and the anesthesiologists and anesthesia equipment are positioned on the left side of the patient. An arterial line and Foley catheter are placed. The patient is placed supine with the head resting freely in the horseshoe head-holder and angled approximately 30° towards the left shoulder as originally described by Laws [40]. This arrangement allows the surgeon to stand comfortably on the patient's right side. The head is inclined in a neutral plane (0°) relative to the floor for sellar lesions; for suprasellar lesions, 10–15° of neck extension is used, and for infrasellar and clival lesions 10–15° of neck flexion is used.

Surgical navigation for trajectory guidance is recommended for all endonasal cases. Although C-arm fluoroscopy is adequate for most pituitary adenomas and Rathke's cleft cysts, in more recent years, frameless surgical navigation (VectorVision cranial; BrainLab, Westchester, IL) has been used for all cases. The perinasal and right lower abdominal areas are sterilely prepped and draped. No nasal mucosal decongestants are used.

15.2.3 Nasal Portion and Sphenoidotomy

The initial portion of the procedure is performed with the operating microscope and a hand-held speculum. The nostril chosen for the approach is based largely upon tumor location as defined by the patient's preoperative MRI scan. For tumors projecting more to one side of the sella, the contralateral nostril is used, given that exposure across the midline to the contralateral sella and cavernous sinus area is consistently wider than to the ipsilateral side. This rule applies even in the vast majority of patients with marked septal deviations. In patients with relatively midline tumors, the right nostril is typically chosen because the surgeon stands on the patient's right side and this will afford a more comfortable operating position for the surgeon. Although a relaxing alar incision was used in a small minority (<5%) of cases in our early experience, given the availability of smaller and thinner specula, it is no longer necessary.

The approach is begun with a hand-held speculum being passed into the anterior nostril to identify the inferior and middle turbinates. The speculum is then gently passed along the trajectory of the middle turbinate. Care should be taken to minimize trauma to the anterior and midnasal septum as well as the turbinates. The speculum blades gently displace the middle turbinate laterally and pass further into the nasal cavity to expose the junction of the keel of the sphenoid and the posterior nasal septum. After confirming the correct trajectory to the sella with fluoroscopy or surgical navigation, the posterior septal mucosa is cauterized with a bipolar in a vertical swath and a vertical mucosal incision is made extending for approximately 2 cm with a Cottle elevator. The mucosa is elevated and reflected laterally to expose the midline keel of the sphenoid bone and ipsilateral sphenoid ostium, which is typically superior–lateral to the equator of the keel at the 10 o'clock or 2 o'clock position. The posterior nasal septum is then displaced off the midline by the distal tips of the hand-held speculum to expose the contralateral side of the keel. The Cottle elevator is used to further reflect this contralateral mucosa to expose the other sphenoid ostium.

Once the sphenoid keel and ostia are exposed, the hand-held speculum is removed and replaced by a self-retaining endonasal speculum, typically 60–70 mm in length (Mizuho America). Alternatively, the hand-held speculum can act as a sleeve for the self-retaining endonasal speculum. After the endonasal speculum is placed, the two halves of the hand-held speculum are removed in two separate pieces to minimize mucosal trauma. The distal speculum blades should straddle the sphenoid keel and the nasal end of the speculum should be flush with the nostril. The sphenoid keel should be clearly exposed bilaterally with the ostia seen at approximately 10 o'clock and 2 o'clock within the circumference of the speculum. If the ostia are seen higher than this, the speculum trajectory is likely too inferior and aiming under the sella which can be confirmed with surgical navigation.

A wide sphenoidotomy is then performed with pituitary and Kerrison rongeurs. Sphenoid bone and mucosal removal should extend beyond the lateral edges of the ostia bilaterally and allow visualization of the

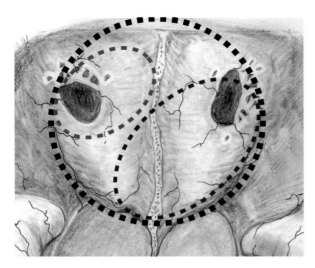

Fig. 15.2 Illustration of the sphenoid keel showing the optimal sphenoidotomy (black opening) needed to achieve adequate access into the sphenoid sinus and to most sellar lesions. The red and blue oval openings represent suboptimal and restricted sphenoidotomies seen in patients undergoing reoperation. (From Mattozo et al. [37])

Mucosa over the sella is removed, but the remaining sphenoid sinus mucosa is left undisturbed. The bony sellar face is then removed from cavernous sinus to cavernous sinus and from the sellar floor inferiorly to the tuberculum sella superiorly with a Kerrison rongeur or in some instances a high-speed diamond bit drill. In patients with large invasive tumors, the sellar bone may be markedly thinned or absent and tumor may be directly under mucosa or under attenuated or absent sellar dura.

15.2.5 Cavernous Carotid Localization

After adequate sellar bone removal and before dural opening, a bayoneted microDoppler probe is used to insonate for the cavernous carotid arteries bilaterally. Suitable probes include the 10-MHz ES-100X MiniDop with NRP-10H bayonet probe (Koven, St. Louis, MO) or the 20-MHz Surgical Doppler (Mizuho America, Beverly, MA). As previously described, the probe is placed initially at the edge of the bony opening

tuberculum sella and sellar floor. Given that the spheno-palatine arteries run in the posterior inferior nasal mucosa at a position of approximately 8 o'clock and 4 o'clock (Fig. 15.2), it is best to displace this mucosa laterally with the speculum or to cauterize it prior to removing it to avoid injuring the artery with a Kerrison or pituitary rongeur. This bleeding, however, can be stopped relatively easily with bipolar or monopolar cautery.

15.2.4 Sellar Exposure

After the sphenoidotomy is completed, the face of the sella turcica is identified. It is important at this point to correlate the intraoperative view of any intrasphenoidal bony septations with septations seen on the patient's preoperative MRI scan. Particular note should be made on the coronal images of where these septations reach the posterior wall of the sphenoid sinus relative to the carotid arteries, pituitary gland and tumor, and on sagittal views where such septations reach the planum or sella. Septations that end on the sellar face are removed with a rongeur down to the sella; those that end over a carotid artery should be removed with care and excessive torque on the bone fragments should be avoided.

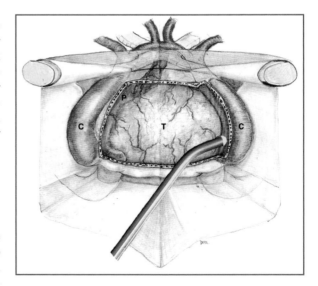

Fig. 15.3 Illustration showing a right endonasal view of the sella containing a macroadenoma that projects more to the left with the normal gland compressed along the right side of the sella. The sellar bone has been removed and, as is often the case, removal of the contralateral bone on the left is somewhat more extensive than on the right, leaving the medial edge of the left cavernous internal carotid artery exposed. The microDoppler probe is being used to localize the left cavernous internal carotid artery and to guide the appropriate location for dural opening (*C* cavernous internal carotid artery, *P* pituitary gland, *T* tumor). (From Dusick et al. [29])

at 90° to the dura [29]. If faint or no audible flow is present, the probe is angled more laterally aiming under the bone edge, and in most cases, the carotid flow will become louder (Fig. 15.3). The probe is then moved superiorly and inferiorly to further determine the course of the carotid which typically courses more medially in the superior sellar area. In most patients, the carotids have their most medial course superiorly near the tuberculum sella just before they pass through the dural ring to enter the subarachnoid space. If no Doppler flow is evident, then additional bone can be removed laterally to maximize sellar exposure. If audible flow is still not evident, consideration should be given to whether there is a technical problem with the probe, which can occur on occasion.

15.2.6 Dural Opening

A wide sellar dural is opening is performed with a straight microblade (Mizuho America) in a U-shaped fashion, avoiding the area of greatest audible Doppler flow [29]. Ideally, the initial dural opening should not transgress the pituitary gland or adenoma. After the ini-

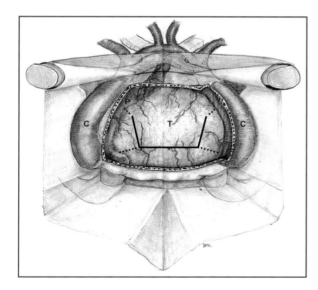

Fig. 15.4 Illustration showing the initial sellar dural opening in a U-shaped fashion (*solid line*) which is performed with a straight microblade as shown in Fig. 15.5, and the subsequent lateral dural openings (*dashed lines*) that may be utilized for additional exposure, and which should be performed with a right-angled microhook blade or angled microscissors (*C* cavernous internal carotid artery, *P* pituitary gland, *T* tumor). (From Dusick et al. [29])

tial opening, angled microdissectors are used to separate the dura from the underlying tumor and pituitary gland. The dural opening is then enlarged superiorly, inferiorly and laterally as needed with the use of a right-angle microhook blade or curved microscissors, which allow the cutting force of the blade to be directed away from the sellar and cavernous sinus structures [29] (Fig. 15.4). Care should be taken not to extend the dural opening too far superiorly in patients with microadenomas who often have a shallow sella and low-lying diaphragma sellae; such an opening can result in an early CSF leak. Laterally, the opening should generally extend to within 1–2 mm of the medial wall of the cavernous sinus. Low pressure cavernous sinus venous bleeding is generally easily controlled using Surgifoam (Ethicon, Johnson & Johnson Co., Piscataway, NJ) or Gelfoam (Pfizer, New York, NY) as needed.

15.2.7 Adenoma Removal

A selective and complete adenomectomy with preservation or improvement of pituitary gland function should be the goal in patients undergoing adenoma removal. In many instances, the tumor pseudocapsule can be identified and a plane established between the adenoma and normal gland. Using microdissectors, irrigation and gentle traction on the pseudocapsule, such adenomas can often be removed completely with preservation of the pseudocapsule as described by Oldfield and Vortmeyer [41]. However, many if not most large macroadenomas are quite soft and require initial internal debulking with ring curettes and suction. After so doing, the tumor "rind" with an intact pseudocapsule can be gently separated away from the normal gland and diaphragma sellae. For the occasional firm or rubbery adenoma, initial debulking with curved and straight pistol-grip microscissors may be needed. Adenomas with suprasellar extension should be debulked inferiorly first, followed by removal of the suprasellar component. This sequence allows the suprasellar tumor to in part deliver itself from above and may minimize the likelihood of causing an early CSF leak. For large macroadenomas, it is essential to confirm descent of the diaphragma sellae as an indication that a complete tumor removal has been accomplished. Probing the folds of the diaphragma with 45° and 90° up-angled ring curettes bilaterally, posteriorly and anteriorly will help dislodge residual tumor in these areas. To further encourage downward descent of the suprasellar tumor, the anesthesiologist can induce a Valsalva maneuver to transiently increase intracranial pressure.

Since most macroadenomas, even with a large suprasellar extension, are contained by a thinned but largely intact diaphragma sellae, the diaphragma sellae should completely invert and fall into the enlarged sella once complete tumor removal is accomplished. A useful check for assessing completeness of removal of such suprasellar adenomas comes from reviewing the preoperative sagittal MRI scan. If an imaginary line is drawn from the planum across the tumor to the posterior dorsum sella (where the diaphragma has its points of attachment), the volume of suprasellar tumor seen on the MRI scan above this line should correspond to the volume created by the complete inversion of the diaphragma into the sellar space seen at surgery. If this "mirror image" descent of the diaphragma sellae is not seen intraoperatively and only a partial descent of the diaphragma is noted, residual tumor is likely present.

For tumors with obvious or possible cavernous sinus invasion, one should attempt to visualize the medial cavernous sinus wall. A microscopic view of the cavernous sinus contralateral to the nostril of approach can often be achieved provided enough lateral sellar bone has been removed and a short endonasal speculum (60–70 mm) is in position. Under direct visualization, in some instances, what appeared to be cavernous sinus invasion on the MRI scan may only be tumor compression of the medial cavernous sinus wall [42, 43]. However, in many cases, after the sellar tumor has been removed, a defect in the medial cavernous sinus wall is seen. Tumor in the medial cavernous sinus can often be removed or at least effectively debulked using gentle suction and angled ring curettes which have smooth outer edges. Given the potential for injury to the cavernous carotid and the abducens nerve lateral to the carotid, aggressive curetting or grasping of tumor tissue along or lateral to the carotid artery should be avoided.

15.2.8 Endoscopic Assistance to Maximize Tumor Removal

Once tumor removal is as complete as possible with the microscope, the 0°, 30° and 45° angled endoscopes can be utilized to further assess for residual tumor, particularly in patients with macroadenomas extending into the suprasellar or cavernous sinus regions. This endoscopic "look" is especially helpful where the diaphragma sellae may not have descended fully into the

sella and in extended approach procedures for nonadenomatous lesions as described below. In the majority of such cases, the endoscope will reveal additional suprasellar tumor hindering a full descent of the diaphragma. Removal of such tumor remnants can often be performed directly with the endoscope using angled suctions, tumor grasping forceps or ring curettes, or with microscopic visualization and angled ring curettes. Similarly, endoscopic visualization of the medial cavernous sinus will often allow additional tumor to be removed that was not visualized or inaccessible with the operating microscope.

Endoscopic visualization and tumor removal is best performed with a three-hand technique in which the assistant holds and drives the endoscope and the surgeon holds the suction and a ring curette or tumor grasping forceps. Alternatively, one can use a fixed endoscope holder, but this provides less maneuverability and flexibility compared with a surgical assistant. The endonasal speculum can also be removed allowing a binostril approach; the endoscope can then be placed in one nostril and the working instruments in the opposite nostril, further reducing instrument conflict and crowding.

15.2.9 Extended Approach Modifications

Several important modifications are employed for reaching suprasellar, infrasellar and cavernous sinus lesions [30, 33, 36]. Surgical navigation and endoscopy is recommended in all such cases. To maximize maneuverability of the endoscope and other instruments, it is important to perform a wider and taller sphenoidotomy than for isolated sellar lesions; the sphenoidotomy should extend to the ethmoid roof superiorly and to the level of the floor of the sphenoid sinus inferiorly. A short (60 mm) up-angled or down-angled trapezoidal speculum is used to provide greater suprasellar or infrasellar exposure and to facilitate use of the endoscope [30]. To gain full advantage of these short specula, 1 to 2 cm of posterior nasal septum and all lateral obstructing bone or soft tissue along the keel is also removed.

15.2.9.1 Suprasellar and Planum Lesions

With increasing experience, the endonasal approach can be used to remove a variety of nonadenomatous suprasellar tumors such as craniopharyngiomas (particularly those in the retrochiasmal space), supraglandular Rathke's cleft cysts and smaller tuberculum sella meningiomas (under 30–35 mm in diameter and without far lateral extension). For such tumors, the patient is positioned with neck extension of 10–15° from neutral which affords a more comfortable operating position for the surgeon. As previously described [33], a low-profile high-speed drill (Micromax; Anspach, Palm Beach Gardens, FL) with a 2- or 3-mm diamond bit is used to remove the tuberculum sella and posterior planum. Care should be taken not to extend the bony opening too far laterally at the level of the optic canals which are the width-limiting structures at this level. Most of these lesions are more fibrous, rubbery, or partially calcified, and require sharp dissection with curved and straight microscissors along arachnoid planes. In patients with intact pituitary function, preservation of function is typically possible in those with supraglandular Rathke's cleft cysts and tuberculum sellae meningiomas, but is often not possible in patients with craniopharyngiomas, particularly those that engulf the pituitary stalk [44]. After tumor debulking, the tumor capsule is dissected away from arachnoid attachments using sharp dissection and gentle traction. Tumor remnants that are densely adherent to the infundibulum, the optic apparatus or perforating vessels from the supraclinoid carotid or anterior cerebral complex should be left behind to avoid new neurological or hormonal deficits.

15.2.9.2 Clival Lesions and Cavernous Sinus Lesions

Given that most clival chordomas have their epicenter medial to the cavernous carotid arteries, they can typically be removed or debulked through an endonasal approach. As we recently described, to remove such chordomas in the infrasellar and cavernous sinus regions, a wide sphenoidotomy is carried to the floor of the sphenoid sinus [36]. A short (60-mm) down-angled endonasal trapezoidal speculum is used as the working channel. Given the tendency of clival chordomas to distort the course of the petrous, vertical and cavernous portions of the carotid arteries, the microDoppler probe and surgical navigation are used to help localize these vessels before and during tumor removal. Given the invasive nature of clival chordomas, complete microscopic tumor removal is rarely possible. However, in the presence of intradural chordoma extension, the dura should be opened further to maximize tumor removal under both microscopic and endoscopic visualization [36].

For removal of tumors with extensive cavernous sinus invasion such as invasive pituitary adenomas or clival chordomas, one can approach these lesions from the contralateral nostril or from the ipsilateral nostril after resecting the ipsilateral middle turbinate. By removing the middle turbinate, the lateral speculum blade can expand more widely, allowing a greater removal of the ipsilateral sphenoid keel and providing direct cavernous sinus exposure lateral to the ipsilateral cavernous carotid artery. For tumors with extensive bilateral involvement, a binostril approach can be used. For descriptions of the removal of other tumor types such as Rathke's cleft cysts, sphenoid sinus carcinomas and intradural retroclival epidermoid tumors reference should be made to our recent publications [33, 35, 45].

15.2.10 Intrasellar Hemostasis

After tumor removal, hemostasis is obtained with hemostatic agents including Surgifoam (Ethicon, Johnson & Johnson Co., Piscataway, NJ) and full-strength hydrogen peroxide. The peroxide is irrigated directly into the sphenoid sinus and sella for up to 5 minutes. Its use appears safe from the standpoint of pituitary hormonal function as we have recently demonstrated, and it may have additional tumoricidal effects on residual microscopic foci of adenoma [46]. However, it should not be used if there is a large diaphragmatic defect present which would allow it to track into the subarachnoid space. In cases in which there is persistent oozing, one should further inspect the sella with the endoscope to look for residual tumor. Of six patients with postoperative hematomas in our series requiring a return to the operating room, four (67%) were patients with a large macroadenoma (30 mm or greater in maximal diameter) who in retrospect had residual tumor remnants left at the initial operation; these remnants presumably continued to ooze, prompting urgent reoperation within 12 hours of the first surgery.

15.2.11 Skull Base Reconstruction and CSF Leak Repair

As recently described [47], skull base reconstruction and CSF leak repair are tailored to the size of the CSF leak and bony and dural defect. Prior to reconstruction, an assessment of the size of diaphragmatic defect is performed. If no obvious defect is seen, a Valsalva maneuver is induced to help visualize an occult or small (grade 1) CSF leak emanating through a small diaphragmatic defect.

All repairs involve the use of collagen sponge (Duragen, Helistat or Instat), as part of the repair which acts as a scaffolding for fibroblast in-growth and a vascularized dural replacement [48–51].

In patients with no CSF leak (grade 0), a single layer of minimally moistened collagen sponge placed over the exposed diaphragma sellae, pituitary gland and sellar dura is typically used as the only repair material. For most small (grade 1) CSF leaks, the repair includes intrasellar collagen sponge with an intrasellar, extradural buttress of titanium mesh or Medpor TSI (transsphenoidal sellar implant; Porex Corporation, Fairburn, GA) and a second outer layer of collagen

placed over the buttress and adjacent sellar and sphenoid bone. The repair is typically held in position with a small amount of tissue glue (BioGlue or DuraSeal). For medium (grade 2) CSF leaks or grade 1 leaks with a large intrasellar dead space, the repair includes an intrasellar abdominal fat graft, a layer of collagen sponge followed by a buttress of titanium mesh or a Medpor plate placed in the intrasellar extradural space. Additional fat is typically placed over the sella followed by another layer of collagen; the construct is held in position with tissue glue.

In some recent cases of grade 1 and 2 leaks, no buttress has been used, and instead the repair with collagen sponge with or without a fat graft has been reinforced only with tissue glue which is itself relatively rigid.

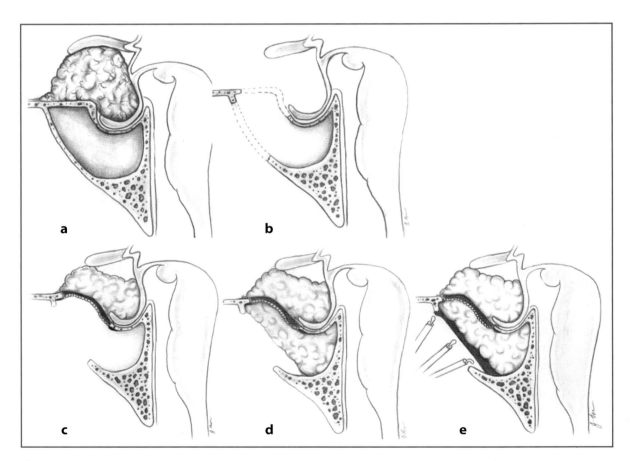

Fig. 15.5 Grade 3 repair of the skull-base defect after tumor removal: **a** tuberculum sellae meningioma; **b** after tumor removal and before repair; **c** intrasellar and suprasellar fat is placed followed by a layer of collagen sponge (*red*) placed over the fat; a titanium mesh buttress is placed in the intrasellar extradural space, wedged inferiorly into the bony lip of the sella and wedged superiorly into the bony defect of the posterior planum sphenoidale; **d** additional fat is placed over the mesh in the sphenoid sinus; **e** this is followed by another layer of collagen sponge then tissue glue. (From Esposito et al. [47])

Such patients are also placed on Diamox (acetazo-lamide) 250 mg every 8 hours for 48 hours after surgery to reduce CSF production. Although this is anecdotal, to date, we have had no failures with this more simplified repair method. To further assess the adequacy of the repair, prior to placing tissue glue, the anesthesiologist is asked to perform a Valsalva maneuver to raise the patient's intracranial pressure; should there be CSF streaming around the repair or movement of the buttress, the repair should be revised.

For large (grade 3) defects, typically seen with extended suprasellar or transclival approaches, the repair construct is similar to that for the grade 2 repair, and a lumbar drain for CSF diversion is also placed for 48 hours (Fig. 15.5). Grade 3 leaks, however, are uncommon after adenoma removal, unless they are extensively invasive above the diaphragma sellae. It is important to note that use of tissue glue in this repair paradigm is not for stopping egress of CSF per se, but more to prevent migration of the construct materials (fat and collagen) away from the sella [52].

15.2.12 Nasal Closure

Once sellar reconstruction is complete, the endonasal speculum is removed and the hand-held speculum is again used to explore both the operated and nonoperated nasal cavities with the microscope. In most instances, there may be mild venous oozing from along the nasal septum, inferior turbinate or middle turbinate. Such mucosal bleeding is stopped with Surgifoam or bipolar cautery. Nasal hemostasis should be relatively complete to minimize the amount of blood the patient will swallow during the first few hours after surgery which can otherwise result in nausea and vomiting. The middle turbinate on the side of the approach, which is out-fractured by the speculum at the start of the procedure, is medialized toward the nasal septum; this minimizes the chance of development of a maxillary sinus mucocele.

Finally, using the hand-held speculum in the contralateral nostril, the nasal septum is returned to the midline. No nasal packing is used; a small gauze "moustache" dressing is placed over the nostrils. To minimize the likelihood of a postoperative CSF leak, nasal epistaxis or intrasellar bleeding, excessive coughing on the endotracheal tube should be avoided during extubation and blood pressure should be carefully monitored and controlled in the early postoperative period.

15.2.13 Postoperative Care

Most patients undergoing adenoma or Rathke's cleft cyst removal are admitted to a non-ICU bed and their arterial line is removed before leaving the recovery room. For the first postoperative night, patients are given a humidified face tent and decongestants are available upon request. Saline nasal spray is provided for a week after surgery and used based on patient preference. The Foley catheter is removed on the morning of postoperative day one and patients are encouraged to ambulate.

All patients with pituitary-related lesions are followed in-hospital by an endocrinologist. Patients are monitored for diabetes insipidus based on urine output and urine specific gravity. Adrenal function is monitored by measuring a.m. serum cortisol and ACTH levels on the mornings of postoperative days one and two. For patients with acromegaly, a prolactinoma or Cushing's disease, growth hormone, prolactin and cortisol/ACTH levels are followed on postoperative days one and two to document early remission based on subnormal hormone levels [38, 39]. Most patients are discharged home on postoperative day 2 and have a serum sodium level checked on postoperative day 4 or 5 to monitor for delayed hyponatremia [53, 54]. The first postoperative visit is at 2 to 3 weeks after surgery with a follow-up visit at 3 months after surgery, including a complete pituitary hormonal evaluation. An early postoperative MRI or CT scan is typically performed within 2 days of surgery for patients with a macroadenoma or another larger tumor. The next follow-up MRI scan is usually performed at 3 months after surgery.

15.3 Discussion

The major advantage of the direct endonasal approach over the sublabial transsphenoidal approach is the obviation of mucosal tunnels and nasal packing, resulting in a rapid and less-painful patient recovery [34, 38]. The major disadvantage of this approach is restricted visualization and maneuverability imposed by the endonasal speculum and the tunnel vision of the operating microscope. To minimize these limitations and to maximize parasellar access, several strategies are recommended. These include:

1. Approach from the nostril contralateral to the greatest degree of tumor extension.
2. Perform a wide sphenoidotomy that incorporates both sphenoid ostia.

3. Use a short endonasal speculum (60–70 mm) to maximize maneuverability and visualization.

4. Perform a wide sellar bony opening that extends to the edges of the cavernous sinus bilaterally and to the tuberculum sella superiorly.

5. Confirm adequate but safe lateral bony removal with the microDoppler or surgical navigation prior to dural opening.

6. Use endoscopy to insure as complete and safe a removal as possible, particularly for tumors extending beyond the confines of the sella.

Regarding the endonasal approach with the operating microscope versus the purely endoscopic approach, three issues are important to consider: nasal recovery, removal of functional adenomas, and removal of suprasellar, cavernous sinus or clival lesions. Regarding nasal recovery, based on our experience and other reports, there appears to be little difference in the degree of rhinological trauma and patient recovery after the direct endonasal approach with the operating microscope versus the purely endoscopic approach [34, 38, 55, 56]. In both instances, patients typically recover rapidly and relatively completely with few long-term nasal complaints.

Regarding completeness of tumor removal of a hormonally active adenoma with the endoscope versus the microscope, the optimal approach is unclear. The success rate of the surgery in such cases is at least in part heavily dependent upon the skill and experience of the surgeon, regardless of technique. For now, removal of functional microadenomas or small macroadenomas, the microscopic approach remains the gold-standard with numerous publications indicating long-term remission rates of 80–95% for patients with microprolactinomas, Cushing's disease and acromegaly [41, 57–

60]. There are fewer data available for the purely endoscopic approach, but it appears that remission rates with this approach are improving, particularly at centers with a focused interest in endoscopy [61–64]. It is likely that in experienced hands, the purely endoscopic approach will rival the microscopic approach in terms of remission rates for functional pituitary adenomas.

Regarding removal of parasellar tumors such as craniopharyngiomas, tuberculum sellae meningiomas, clival chordomas and invasive adenomas, it is increasingly clear that the endoscope is essential for maximizing safe tumor removal [36, 63, 65–72]. Purely microscopic removal of such tumors without endoscopic assistance is not recommended.

15.4 Conclusion

In summary, the direct endonasal approach with the operating microscope provides an effective minimally invasive route for removal of parasellar tumors. The use of this approach for removal of more challenging tumors such craniopharyngiomas, tuberculum sellae meningiomas and clival chordomas should be attempted only after gaining considerable experience with simpler sellar lesions such as adenomas and Rathke's cleft cysts, and should be done with endoscopic assistance. For those using the extended endonasal approach, the microscopic surgeon must be willing to take advantage of the expanded visualization provided by the endoscope and face the learning curve that goes with it in a cautious and incremental way that insures patient safety.

References

1. Cohen-Gadol AA, Liu JK, Laws ER Jr (2005) Cushing's first case of transsphenoidal surgery: the launch of the pituitary surgery era. J Neurosurg 103:570–574
2. Hardy J (1969) Transphenoidal microsurgery of the normal and pathological pituitary. Clin Neurosurg 16:185–217
3. Liu JK, Das K, Weiss MH et al (2001) The history and evolution of transsphenoidal surgery. J Neurosurg 95:1083–1096
4. McDonald TJ, Laws ER (1982) Historical aspects of the management of pituitary disorders with emphasis on transsphenoidal surgery. In: Laws E, Randall R, Kern E (eds) Management of pituitary adenomas and related lesions: with emphasis on transsphenoidal microsurgery. Appleton-Century-Crofts, New York, pp 1–13

5. Black PM, Zervas NT, Candia GL (1987) Incidence and management of complications of transsphenoidal operation for pituitary adenomas. Neurosurgery 20:920–924
6. Ciric I, Mikhael M, Stafford T et al (1983) Transsphenoidal microsurgery of pituitary macroadenomas with long-term follow-up results. J Neurosurg 59:395–401
7. Ebersold MJ, Quast LM, Laws ER Jr et al (1986) Long-term results in transsphenoidal removal of nonfunctioning pituitary adenomas. J Neurosurg 64:713–719
8. Fahlbusch R, Buchfelder M, Muller OA (1986) Transsphenoidal surgery for Cushing's disease. J R Soc Med 79:262–9
9. Kern EB, Pearson BW, McDonald TJ, Laws ER Jr (1979) The transseptal approach to lesions of the pituitary and parasellar regions. Laryngoscope 89:1–34
10. Randall RV, Laws ER Jr, Abboud CF et al (1983) Transsphenoidal microsurgical treatment of prolactin-producing pitu-

itary adenomas. Results in 100 patients. Mayo Clin Proc 58:108–121

11. Weiss MH (1977) Surgery of the pituitary gland. Bull Los Angeles Neurol Soc 42:190–200

12. Wilson CB (1984) A decade of pituitary microsurgery. The Herbert Olivecrona lecture. J Neurosurg 61:814–833

13. Wilson CB, Dempsey LC (1978) Transsphenoidal microsurgical removal of 250 pituitary adenomas. J Neurosurg 48:13–22

14. Ciric I, Ragin A, Baumgartner C, Pierce D (1997) Complications of transsphenoidal surgery: results of a national survey, review of the literature, and personal experience. Neurosurgery 40:225–236

15. Cooke RS, Jones RA (1994) Experience with the direct transnasal transsphenoidal approach to the pituitary fossa. Br J Neurosurg 8:193–196

16. Eisele DW, Flint PW, Janas JD et al (1988) The sublabial transseptal transsphenoidal approach to sellar and parasellar lesions. Laryngoscope 98:1301–1308

17. Griffith HB, Veerapen R (1987) A direct transnasal approach to the sphenoid sinus. Technical note. J Neurosurg 66:140–142

18. Schoem SR, Khan A, Wilson WR, Laws ER (1997) Minimizing upper lip and incisor teeth paresthesias in approaches to transsphenoidal surgery. Otolaryngol Head Neck Surg 116:656–661

19. Sharma K, Tyagi I, Banerjee D et al (1996) Rhinological complications of sublabial transseptal transsphenoidal surgery for sellar and suprasellar lesions: prevention and management. Neurosurg Rev 19:163–167

20. Sherwen PJ, Patterson WJ, Griesdale DE (1986) Transseptal, transsphenoidal surgery: a subjective and objective analysis of results. J Otolaryngol 15:155–160

21. Badie B, Nguyen P, Preston JK (2000) Endoscopic-guided direct endonasal approach for pituitary surgery. Surg Neurol 53:168–172

22. Das K, Spencer W, Nwagwu CI et al (2001) Approaches to the sellar and parasellar region: anatomic comparison of endonasal-transsphenoidal, sublabial-transsphenoidal, and transethmoidal approaches. Neurol Res 23:51–54

23. Kawamata T, Iseki H, Ishizaki R, Hori T (2002) Minimally invasive endoscope-assisted endonasal trans-sphenoidal microsurgery for pituitary tumors: experience with 215 cases comparing with sublabial trans-sphenoidal approach. Neurol Res 24:259–265

24. Koren I, Hadar T, Rappaport ZH, Yaniv E (1999) Endoscopic transnasal transsphenoidal microsurgery versus the sublabial approach for the treatment of pituitary tumors: endonasal complications. Laryngoscope 109:1838–1840

25. Nasseri SS, Kasperbauer JL, Strome SE et al (2001) Endoscopic transnasal pituitary surgery: report on 180 cases. Am J Rhinol 15:281–287

26. Sheehan MT, Atkinson JL, Kasperbauer JL et al (1999) Preliminary comparison of the endoscopic transnasal vs the sublabial transseptal approach for clinically nonfunctioning pituitary macroadenomas. Mayo Clin Proc 74:661–670

27. Cavallo LM, Messina A, Cappabianca P et al (2005) Endoscopic endonasal surgery of the midline skull base: anatomical study and clinical considerations. Neurosurg Focus 19:E2

28. Cavallo LM, Prevedello D, Esposito F et al (2008) The role of the endoscope in the transsphenoidal management of cystic lesions of the sellar region. Neurosurg Rev 31:55–64

29. Dusick JR, Esposito F, Malkasian D, Kelly DF (2007) Avoidance of carotid artery injuries in transsphenoidal surgery with the Doppler probe and micro-hook blades. Neurosurgery 60:322–328

30. Fatemi N, Dusick JR, Malkasian D et al (2008) A short trapezoidal speculum for suprasellar and infrasellar exposure in endonasal transsphenoidal surgery. Neurosurgery 62(5 Suppl 2):ONS329–ONS330

31. Jagannathan J, Prevedello DM, Ayer VS et al (2006) Computer-assisted frameless stereotaxy in transsphenoidal surgery at a single institution: review of 176 cases. Neurosurg Focus 20:E9

32. Prevedello DM, Doglietto F, Jane JA Jr et al (2007) History of endoscopic skull base surgery: its evolution and current reality. J Neurosurg 107:206–213

33. Dusick JR, Esposito F, Kelly DF et al (2005) The extended direct endonasal transsphenoidal approach for nonadenomatous suprasellar tumors. J Neurosurg 102:832–841

34. Dusick JR, Esposito F, Mattozo CA et al (2006) Endonasal transsphenoidal surgery: the patient's perspective – survey results from 259 patients. Surg Neurol 65:332–341

35. Esposito F, Becker DP, Villablanca JP, Kelly DF (2005) Endonasal transsphenoidal transclival removal of prepontine epidermoid tumors: technical note. Neurosurgery 56:E443

36. Fatemi N, Dusick JR, Gorgulho AA et al (2008) Endonasal microscopic removal of clival chordomas. Surg Neurol 69:331–338

37. Mattozo CA, Dusick JR, Esposito F et al (2006) Suboptimal sphenoid and sellar exposure: a consistent finding in patients treated with repeat transsphenoidal surgery for residual endocrine-inactive macroadenomas. Neurosurgery 58:857–865

38. Zada G, Kelly DF, Cohan P et al (2003) Endonasal transsphenoidal approach for pituitary adenomas and other sellar lesions: an assessment of efficacy, safety, and patient impressions. J Neurosurg 98:350–358

39. Esposito F, Dusick JR, Cohan P et al (2006) Clinical review: early morning cortisol levels as a predictor of remission after transsphenoidal surgery for Cushing's disease. J Clin Endocrinol Metab 91:7–13

40. Laws ER (1995) Transsphenoidal approach to pituitary tumors. In: Schmidek H, Sweet W (eds) Operative neurosurgical techniques: indications, methods, and results, vol 1, 3rd edn. WB Saunders, Philadelphia, pp 283–292

41. Oldfield EH, Vortmeyer AO (2006) Development of a histological pseudocapsule and its use as a surgical capsule in the excision of pituitary tumors. J Neurosurg 104:7–19

42. Yokoyama S, Hirano H, Moroki K et al (2001) Are nonfunctioning pituitary adenomas extending into the cavernous sinus aggressive and/or invasive? Neurosurgery 49:857–862

43. Yoneoka Y, Watanabe N, Matsuzawa H et al (2008) Preoperative depiction of cavernous sinus invasion by pituitary macroadenoma using three-dimensional anisotropy contrast periodically rotated overlapping parallel lines with enhanced reconstruction imaging on a 3-tesla system. J Neurosurg 108:37–41

44. Dusick JR, Fatemi N, Mattozo CA et al (2008) Pituitary function after endonasal surgery for nonadenomatous

parasellar tumors: Rathke's cleft cysts, craniopharyngiomas, and meningiomas. Surg Neurol 70:482–490

45. Esposito F, Kelly DF, Vinters HV et al (2006) Primary sphenoid sinus neoplasms: a report of four cases with common clinical presentation treated with transsphenoidal surgery and adjuvant therapies. J Neurooncol 76:299–306

46. Mesiwala AH, Farrell L, Santiago P et al (2003) The effects of hydrogen peroxide on brain and brain tumors. Surg Neurol 59:398–407

47. Esposito F, Dusick JR, Fatemi N, Kelly DF (2007) Graded repair of cranial base defects and cerebrospinal fluid leaks in transsphenoidal surgery. Neurosurgery 60:295–303

48. Kelly DF, Oskouian RJ, Fineman I (2001) Collagen sponge repair of small cerebrospinal fluid leaks obviates tissue grafts and cerebrospinal fluid diversion after pituitary surgery. Neurosurgery 49:885–889

49. Kleinman HK, Klebe RJ, Martin GR (1981) Role of collagenous matrices in the adhesion and growth of cells. J Cell Biol 88:473–485

50. Narotam PK, Van Dellen JR, Bhoola K, Raidoo D (1993) Experimental evaluation of collagen sponge as a dural graft. Br J Neurosurg 7:635–641

51. Narotam PK, van Dellen JR, Bhoola KD (1995) A clinicopathological study of collagen sponge as a dural graft in neurosurgery. J Neurosurg 82:406–412

52. Dusick JR, Mattozo CA, Esposito F, Kelly DF (2006) BioGlue for prevention of postoperative cerebrospinal fluid leaks in transsphenoidal surgery: a case series. Surg Neurol 66:371–376

53. Kelly DF, Laws ER Jr, Fossett D (1995) Delayed hyponatremia after transsphenoidal surgery for pituitary adenoma. Report of nine cases. J Neurosurg 83:363–367

54. Zada G, Liu CY, Fishback D et al (2007) Recognition and management of delayed hyponatremia following transsphenoidal pituitary surgery. J Neurosurg 106:66–71

55. Cappabianca P, Cavallo LM, Colao A, de Divitiis E (2002) Surgical complications associated with the endoscopic endonasal transsphenoidal approach for pituitary adenomas. J Neurosurg 97:293–298

56. Cappabianca P, Cavallo LM, Colao A et al (2002) Endoscopic endonasal transsphenoidal approach: outcome analysis of 100 consecutive procedures. Minim Invasive Neurosurg 45:193–200

57. Chen JC, Amar AP, Choi S et al (2003) Transsphenoidal microsurgical treatment of Cushing disease: postoperative assessment of surgical efficacy by application of an overnight low-dose dexamethasone suppression test. J Neurosurg 98:967–973

58. Krieger MD, Couldwell WT, Weiss MH (2003) Assessment of long-term remission of acromegaly following surgery. J Neurosurg 98:719–724

59. Locatelli M, Vance ML, Laws ER (2005) Clinical review: the strategy of immediate reoperation for transsphenoidal surgery for Cushing's disease. J Clin Endocrinol Metab 90:5478–5482

60. Tyrrell JB, Lamborn KR, Hannegan LT et al (1999) Transsphenoidal microsurgical therapy of prolactinomas: initial outcomes and long-term results. Neurosurgery 44:254–261

61. Cappabianca P, Alfieri A, Colao A et al (1999) Endoscopic endonasal transsphenoidal approach: an additional reason in support of surgery in the management of pituitary lesions. Skull Base Surg 9:109–117

62. Cappabianca P, Cavallo LM, de Divitiis E (2004) Endoscopic endonasal transsphenoidal surgery. Neurosurgery 55:933–940

63. Frank G, Pasquini E (2006) Endoscopic endonasal cavernous sinus surgery, with special reference to pituitary adenomas. Front Horm Res 34:64–82

64. Netea-Maier RT, van Lindert EJ, den Heijer M et al (2006) Transsphenoidal pituitary surgery via the endoscopic technique: results in 35 consecutive patients with Cushing's disease. Eur J Endocrinol 154:675–684

65. de Divitiis E, Cavallo LM, Cappabianca P, Esposito F (2007) Extended endoscopic endonasal transsphenoidal approach for the removal of suprasellar tumors: part 2. Neurosurgery 60:46–58

66. Dumont AS, Kanter AS, Jane JA Jr, Laws ER Jr (2006) Extended transsphenoidal approach. Front Horm Res 34:29–45

67. Frank G, Pasquini E, Doglietto F et al (2006) The endoscopic extended transsphenoidal approach for craniopharyngiomas. Neurosurgery 59:ONS75–ONS83

68. Jane JA Jr, Han J, Prevedello DM et al (2005) Perspectives on endoscopic transsphenoidal surgery. Neurosurg Focus 19:E2

69. Kassam A, Snyderman CH, Mintz A et al (2005) Expanded endonasal approach: the rostrocaudal axis. Part I. Crista galli to the sella turcica. Neurosurg Focus 19:E3

70. Kassam A, Thomas AJ, Snyderman C et al (2007) Fully endoscopic expanded endonasal approach treating skull base lesions in pediatric patients. J Neurosurg 106:75–86

71. Laufer I, Anand VK, Schwartz TH (2007) Endoscopic, endonasal extended transsphenoidal, transplanum transtuberculum approach for resection of suprasellar lesions. J Neurosurg 106:400–406

72. Laws ER, Kanter AS, Jane JA Jr, Dumont AS (2005) Extended transsphenoidal approach. J Neurosurg 102:825–827

Transsphenoidal Approaches: Microscopic

16

Ian F. Dunn and Edward R. Laws

16.1 Introduction

Shaped by the brilliant insight of individual surgeons and technological innovation, the microscopic transsphenoidal approach to the sellar and parasellar regions is a fascinating chronicle in surgical history whose evolution continues unabated. Indeed, although subtemporal, transfacial, and frontal transcranial routes were propounded at the turn of the 20th century, only the transsphenoidal route has endured as the preferred approach to the overwhelming majority of sellar and parasellar lesions.

Transsphenoidal approaches to the sella were preceded by transcranial surgical attempts to gain access to the region. Fedor Krause of Berlin described the details of a frontal transcranial approach to the sella in 1905; varying modifications of frontal and subtemporal approaches by such pioneering surgeons as Sir Victor Horsley, Walter Dandy, and Harvey Cushing followed [1]. The morbidity of these transcranial approaches, however, catalyzed the development of extracranial approaches to the sella. Schloffer reported the first transsphenoidal approach to the sella in 1907 [2], followed by von Eiselsberg [3] and Kocher [4]; their approaches required external rhinotomy incisions. Endonasal and sublabial approaches performed without a disfiguring rhinotomy incision were soon introduced by Hirsch [5] and Halstead [6], respectively, en route to Cushing's introduction of his sublabial submucosal transseptal approach [7]. Although Cushing famously abandoned transsphenoidal surgery in favor of transcranial techniques in 1927, transsphenoidal approaches were sustained and refined by Norman Dott, his trainee Gerard Guiot—who would introduce fluoroscopy—and Jules Hardy, whose titanic contributions included the introduction of the operating microscope and the concept of the microadenoma to transsphenoidal surgery [5].

Since its inception, the microscopic transsphenoidal approach has undergone several modifications: the sublabial approach has given way to primary endonasal techniques, which have become increasingly direct; frameless stereotaxy has been routinely adopted; and the corridors accessible through the transsphenoidal approach have been extended and, as reviewed elsewhere, the endoscope has added significantly to the armamentarium of the transsphenoidal surgeon [8]. Fundamentally, these are skull-base approaches emphasizing wide bony exposure, microsurgical techniques and microdissection.

In this chapter, we review the essential practical details of the microscopic transsphenoidal approaches with a focus on surgical technique, drawing on the personal series of over 5,000 transsphenoidal operations performed by the senior author (E.R.L.).

16.2 Special Considerations

Several variations of the microscopic transsphenoidal approach have been described. Among these are the transnasal and sublabial submucosal transseptal, transnasal septal displacement/septal pushover, and the direct sphenoidotomy [9, 10]. Preoperative considera-

I.F. Dunn (✉)
Dept of Neurosurgery, Brigham and Women's Hospital
Harvard Medical School, Boston, MA, USA

P. Cappabianca et al. (eds.), *Cranial, Craniofacial and Skull Base Surgery.*
© Springer-Verlag Italia 2010

tions in the microscopic transsphenoidal approach include anatomic and lesional characteristics which influence the choice of surgical corridor, along with more general considerations which apply to all transsphenoidal approaches. Anatomic factors of note include the size of the nose and nostril; the presence of septal deviation, lateral spurs, or perforation, and a history of septal surgery; the presence of ongoing sinus disease or infection; the size of the sphenoid sinus; and, germane to sublabial approaches, the presence of dentures, capped teeth, or root canal surgery involving the anterior incisors [11]. Any significant laterality in cavernous sinus or suprasellar tumor extension may influence which nostril is used for entry, or if any modifications of the transsphenoidal approach are made, as a "cross-court" approach in such lesions is sometimes preferred [12].

Other preoperative considerations aimed at maximizing the safety of the procedure and its potential complications include ensuring that adequate endovascular support is available in case of carotid artery injury [13] and that any image guidance platforms to be used are precise, accurate and fully functional.

16.3 Surgical Technique

16.3.1 General

The microscopic transsphenoidal technique has continued to evolve over the past three decades with a wide range of indications (Table 16.1). Sublabial approaches have largely been replaced by more direct transnasal approaches in most centers, with notable exceptions reviewed below. Common transnasal microscopic transsphenoidal approaches include the transseptal submucosal technique, the septal displacement ("septal pushover"), and the direct sphenoidotomy [11, 12, 14–17]. Essentially, the location of the initial incision within the nose and the resultant width of the sellar exposure distinguish these approaches. The most traditional of the endonasal approaches is the transseptal submucosal approach, initiated with a hemitransfixion incision made just inside the nose. In the septal pushover, the incision is made more posteriorly, at the junction of the osseous and cartilaginous septum. The direct sphenoidotomy is initiated even more posteriorly, at the rostrum of the sphenoid. Potential advantages of a deeper nasal incision include the avoidance of anterior septal complications and postoperative discomfort; disadvantages in-

Table 16.1 Lesions accessed through the transsphenoidal approach

Type of lesion
Tumors of adenohypophyseal origin
Pituitary adenoma
Pituitary adenoma–neuronal choristoma (pituitary adenoma–gangliocytoma)
Pituitary carcinoma
Tumors of neurohypophyseal origin
Granular cell tumor
Astrocytoma of posterior lobe or stalk, or both (rare)
Tumors of nonpituitary origin
Craniopharyngioma
Germ-cell tumors
Glioma (hypothalamic, optic nerve or chiasm, infundibulum)
Meningioma
Chordoma
Rare tumors of nonpituitary origin
Chondroma
Esthesioneuroblastoma
Giant-cell tumor of bone
Glomangioma
Hemangiopericytoma
Hemangioblastoma
Lipoma
Leiomyosarcoma
Lymphoma
Melanoma
Myxoma
Paraganglioma
Postirradiation neoplasms
Rhabdomyosarcoma
Sarcoma (chondrosarcoma, osteosarcoma, fibrosarcoma)
Schwannoma
Cysts, hamartomas, and malformations
Rathke's cleft cyst
Arachnoid cyst
Epidermoid cyst
Dermoid cyst
Hypothalamic hamartoma
Empty sella syndrome
Metastatic tumors
Carcinoma
Plasmacytoma
Lymphoma
Leukemia
Inflammatory conditions
Pyogenic infection or abscess
Granulomatous infections
Mucocele
Lymphocytic hypophysitis
Sarcoidosis
Langerhans cell histiocytosis
Giant-cell granuloma
Vascular lesions
Saccular aneurysm (intracavernous carotid, supraclinoid carotid, anterior communicating artery complex, basilar artery tip)
Cavernous angioma

clude a slightly diminished width of exposure and an off-midline trajectory.

Below, we review the practical aspects of these approaches, emphasizing patient positioning and preparation; adjunctive imaging; the technical aspects of the surgical approaches; and the concept of the extended transsphenoidal approach.

16.3.2 Patient Positioning

Patient positioning is critical in transsphenoidal surgery and is identical in the submucosal and endonasal variants. Important tenets are the adherence to a standard method of positioning to ensure recognition of the midline and to provide a comfortable and ergonomic position for the operating surgeon [15]. The patient is prepared so that the surgeon will stand to the supine patient's right, with the patient's head angled and body turned so that the surgeon is operating without leaning over to the right. To accomplish this, we place the patient with the right shoulder at the upper right-hand corner of the table to facilitate placement of the head in the Mayfield headrest (Fig. 16.1). We then elevate the thorax 25–30° while gently flexing the knees, confer-

ring a semirecumbent or lawn-chair position with the head above the heart to reduce venous pressure and to allow venous blood to drain from the sphenoid and sella. This reduction in venous bleeding is particularly important in patients with Cushing's disease and in surgery for microadenomas.

We next flex the head laterally 20–30° to the left with the left ear toward the left shoulder so that the patient is looking toward his or her right shoulder. Once laterally flexed, the head is positioned so that the surgeon's view into the nose aims toward the sella. A reliable way to achieve this in most patients is to ensure that the nasal dorsum is parallel to the floor (Fig. 16.1). The head can then either be supported by a Mayfield horseshoe headrest—having as its main advantage the ability to subtly manipulate the head position during surgery—or placed in rigid three-point fixation, which we do now routinely in order to employ frameless stereotactic image guidance during surgery [18–20]. We then tilt the bed slightly to the right to allow the surgeon to operate sitting or standing looking straight ahead as opposed to leaning over the patient. Tilting may also help when positioning patients with cervical spondylosis in whom lateral neck flexion is difficult [9, 15]. The right arm is then tucked away unobtrusively.

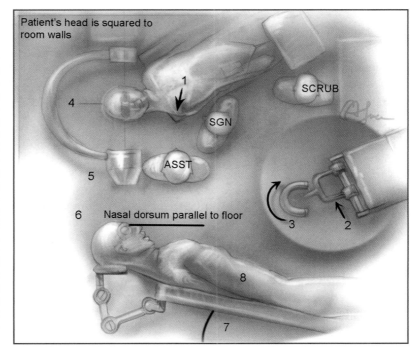

Fig. 16.1 Patient positioning and surgical team; our scrub now stands across the patient from the surgeon for ease of instrument passing. *1* The patient's right shoulder is positioned in the top right-hand corner of the operative table. *2* The headrest frame is positioned to the far left. *3* The horseshoe headrest is rotated so that the patient's head is oriented toward the surgeon. *4* and *5* The patient's head is oriented at a right angle to the walls of the room to facilitate lateral intraoperative videofluoroscopy on the draped patient. *6* The head is positioned so that the trajectory is toward the sella. This is most easily accomplished by positioning the neck such that the dorsum of the nose is parallel with the floor. *7* The beach-chair position is used with the table angled approximately 20°. *8* The patient's right hand is carefully positioned so that it is located unobtrusively under the buttocks. *SGN* surgeon, *ASST* assistant

Once the patient is positioned on the table and in the headrest, we move the operating room table so that the sides of the patient's head are parallel to the walls of the room. In addition to establishing an identical geometric sense for each case, this head positioning is especially useful for radiology technicians or other staff to gauge head position when aligning fluoroscopic C-arm machinery during surgery.

It should be recognized that some very accomplished pituitary surgeons utilize a modified cleft palate position for the patient, whose neck is extended, and stand at the head of the table with a direct downwards microscopic view of the sella.

16.3.3 Surgical Team Positioning

The assisting surgeon is to the left of the operating surgeon, viewing through the observer objective on the microscope (Fig. 16.1). The scrub nurse is positioned across the patient from the operating surgeon so that instruments are easily exchanged while the principal surgeon remains in the operative position. The anesthesia team is based at the foot of the patient. The microscope enters from the left of the surgeon, while the image guidance system may be positioned on the left side of the patient across from the surgeon.

16.3.4 Patient Preparation

Preparation for surgery comprises preparing the face, nares, and umbilical region; inserting a lumbar drain if indicated; and administering antibiotics and cortisol support if preoperative testing reveals steroid deficiency. We prepare the skin of the face with an aqueous antiseptic solution. To help minimize nasal mucosal bleeding during the approach, we apply topical vasoconstrictors and inject local anesthetic solution. We spray oxymetolazine (Afrin) into the nose before induction and then pack both nostrils with cotton pledgets soaked in 5% cocaine inserted with bayonets through a nasal speculum, and leave these in for 10–15 minutes. During this time, the remainder of the patient preparation is performed. We prepare the abdomen in the subumbilical region for a possible incision to obtain a small fat graft; the incision is usually made in the fold just below the umbilicus and is about 2 cm in length. For patients with lesions with large suprasellar exten-

sions which may be driven down by injecting air or saline intrathecally, a lumbar drain may be placed at this time.

Ordinarily one dose of a broad-spectrum antibiotic is given, and if the patient is deficient in cortisol prior to surgery, steroid support in the form of hydrocortisone, usually 100 mg intravenous Solu-Cortef, is given at the beginning of surgery. Cortisol support is continued as indicated in the postoperative period, but antibiotics are given ordinarily as just one dose unless the nose is packed for a prolonged period.

16.3.5 Adjunctive Navigation

16.3.5.1 Image Guidance

The most widely used intraoperative imaging device is the C-arm videofluoroscope. Most often, a lateral image confirms the appropriate trajectory to the sella turcica and is also used to confirm its superior and inferior confines. Knowing the superior and inferior limits of the sella turcica allows the surgeon to confirm adequate exposure and prevents unnecessary opening of the planum sphenoidale and cerebrospinal fluid leakage. The advantage of using a standard fluoroscope is its simplicity and accuracy. Its disadvantages are the radiation exposure and its inability to depict soft tissue anatomy, including the tumor and neurovascular structures [10].

The proximity of sellar and parasellar masses to the optic apparatus and carotid arteries demands absolute surgical precision in the approach to this region. The increasing sophistication of image-guidance platforms allowing highly accurate and precise instrument tracking on a coregistered preoperative magnetic resonance imaging (MRI) scan has influenced our and others' practices, and we now perform virtually every transsphenoidal operation with the aid of frameless stereotaxy. Several image guidance platforms are available which require coregistration of the patient's anatomy with a preoperative CT or MR image. The particular system we employ requires the fixation of a rigid arm to the Mayfield headrest, which we angle off to the left side of the patient's head. Its main utility is in the initial stages of the transsphenoidal approach to the sella, as such systems provide very accurate information regarding operative trajectory and adherence to the midline, and proximity to the sphenoid, sella, and carotids. The sagittal view is especially helpful in tracking the trajectory to the sphenoid and sellar face, while the coronal and axial views are useful in verifying proximity to the midline and helping to prevent errant entry into the cavernous sinus or carotid arteries [18, 19, 21].

While frameless systems rely on preoperatively acquired image data, intraoperative MRI (iMRI) systems providing real-time images have been used in transsphenoidal surgery [22–26]; their main benefit is in immediate assessment of the extent of resection, particularly in cases with suprasellar extension. One formidable barrier to the widespread use of iMRI is the tremendous outlay costs in its establishment [25, 27]. This, coupled with the rapid evolution of panoramic endoscopic technology, may conspire to confine iMRI-guided transsphenoidal surgery to select centers.

16.3.5.2 Doppler Probe

Another useful adjunct in an attempt to avoid cavernous carotid injury is a bayoneted microDoppler probe [22, 26] such as a 20-MHz surgical Doppler probe (Mizuho America, Beverly, MA). Although the absence of a reliable positive internal control has tempered its widespread use, it can still be a helpful tool in identifying the carotid arteries prior to incising the sellar dura and during removal of lateral portions of sellar lesions.

Tools such as this may be increasingly applicable as centers adopt more direct transsphenoidal approaches (e.g., septal pushover, direct sphenoidotomy) which tend to provide a surgical trajectory just off the midline, with a more restricted exposure. Moreover, the promulgation of extended endoscopic approaches—wherein wider sellar exposures are sought for an expanding range of cranial base lesions—may render the carotids more vulnerable. One may also choose to use an intraoperative Doppler probe when the preoperative studies demonstrate carotids with unusually medial courses.

16.3.6 Surgical Approaches

The transsphenoidal corridor is accessed by either a transnasal or a sublabial approach. Although the sublabial route was once the preferred approach to the sella, transnasal approaches have supplanted the sublabial approach for most transsphenoidal surgeons. Trends in transsphenoidal surgery have included a shift

towards endonasal approaches featuring increasingly direct approaches to the sphenoid. Below, we divide the microscopic transsphenoidal operation into distinct phases, emphasizing similarities and differences between approaches when necessary:

1. The nasal phase, from initial sublabial or endonasal incision to entry into the sphenoid sinus.
2. The sphenoid phase, from entry into the sphenoid sinus to the sellar dura.
3. The sellar phase, from opening of the sellar dura to lesion resection to establishment of hemostasis and preparation for closure.
4. Reconstruction and closure phase.

16.3.6.1 Nasal Phase

This phase in the operation comprises the surgical maneuvers required to establish a corridor to the sphenoid sinus. The nasal cavity may be entered directly (transnasal) or through a sublabial approach. Through either of these approaches, a submucosal transseptal approach may be used to approach the sphenoid. We also discuss the more direct transnasal approaches to the sphenoid, the transnasal septal displacement ("septal pushover") and direct sphenoidotomy.

Transnasal Submucosal Transseptal Approach

This approach requires considerable submucosal dissection, the main advantage of which is broad septal mobilization, a wide surgical corridor, and strict fidelity to the midline. Sinonasal complications and postoperative discomfort associated with the submucosal transseptal approaches and the refinement of more direct approaches to the sphenoid have lessened the popularity of submucosal transseptal approaches. The nasal packing usually required to prevent submucosal septal hematoma causes facial pain and headache in as many as 35% of patients, and the procedures can cause rhinological complaints including alveolar numbness, anosmia, saddle nose deformity, and nasal septal perforations [28–30].

To diminish bleeding during the submucosal dissection, we inject 10–20 cm3 of 0.5% xylocaine with 1:200,000 epinephrine along the inferior and lateral aspects of the nasal septum with an attempt to dissect the nasal mucosa away from the cartilaginous septum with the injection. The transseptal approach begins with a right-sided hemitransfixion incision in the right nostril with the columella retracted to the patient's left, facil-

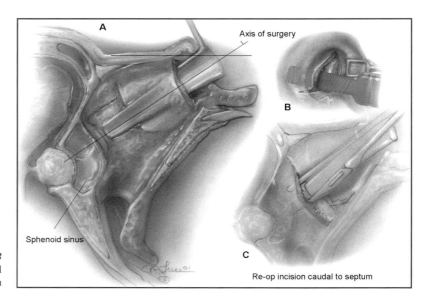

Fig. 16.2 Endonasal approaches. *A* and *B* submucosal endonasal approach, *C* septal displacement approach, *Re-op* reoperation

itating the dissection of the right anterior nasal mucosal tunnel away from the septum [9] (Fig. 16.2). The inferior border of the cartilaginous septum is exposed with sharp dissection, and one side of the septum is exposed submucosally with a combination of sharp and blunt dissection, thereby creating the anterior tunnel. The dissection continues posteriorly, elevating the nasal mucosa away from the cartilaginous septum back to the junction with the bony septum. A vertical incision is then made at this junction, and bilateral posterior submucosal tunnels are created on either side of the perpendicular plate of the ethmoid. The articulation of the cartilaginous septum with the maxilla is then dissected free, and the inferior mucosal tunnel on the opposite side is raised so that the cartilaginous septum can be displaced laterally without creating inferior mucosal tears. A self-retaining nasal speculum can then be introduced to straddle the perpendicular plate of the ethmoid, exposing the face of the sphenoid sinus. If the nostril is too small to accommodate a standard speculum, an inferior extension of the hemitransfixion incision within the alar ring or a relaxing right alotomy may be performed.

Sublabial Submucosal Transseptal Approach

This approach, used by Cushing and promulgated by Dott, Hardy, and Guiot [1, 31], has as its main advantages a wide surgical corridor and straight midline tra-

jectory, with the disadvantage of its complex surgical anatomy and potential complications of numbness of the upper lip and teeth. We tend to reserve the sublabial approach for patients with small nostrils, particularly children, or for massive tumors or extended approaches.

The sublabial approach begins with a transverse submucosal gingival sublabial incision from canine to canine and dissection from the maxillary ridge and the anterior nasal spine until the inferior aspect of the piriform aperture is exposed [9] (Fig. 16.3). Excessive cautery should be avoided as the upper teeth can be devitalized. Working from the lateral border medially, the two inferior nasal tunnels are created by dissecting the mucosa away from the superior surface of the hard palate. The caudal end of the nasal septum is carefully dissected and a right anterior tunnel is created along the right side of the nasal septum. With sharp dissection, the right anterior endonasal submucosal tunnel and the right inferior tunnels are connected, and the entire right side of the nsasal septum is exposed back to the perpendicular plate of the ethmoid. Using firm, blunt dissection along the right side of the base of the nasal septum, the cartilaginous portion of the septum is dislocated at its junction with the perpendicular plate of the ethmoid and vomer and is reflected to the left, and a left posterior mucosal tunnel is developed along the left side of the bony septum. At this point it should be possible to insert the transsphenoidal retractor, with care taken to place all tears in the nasal mucosa lateral

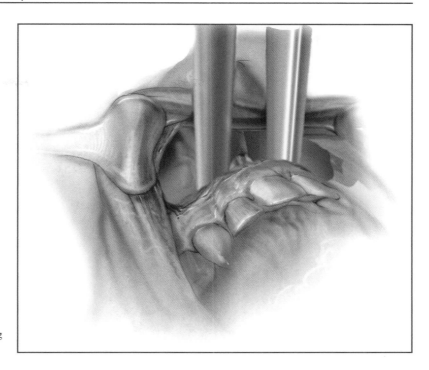

Fig. 16.3 Sublabial approach showing nasal speculum inserted

to the retractor blades. The turbinates will collapse as the retractor is opened. Once the retractor is in place, the submucosal dissection is carried up to the rostrum of the sphenoid, and the retractor is repositioned.

An alternative approach allows the surgeon to couple the ease of performing the submucosal dissection through an endonasal hemitransfixion incision with the wide exposure afforded by the sublabial approach. In this modification, the submucosal dissection can be performed first endonasally, followed by the sublabial incision, entering an already dissected nasal cavity [15].

Septal Displacement ("Septal Pushover")

In our practice, the transnasal septal displacement or "septal pushover" technique has replaced sublabial or transnasal submucosal transseptal approaches almost entirely. In place of the more traditional anteriorly placed hemitransfixion incision, we place an initial incision more posteriorly, at the junction of the bony and cartilaginous septum, to avoid extensive submucosal dissection along the anterior septum (Fig. 16.4). This approach was initially adopted for patients undergoing repeat transsphenoidal operations in which the nasal mucosa is often densely adherent and scarred to the

cartilaginous septum [16]. However, this approach provides a rapid exposure of the sphenoid rostrum in first-time transsphenoidal procedures as well [15], counting among its advantages a reduction in septal complications.

In the septal pushover technique, a vertical incision is made along the border of the cartilaginous septum and the perpendicular plate of the ethmoid. The incision is then angled anteriorly in the horizontal plane along the junction of the cartilaginous septum and the nasal ridge, allowing the cartilaginous septum to be mobilized laterally. Submucosal dissection is then carried caudally on either side of the bony septum toward the sphenoid rostrum, and then the transsphenoidal retractor may be placed, with the sphenoid rostrum in the midline. At the end of the operation, the cartilaginous septum is repositioned in the midline, and no attempt is made to close the mucosal incisions.

The endonasal septal pushover is our approach of choice in microscopic transsphenoidal surgery; it is fast, greatly reduces the risk of septal complications, and diminishes the need for uncomfortable nasal packing. One caveat is that the exposure may be mildly compromised as the septum cannot be mobilized as dramatically as in the endonasal or sublabial transseptal approaches.

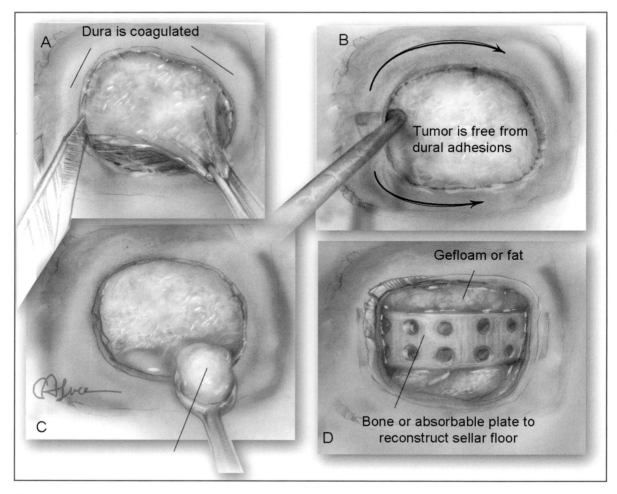

Fig. 16.4 Steps of tumor resection. *A* dural incision. *B* subdural plane developed. *C* sequential removal of tumor inferiorly, laterally, then superiorly. *D* reconstruction of sella with fat or Gelfoam pieces buttressed by a bioabsorbable plate

Direct Sphenoidotomy

Another option which reaches the sphenoid even more directly is a direct sphenoidotomy [14, 17]. In this approach, an incision is made right at the junction of the bony nasal septum and the sphenoid rostrum, and the posterior part of the septum just in front of the sphenoid sinus is deflected laterally, exposing the face of the sphenoid. The approach is similar to the septal pushover with a more posteriorly placed incision, with similar attendant advantages and drawbacks.

The mucosal incision is made at the junction of the nasal septum and the rostrum of the sphenoid. To provide working space, the middle turbinate is outfrac-

tured, and the mucosa-covered septum is translated laterally by the blade of a nasal speculum. Mucosal flaps are made over the sphenoid rostrum and the sphenoid ostia are identified bilaterally. The vomer and perpendicular plate of the ethmoid are not widely exposed, so bone is often not available for reconstructing the sellar floor. A variant of the direct sphenoidotomy retaining the wide exposure of the sublabial approach has recently been described [32].

A potential drawback to this procedure is the narrow exposure and the off-midline trajectory. Indeed, series reporting the use of the microscopic direct sphenoidotomy indicate that a relaxing alar incision had to be performed in as many as 20% of cases [17]. We have continued to prefer the septal pushover to the direct approach owing to the ability to lateralize the cartilaginous septum in the pushover technique, affording nearly the same exposure as the standard endonasal submucosal transseptal approach. The direct sphenoidotomy, however, is used extensively in endoscopic approaches, described elsewhere.

16.3.6.2 Sphenoid Phase

Having reached the anterior face of the sphenoid sinus by one of the described routes, C-arm fluoroscopy or image guidance is used to verify the trajectory and midline orientation. Portions of the bony nasal septum in the field should be resected with a Lillie-Koffler forceps or a Ferris-Smith punch. Any cartilage or bone resected is preserved for possible use during closure. This done, the surgical field comprises the keel of the vomer and face of the sphenoid centrally, with the sphenoid ostia on either side. Fracturing into the sphenoid sinus is usually possible by grasping the vomer with forceps or a punch, or with a chisel if necessary. The mucosa in the sinus is resected with a cup forceps to reduce bleeding and the risk of postoperative mucocele. Overspreading of the speculum can cause maxillary, sphenoid, or optic foramen fracture and may cause permanent face numbness in the first and second distributions of the Vth nerve, or damage to the lacrimal ducts [15].

It is again important to confirm the position and trajectory of the speculum by C-arm fluoroscopy or neuronavigational image guidance. Once in the sinus, it is critical to appreciate the compartmentalization of the sphenoid sinus and to correlate intraoperative findings with preoperative imaging. The operative procedures within the sphenoid sinus begin with removing the sphenoid septations; it is essential to note that septations not uncommonly lead toward one or the other of the carotid canals. The sphenoid exposure is then widened with an angled Kerrison punch. A wide exposure, as is done with the endoscopic approach, visualizing the carotid canals, the clivus, the opticocarotid recesses when possible, and the planum sphenoidale, is ideal.

Prior to opening the sella, the trajectory and midline orientation are again verified. This done, the sella is then opened, fracturing the thin floor using a chisel or, in cases where the sellar face is very thin, a blunt nerve hook. The opening is expanded with 1- and 2-mm Kerrison punches to expose the dura widely. In most cases the entire sellar floor is removed, and lateral exposure

is carefully carried out until the margin of the cavernous sinuses can be seen. Restraint is used with superior exposure as the dura is adherent to the region on the tuberculum sellae, and there may be an arachnoid diverticulum behind the dura at the upper margin of the sella. The microscope is adjusted to an objective distance of 350 to 375 mm so that the sella occupies the entire field of view and also allowing easy passage of instruments between the microscope and the sella [15].

The dura is evaluated grossly for the possibility of invasion by tumor, for the presence of a helpful characteristic midline vessel, and for the venous channels that may occur in the dura, particularly the superior and inferior circular sinuses. When necessary the dura can be cauterized either with monopolar or bipolar cautery.

16.3.6.3 Sellar Phase

The anatomical hazards to bear in mind prior to opening the dura are the cavernous sinuses and carotids laterally, the intercavernous sinuses at the tuberculum superiorly and the floor of the sella inferiorly, and the venous sinuses which may run between the two leaves of sellar dura. Surgery begins by coagulating and opening the dura. Fine needle aspiration may be wise if there is any chance that the lesion could be an aneurysm or an empty sella. The dura is then opened with a suitable blade. Usually we use a rectangular excision of the dura for large tumors (macroadenomas) and a cruciate or "x" type incision for smaller tumors that do not invade the dura. A specimen of dura may be sent to pathology for evaluation for microscopic dural invasion. Use of a bayoneted microDoppler probe to ascertain the location of each carotid is helpful if the preoperative studies suggest overly medialized carotid arteries. The dural opening is carefully extended, avoiding injury to the carotid and entry into the cavernous sinuses laterally.

Once the dura is open, an initial helpful step is to establish a careful subdural plane using a blunt hook or a small curette [15]. One can then identify and excise the lesion using an extracapsular technique when this is feasible or by working within the lesion and resecting it from surrounding structures when it is not. Portions of macroadenomas are removed sequentially. The surgeon should remove the inferior and lateral aspects of the tumor first, allowing suprasellar extension to drop into the operative field. Palpation of the far lateral reaches of the sella should be done with blunt curettes in order to minimize injury to the carotid and cranial nerves. Central and superior resection first may deliver the diaphragma sella into view, hiding remaining tumor and perhaps increasing the risk of a CSF leak. Suprasellar tumor can be delivered by the injection of air through a lumbar drain or by using a Valsalva maneuver or with bilateral jugular compression. During this phase, a careful evaluation for the possible presence of a spinal fluid leak is done, recognizing that dark black "strings" in the blood within the sella may indicate the presence of spinal fluid. Every effort should be made to protect and preserve the normal anterior and posterior pituitary gland, for which good visualization and careful hemostasis are critical.

Hemostasis is carefully achieved in the sellar region, with bipolar cautery for the dural margins, Gelfoam packing for the cavernous sinuses, and bipolar cautery for visible tumor feeding vessels. Bone wax worked with micropatties is used for bleeding edges of the sphenoid, clivus and sella. Occasionally, a topically applied hemostatic agent such as Floseal (Baxter, Deerfield, IL), crosslinked gelatin and thrombin mix, is an especially useful adjunct to conventional methods of hemostasis [33].

16.3.6.4 Reconstruction/Closure

This phase begins with a careful inspection for the presence of CSF leaks—these can occur during all types of intrasellar explorations. If a CSF leak is present or suspected, a fat graft is obtained from a subumbilical incision, prepared as described below. The fat is cut into appropriately sized pieces soaked in 10% chloramphenicol solution, patted on a cotton ball in order to incorporate a few wisps of cotton fiber (which provoke a fibrotic reaction), and the fat is then rolled in Avitene (Davol, Cranston, RI) hemostatic collagen powder. The fat is packed into the sellar cavity, avoiding excessive packing but placing enough to occlude the sella, to prevent spinal fluid leakage, and to achieve hemostasis. The sellar floor is then reconstructed. One can use bone from the initial operative phase or artificial constructs such as a MedPor (Porex, Neman, GA) tailored plate [15, 34]. The MedPor plate is a thin polyethylene plate with a perpendicularly oriented tab to facilitate implant placement and maneuvering; its micropores allow tissue ingrowth and it features a very low signal intensity on MRI [34]. This is placed epidurally if a CSF leak was present and otherwise is placed intradurally; other groups also stress the importance of the extradural layer in preventing CSF leaks [35].

Blood and surgical debris are carefully suctioned from the sphenoid cavity and the nasopharynx prior to closure, and if no packing is necessary, the turbinates are then medialized. We place Merocel nasal packs in patients who have undergone submucosal dissection or in whom hemostasis was challenging. The abdominal incision is closed with subcuticular technique. The oropharynx is carefully suctioned prior to extubation of the patient.

16.3.7 Summary of Conventional Approaches

The transseptal and septal displacement approaches performed endonasally or sublabially should be learned by all transsphenoidal surgeons so that they may consider the advantages and disadvantages of each approach. The sublabial approach, although replaced in most centers by endonasal approaches, maintains the anatomic midline and is especially indicated when a patient's anatomy precludes an endonasal approach and when a particularly wide exposure and view is necessary during surgery. As such, it is particularly indicated in patients with small nasal apertures, in pediatric patients, and in patients with large tumors with significant extension into the cavernous sinuses and clivus which may be inadequately visualized through an endonasal approach. We often use a sublabial approach in our extended cases.

The transseptal approach, discarded by many due to the risk of anterior septal perforation and the need for uncomfortable postoperative nasal packing, tends to direct the surgeon to a truer midline with a less restricted corridor because of the wider mobilization of the nasal septum. The septal pushover has replaced the transseptal approach in our practice as it features a faster exposure and closure and can be used in patients with septal pathology or prior septal surgery. Mobilization of the cartilaginous septum retains the advantage of the transseptal approaches while minimizing septal mucosal dissection and its complications.

16.3.7.1 Boundaries of the Microscopic Transsphenoidal Approaches: Extended Approaches

The boundaries of the standard microscopic transsphenoidal approaches described above have been extended in recent years (reviewed in references [36–38]) to expose the anterior skull base (transtuberculum/transplanum), the cavernous sinus (transcavernous), the inferior clivus (transclival), and the supradiaphragmatic space (transdiagphragmatic). These modifications are often combined and have expanded the range of lesions accessible through the transsphenoidal corridor. Perhaps the most widely used extension of the standard transsphenoidal approach is the transsphenoidal transtuberculum sellae/transplanum approach, originally described by Weiss [39] but since refined and employed for resection of craniopharyngiomas, tuberculum sellae meningiomas, Rathke's cleft cysts, and other lesions with suprasellar, parasellar, and/or anterior cranial base extension [15, 36, 38, 40–44] with or without sellar expansion.

We occasionally use a lumbar drain on our extended cases which allows insufflation of air intraoperatively as well as CSF diversion during the postoperative period. In contrast to our traditional sellar approach in which the head is positioned such that the dorsum of the nose is parallel to the floor, the head is extended slightly to allow a more direct view towards the planum. Under frameless stereotactic guidance, an endonasal or sublabial approach to the sphenoid is taken; we favor the sublabial approach in extended cases owing to the wider exposure and truer adherence to the midline it affords. A wide sphenoid opening and sellar opening are created. The tuberculum and planum are then removed with either a high-speed drill or combination of Kerrison punches to complete the rostral-caudal exposure; the lateral exposure usually does not exceed 1.5 cm to avoid carotid and optic nerve injury [37]. Dural opening follows; particular attention is paid to the superior intercavernous sinus which is frequently recalcitrant to simple bipolar cautery should it be entered. The sellar dura is opened parallel and just inferior to the superior intercavernous sinus, after which clips are placed across the sinus which can then be cut. In some cases the intercavernous sinus can be controlled by Surgicel carefully placed at the margins. The dura of the anterior cranial fossa is then opened.

Following dural opening, the pituitary gland is identified and protected, followed by sharp arachnoid dissection and identification of the tumor capsule. For cases in which an intrasellar mass with a suprasellar component has expanded the volume of the sella, the diaphragm may be violated intentionally to access the suprasellar tumor capsule, enabling an extracapsular dissection of midline lesions extending from the sella [45]. Once identified, the planes between the tumor and optic

nerves, chiasm, and stalk may be identified and developed; internal tumor decompression may simplify microsurgical dissection off these structures. In approaches such as these which push the boundaries of the strictly microscopic approach, neuroendoscopes of varying angulation enhance deep and lateral views and have proved indispensable in the inspection of local anatomy and the assessment of the extent of tumor resection.

Closure and sellar reconstruction are critical as our rates of CSF leak have tended to be higher in the extended approach (11%) [37]. We try to close the dural defect with a synthetic dural substitute and the bony defect with septal bone or a titanium or polymer plate placed extradurally. The use of septal mucosal flaps or mucoperichondrial flaps from the turbinate is helpful in some cases. We supplement our closure as outlined above by packing the sphenoid with fat.

16.3.8 Special Surgical Considerations

16.3.8.1 Cushing's Disease

The sellar phase of the microscopic transsphenoidal operation for Cushing's disease features several specific modifications, and preoperative certainty of this diagnosis is critical prior to surgery. As sellar imaging and inferior petrosal sinus sampling are imperfect in their estimation of tumor location, a systematic dissection of sellar contents is sometimes required [15]. Subtle changes in tissue texture or color may suggest an adenoma. Failing this, the gland itself is incised horizontally and inspected, followed by the lateral aspects of the gland and, if still unsuccessful, the posterior pituitary. Damage to the superior rim of residual normal pituitary and traction on the pituitary stalk is avoided. Should these maneuvers and cavernous sinus exploration fail, a subtotal hypophysectomy may be performed in adult patients with no fertility concerns.

16.3.8.2 Acromegaly

The surgeon should be aware that patients with acromegaly have thicker bone, larger and more tortuous carotid arteries and blood vessels in general, and thicker upper airway tissue conferring greater difficulty with airway maintenance during surgery. We often place nasal breathing trumpets in severely affected patients postoperatively to facilitate adequate ventilation [15].

16.4 Complications

The microscopic transsphenoidal approach is a safe operation with a well-established complication profile (Table 16.2). In a carefully analyzed series of over 2,500 patients who had received transsphenoidal surgery, the mortality rate was 1% and the rate of major complications 3.4% comprising vascular injury and its sequelae, visual loss, cranial nerve injury, CSF leakage, and meningitis. Transient diabetes insipidus occurs in 18% of patients with 2% requiring long-term treatment [46]. Anterior septal perforations are becoming less common as surgeons adopt progressively more direct approaches to the sphenoid sinus.

Table 16.2 Complications of transsphenoidal surgery from the senior author's (E.R.L.) series of 2,562 pituitary adenomas

Complication	Patients
Operative mortality (30 day)	
Hypothalamic injury or hemorrhage	5
Meningitis	2
Vascular injury or occlusion	4
Cerebrospinal fluid leak or pneumocephalus, subarachnoid hemorrhage or spasm, myocardial infarction	1
Postoperative myocardial infarction, postoperative seizure	2
Total	14 (0.5%)
Major morbidity	
Vascular occlusion, stroke, subarachnoid hemorrhage, or spasm	5
Visual loss (new)	11
Vascular injury (repaired)	8
Meningitis (nonfatal)	8
Sellar abscess	1
Sellar pneumatocele	1
Sixth cranial nerve palsy	2
Third cranial nerve palsy	1
Cerebrospinal fluid rhinorrhea	49
Total	86 (3.4%)
Lesser morbidity	
Hemorrhage (intraoperative or postoperative)	9
Postoperative psychosis	5
Nasal septal perforation	16
Sinusitis, wound infection	5
Transient cranial nerve palsy (III or IV)	5
Diabetes insipidus (usually transient)	35
Cribriform plate fracture	2
Maxillary fracture	2
Hepatitis	1
Symptomatic syndrome of inappropriate antidiuretic hormone	37
Total	117 (4.6%)

16.4.1 Complication Avoidance: Postoperative CSF Leakage and Vascular Injury

Intraoperative CSF leakage is common during transsphenoidal surgery, and an adequate repair during surgery is essential to avoid a postoperative leak. Upon confirmation or suspicion of an intraoperative CSF leak, we harvest a fat graft as described above and bathe it in chloramphenicol before gently abrading it with cotton to allow minute inflammation-inducing cotton strands to adhere to the graft. The graft is then rolled in Avitene and placed into the sinus, buttressed by a bioabsorbable plate placed extradurally across the sella. Patients with postoperative CSF leaks are usually taken back promptly to the operating room for exploration, repacking, and reconstruction of the sellar floor.

Iatrogenic injury to the internal carotid artery is arguably the most feared complication of transsphenoidal surgery; exuberant cavernous sinus bleeding and sphenopalatine artery injury are among other vascular complications encountered. Carotid injury occurs in 1–2% of cases, with patients who have had prior craniotomy, transsphenoidal surgery, or radiation therapy at greater risk [13, 47]. Careful study of preoperative imaging to appreciate the course of the carotids and operating from a true midline position are critical. Intraoperative image guidance can help confirm midline positioning during surgery, particularly in reoperations or in other cases where normal anatomy appears distorted. A microDoppler probe can help confirm carotid location. The endoscope may also be used and is especially useful in identifying the course of the carotids after sphenoid sinus entry. Blunt curettes should be used during lateral sellar exploration [13]. Should the carotid be injured during surgery, options include direct repair and nonobliterative packing, with the latter more commonly employed. Immediate angiography should be performed to delineate a possible cavernous–carotid fistula or pseudoaneurysm and a balloon occlusion test performed should the carotid require sacrifice. If the angiogram is normal, it should be repeated in one week. Stent occlusion of false aneurysms in the carotid after transsphenoidal surgery is an evolving concept which may gain traction should longer-term data be promising [48].

16.5 Summary

The product of a century of innovation and surgical refinement, the microscopic transsphenoidal approaches are the first-choice routes to the sella and parasellar region.

Trends in transsphenoidal surgery include the preponderance of increasingly direct endonasal approaches, the routine employment of image guidance platforms, and the extension of sellar approaches to expose the anterior cranial base, cavernous sinuses, inferior clivus, and supradiaphragmatic region. The increasing prevalence of the endoscope in transsphenoidal surgery will only enhance the safety and flexibility of this skull-base approach.

Aknowledgment: The authors are grateful to Craig Luce for his artwork and assistance in final preparation.

References

1. Kanter AS, Dumont AS, Asthagiri AR et al (2005) The transsphenoidal approach. A historical perspective. Neurosurg Focus 18:e6
2. Schloffer H (1907) Erfolgreiche Operationen eines Hypophysentumors auf Nasalem Wege. Wien Klin Wochenschr 20:621–624
3. von Eiselsberg A (1908) The operative cure of acromegaly by removal of a hypophysial tumor. Ann Surg 48:781–783
4. Kocher T (1909) Ein Fall von Hypophysis-Tumor mit operativer Heilung. Dtsch Z Chir 100:13–37
5. Lanzino G, Laws ER Jr (2003) Key personalities in the development and popularization of the transsphenoidal approach to pituitary tumors: an historical overview. Neurosurg Clin North Am 14:1–10
6. Halstead AE (1910) Remarks on the operative treatment of tumors of the hypophysis. With the report of two cases operated on by an oro-nasal method. Trans Am Surg Assoc 28:73–93
7. Cushing H (1914) The Weir Mitchell Lecture. Surgical experiences with pituitary adenoma. JAMA 63:1515–1525
8. Jane JA Jr, Han J, Prevedello DM et al (2005) Perspectives on endoscopic transsphenoidal surgery. Neurosurg Focus 19:E2
9. Elias WJ, Laws ER (2000) Transsphenoidal approaches to lesions of the sella. In: Schmidek HH, Sweet WH (eds) Operative neurosurgical techniques: indications, methods, and results. W.B. Saunders, Philadelphia, pp 373–384
10. Jane JA Jr, Dumont AS, Sheehan JP, Laws ER (2004) Surgical techniques in transsphenoidal surgery: what is the standard of care in pituitary adenoma surgery? Current Opin Endocrinol Diabetes 14:264–270
11. Wilson WR, Khan A, Laws ER Jr (1990) Transseptal approaches for pituitary surgery. Laryngoscope 100:817–819
12. Kern EB, Pearson BW, McDonald TJ, Laws ER Jr (1979) The transseptal approach to lesions of the pituitary and parasellar regions. Laryngoscope 89:1–34
13. Laws ER Jr (1999) Vascular complications of transsphenoidal surgery. Pituitary 2:163–170
14. Griffith HB, Veerapen R (1987) A direct transnasal approach to the sphenoid sinus. Technical note. J Neurosurg 66:140–142
15. Jane JA Jr, Thapar K, Kaptain GJ et al (2002) Pituitary surgery: transsphenoidal approach. Neurosurgery 51:435–442
16. Wilson WR, Laws ER Jr (1992) Transnasal septal displacement approach for secondary transsphenoidal pituitary surgery. Laryngoscope 102:951–953
17. Zada G, Kelly DF, Cohan P et al (2003) Endonasal transsphenoidal approach for pituitary adenomas and other sellar lesions: an assessment of efficacy, safety, and patient impressions. J Neurosurg 98:350–358
18. Elias WJ, Chadduck JB, Alden TD, Laws ER Jr (1999) Frameless stereotaxy for transsphenoidal surgery. Neurosurgery 45:271–275
19. Jane JA Jr, Thapar K, Alden TD, Laws ER Jr (2001) Fluoroscopic frameless stereotaxy for transsphenoidal surgery. Neurosurgery 48:1302–1307
20. McCutcheon IE, Kitagawa RS, Demasi PF et al (2004) Frameless stereotactic navigation in transsphenoidal surgery: comparison with fluoroscopy. Stereotact Funct Neurosurg 82:43–48
21. Jagannathan J, Prevedello DM, Ayer VS et al (2006) Computer-assisted frameless stereotaxy in transsphenoidal surgery at a single institution: review of 176 cases. Neurosurg Focus 20:E9
22. Dusick JR, Esposito F, Malkasian D, Kelly DF (2007) Avoidance of carotid artery injuries in transsphenoidal surgery with the Doppler probe and micro-hook blades. Neurosurgery 60:322–328
23. Fahlbusch R, Ganslandt O, Buchfelder M et al (2001) Intraoperative magnetic resonance imaging during transsphenoidal surgery. J Neurosurg 95:381–390
24. Martin CH, Schwartz R, Jolesz F, Black PM (1999) Transsphenoidal resection of pituitary adenomas in an intraoperative MRI unit. Pituitary 2:155–162
25. Nimsky C, von Keller B, Ganslandt O, Fahlbusch R (2006) Intraoperative high-field magnetic resonance imaging in transsphenoidal surgery of hormonally inactive pituitary macroadenomas. Neurosurgery 59:105–114
26. Yamasaki T, Moritake K, Hatta J, Nagai H (1996) Intraoperative monitoring with pulse Doppler ultrasonography in transsphenoidal surgery: technique application. Neurosurgery 38:95–97
27. Hall WA, Kowalik K, Liu H et al (2003) Costs and benefits of intraoperative MR-guided brain tumor resection. Acta neurochirurgica 85:137–142
28. Sharma K, Tyagi I, Banerjee D et al (1996) Rhinological complications of sublabial transseptal transsphenoidal surgery for sellar and suprasellar lesions: prevention and management. Neurosurg Rev 19:163–167
29. Sherwen PJ, Patterson WJ, Griesdale DE (1986) Transseptal, transsphenoidal surgery: a subjective and objective analysis of results. J Otolaryngol 15:155–160
30. Spencer WR, Levine JM, Couldwell WT et al (2000) Approaches to the sellar and parasellar region: a retrospective comparison of the endonasal-transsphenoidal and sublabial-transsphenoidal approaches. Otolaryngol Head Neck Surg 122:367–369

31. Liu JK, Nwagwu C, Pikus HJ, Couldwell WT (2001) Laparoscopic anterior lumbar interbody fusion precipitating pituitary apoplexy. Acta Neurochir (Wien) 143:303–306

32. Kerr PB, Oldfield EH (2008) Sublabial-endonasal approach to the sella turcica. J Neurosurg 109:153–155

33. Ellegala DB, Maartens NF, Laws ER Jr (2002) Use of FloSeal hemostatic sealant in transsphenoidal pituitary surgery: technical note. Neurosurgery 51:513–515

34. Park J, Guthikonda M (2004) The Medpor sheet as a sellar buttress after endonasal transsphenoidal surgery: technical note. Surg Neurol 61:488–492

35. Cavallo LM, Messina A, Esposito F et al (2007) Skull base reconstruction in the extended endoscopic transsphenoidal approach for suprasellar lesions. J Neurosurg 107:713–720

36. Couldwell WT, Weiss MH, Rabb C et al (2004) Variations on the standard transsphenoidal approach to the sellar region, with emphasis on the extended approaches and parasellar approaches: surgical experience in 105 cases. Neurosurgery 55:539–547

37. Dumont AS, Kanter AS, Jane JA Jr, Laws ER Jr (2006) Extended transsphenoidal approach. Front Horm Res 34:29–45

38. Kouri JG, Chen MY, Watson JC, Oldfield EH (2000) Resection of suprasellar tumors by using a modified transsphenoidal approach. Report of four cases. J Neurosurg 92:1028–1035

39. Weiss MH (ed) (1987) Transnasal transsphenoidal approach. Williams and Wilkins, Baltimore

40. Cappabianca P, Cavallo LM, Colao A et al (2002) Endoscopic endonasal transsphenoidal approach: outcome analysis of 100 consecutive procedures. Minim Invasive Neurosurg 45:193–200

41. de Divitiis E, Cappabianca P, Cavallo LM (2002) Endoscopic transsphenoidal approach: adaptability of the procedure to different sellar lesions. Neurosurgery 51:699–705

42. Frank G, Pasquini E, Mazzatenta D (2001) Extended transsphenoidal approach. J Neurosurg 95:917–918

43. Jho HD, Ha HG (2004) Endoscopic endonasal skull base surgery: Part 1--The midline anterior fossa skull base. Minim Invasive Neurosurg 47:1–8

44. Kato T, Sawamura Y, Abe H, Nagashima M (1998) Transsphenoidal-transtuberculum sellae approach for supradiaphragmatic tumours: technical note. Acta Neurochir (Wien) 140:715–718

45. Kaptain GJ, Vincent DA, Sheehan JP, Laws ER Jr (2008) Transsphenoidal approaches for the extracapsular resection of midline suprasellar and anterior cranial base lesions. Neurosurgery 62:1264–1271

46. Nemergut EC, Zuo Z, Jane JA Jr, Laws ER Jr (2005) Predictors of diabetes insipidus after transsphenoidal surgery: a review of 881 patients. J Neurosurg 103:448–454

47. Ciric I, Ragin A, Baumgartner C, Pierce D (1997) Complications of transsphenoidal surgery: results of a national survey, review of the literature, and personal experience. Neurosurgery 40:225–236

48. Oskouian RJ, Kelly DF, Laws ER Jr (2006) Vascular injury and transsphenoidal surgery. Front Horm Res 34:256–278

Expanded Endoscopic Endonasal Approaches to the Skull Base

17

Daniel M. Prevedello, Amin B. Kassam, Paul A. Gardner,
Ricardo L. Carrau and Carl H. Snyderman

17.1 Introduction

Although endoscopic sinus surgery started in the early 1900s with the work of Hirschmann [1] in 1903 and Escat in 1911 [2], it only progressed after a better understanding of sinonasal physiology was provided by Messerklinger [3], and the development of rod lens systems by Hopkins in the 1960s [1].

Kennedy et al. [4, 5] coined the term functional endoscopic sinus surgery in 1985 and, along with Stammberger [6] and Draf [7], popularized the use of modern endoscopy for the paranasal sinuses in the 1980s. The use of endoscopes in neurosurgery had a diverse evolution. In an attempt to improve visualization, Guiot in 1963 was the first neurosurgeon to use the endoscope in transsphenoidal surgery [1, 8, 9]. However, the endoscopes at that time were archaic and Hardy established the transsphenoidal route with the aid of microscopes in 1967 [1, 9–11].

In late 1970s, Apuzzo et al. [12] and Bushe and Halves [13, 14] reintroduced the endoscope as an adjunct to the microscope for resection of pituitary lesions with extrasellar extension, and they were followed by others [15–20]. However, when the microscope is the primary form of visualization, the speculum limits the working space and the maneuverability of the endoscope and instruments [15–20].

The endoscope was first used as the only visualizing tool in skull-base surgery for pituitary lesions in the early 1990s [1]. In 1992, Jankowski et al. reported their experience with three cases using a pure endoscopic transsphenoidal approach to the sella [21].

Others subsequently confirmed the feasibility of pure endoscopic approaches to the sella [22–25]. Cappabianca, de Divitiis and Cavallo were extremely important in advocating and disseminating the technique to the world [26–36].

As an expected progression, various centers around the world began to perform pure endoscopic approaches to the sella [1, 37]. Although the endoscope offers a panoramic view beyond the sella, endoscopic skull-base surgery was born only after developing an understanding of ventral skull-base anatomy and the development of appropriate instrumentation, made possible by the collaboration between otolaryngologists and neurosurgeons [38–41].

While improved cosmetics are often cited as an advantage of endoscopy, in our opinion, this is a secondary gain. Because of its "flash-light" visualization properties and ability to provide direct access, the key advantage offered by the endoscope is a reduced need to manipulate neural tissue. In particular, direct ventral corridors offer the ability in selected cases to remove lesions without having to cross the plane of cranial nerves and to minimize brain manipulation. These advantages have the potential to decrease morbidity due to less tissue trauma, which may lead to a faster recovery, shortened hospitalization, and decreased cost of medical care.

Since 1998, over 1,000 patients have undergone endoscopic skull-base procedures at the University of Pittsburgh Medical Center for a wide variety of pathologies.

A.B. Kassam (✉)
Dept of Neurological Surgery and Dept of Otolaryngology
University of Pittsburgh School of Medicine, Pittsburgh, PA, USA

P. Cappabianca et al. (eds.), *Cranial, Craniofacial and Skull Base Surgery*.
© Springer-Verlag Italia 2010

17.2 Endoscopic Endonasal Approach

17.2.1 Planning

Frameless stereotactic image guidance is used in all expanded/extended (endoscopic) endonasal approaches to the skull base. Image guidance helps to confirm the visual impression of the surgical anatomy, especially critical neurovascular structures, and to define a targeted resection.

A high-resolution CT angiogram is used for most skull-base procedures, as it allows the simultaneous visualization of osseous, vascular and soft-tissue anatomy. Increasingly, we utilize image fusion of CT and MRI scans to take advantage of the best features of each: CT for the bony anatomy of the cranial base and MRI for intracranial tumor margins. Intraoperative CT is frequently performed and the image guidance system can be updated if necessary.

17.2.2 Operating Room Setup

The surgeons are positioned on the right side of the patient opposite the anesthesia team. The surgical technician or nurse is positioned towards the foot of the table. This arrangement gives the surgeons unrestricted access to the nasal region. Electrical cords and suction tubing are directed away from the surgical field toward the head and foot of the table to minimize interference with surgical instruments.

A pin fixation system is used to reduce intraoperative movement of the head, especially during drilling and neurovascular dissection. The head is fixed, following endotracheal intubation, the vertex tilted to the left with the face turned to the right by 15–20°. The patient should be as close to the right side of the operating table as possible. The table can be angulated in the room such that the foot goes away from the surgeons allowing even more space. However, this angulation is not possible when the surgery is performed with the patient inside the CT scanner.

Neurophysiological monitoring of cortical function (somatosensory evoked potentials) and if necessary brainstem function (brainstem evoked responses) is routinely performed in all cases in which the dura is exposed or dissection near the carotid arteries is performed. Neurophysiological monitoring can identify changes in cerebral blood flow that may occur with changes in blood pressure and alert the anesthesiologist to the need

for adjustments. Cranial nerve electromyography is performed as necessary based on tumor anatomy.

A nasal decongestant, such as oxymetazoline 0.5%, is applied topically to the nasal mucosa using cottonoids. The skin of the external nose and nasal vestibule as well as of the abdomen (fat graft donor site if potentially needed) is prepped with a povidone antiseptic solution. The intranasal space and mucosa are not prepped. The patient is given a third or fourth generation cephalosporin for perioperative antibiotic prophylaxis.

17.2.3 Surgical Exposure

The endoscope is introduced at the "12 o'clock" position of the nostril (usually the right) and is used to retract the nasal vestibule superiorly, therefore elongating the nostril and increasing the available space for other instruments. A suction tip is introduced at the "6 o'clock" position on the ipsilateral side. Dissecting instruments are introduced through the left nasal cavity. A suction irrigation sheath or continual irrigation by an assistant or co-surgeon cleans the lens of the scope and preserves visualization without removing the scope for frequent cleaning. If, for any reason, a bimanual (preferably binarial) approach cannot be pursued then proceeding further is absolutely contraindicated. Additionally, we discourage the use of an endoscopic holder for all endonasal approaches since it decreases maneuverability, slows the dissection process and generates a static two-dimensional picture.

Widening of the nasal corridor is achieved initially by out-fracturing of the inferior turbinates, followed by removal of the right middle turbinate to provide room for the endoscope. Injection of vasoconstrictors is optional and is performed according to the surgeon's preference.

In cases in which a CSF leak is anticipated, a nasoseptal vascularized mucosal flap is elevated during the initial stage of the procedure [42, 43]. In cases in which a CSF leak is unlikely, a sphenoidectomy is performed directly with preservation of a potential pedicle for a nasoseptal flap by preserving the mucosa around the posterior nasal arteries. Thus, at the end of the procedure, a 'rescue flap' can still be elevated.

For creating the flap we use unipolar electrocautery with an insulated needle tip to incise the septal mucosa. Two parallel incisions are performed following the superior and inferior insertions of the septum. One follows the maxillary crest and the parallel incision follows a line 1 cm below the most superior aspect of the septum to preserve the olfactory epithelium and function. These parallel incisions are joined anteriorly by a vertical incision usually placed just rostral to the anterior head of the inferior turbinate (Fig. 17.1). Posteriorly, the superior incision is extended laterally inferior to the natural sphenoid ostium. The inferior incision extends laterally on the superior margin of the choana. Elevation of the mucoperichondrium, using a Cottle dissector, proceeds from anterior to posterior after ascertaining that all incisions have been carried through the periosteum and perichondrium. Elevation of the flap from the anterior face of the sphenoid sinus is completed preserving the vascular pedicle between the sphenoid ostium sinus and choana.

The flap can be stored in the nasopharynx for sellar or suprasellar cases or inside the maxillary sinus after an antrostomy is performed to facilitate dissection at the level of the clivus or cervical spine until the resection is concluded.

The sphenoidotomy is initiated by identifying and enlarging the natural ostium of the sphenoid sinus or by direct removal of the sphenoid rostrum. A Cottle dissector is used to incise and disarticulate the posterior septum from the rostrum of the sphenoid bone. Removal of the bony rostrum is completed using Kerrison rongeurs and/or a surgical drill. Wide bilateral sphenoidotomies are performed extending laterally to the level of the medial pterygoid plates and the lateral wall of the sphenoid sinus (taking care to preserve the flap

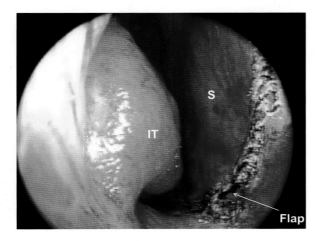

Fig. 17.1 Intraoperative view during endoscopic endonasal surgery at the time of elevation of the nasoseptal flap using a zero-degree endoscope. Note the anterior cut in the mucosa of the septum (*S*) at the level of the head of the inferior turbinate (*IT*)

vascular pedicle as needed), superiorly to the level of the planum sphenoidale, and inferiorly to the floor of the sphenoid sinus. The posterior edge of the nasal septum (1–2 cm) is resected with backbiting forceps or a microdebrider. The posterior septectomy facilitates bilateral instrumentation without displacing the septum into the path of the endoscope, and increases the lateral angulation and range of motion of the instruments. Wide bilateral sphenoidotomies and a posterior septectomy provide bilateral access and visualization of key anatomical structures. This was a critical step initiated by our group a decade ago that formed the foundation of all subsequent endoscopic modules to the skull base described below.

Once the sphenoid sinus is widely exposed and all the septations are drilled, the desired module of the expanded endonasal approach can be pursued.

Two concepts are critical for the endoscopic exposure: bilateral nasal access (binarial) to allow for a two-surgeon, three-/four-hand technique, and the optimized removal of the posterior septum to create a single work cavity. These allow a bimanual dissection technique with dynamic scope movement providing adequate visualization of the surgical field at all times during the surgical procedure with freedom of movement.

17.3 Anatomical Modules

The modules are divided into median (sagittal plane – between the carotid arteries) and paramedian (coronal planes – lateral to the carotid arteries) approaches based on the inherent anatomy of the region. The coronal planes are considered in three levels: anterior, midcoronal and posterior.

17.3.1 Sagittal Plane (Anterior to Posterior)

Transcribriform Approach

The transcribriform approach [41] is defined by the removal of the cribiform plate and anterior skull base to access the anterior fossa through a nasal and ethmoidal corridor. This module extends anteriorly from the posterior ethmoidal arteries up to the level of the crista galli and frontal sinuses. The limits of this module are the laminae papyraceae laterally, the frontal sinus anteriorly and the transition with the planum sphenoidale

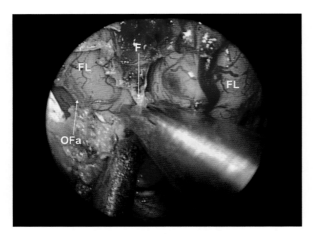

Fig. 17.2 Intraoperative view during an expanded endonasal transcribriform approach for resection of an esthesioneuroblastoma using a zero-degree endoscope. Note the frontal lobes exposed bilaterally (*FL*) at the moment the falx (*F*) is cut in the midline. The orbital-frontal artery (*OFa*) is seen on the surface of the right frontal lobe

posteriorly at the level of the posterior ethmoidal arteries. The most important structures related to this module are the orbits and the anterior cerebral arteries (A2) and their branches (frontoorbital, frontopolar). Complications related to the ethmoidal arteries can also occur. Retrobulbar hematoma is an example of a problem that can occur if they are not well coagulated or clipped during the approach.

Commonly, a transcribriform approach is associated with removal of the planum sphenoidale for resection of large anterior fossa meningiomas. Other pathologies that often require a transcribriform approach are esthesioneuroblastomas and invasive sinonasal malignancies. It is very important to stress that a bilateral transcribriform approach sacrifices olfaction. However, it is likely that the disease in question has already compromised this function in many of the patients. A unilateral approach can be performed for small paramedian lesions with the intention of olfaction preservation.

An intraoperative view during a transcribriform approach for resection of an esthesioneuroblastoma is shown in Fig. 17.2

Transplanum/Transtuberculum Approach

The transplanum/transtuberculum approach [41] is defined by the removal of the planum sphenoidale and tu-

berculum sellae. The optic canals mark the lateral limits for the transplanum approach. Anteriorly, the bony resection is limited to the level of the posterior ethmoidal arteries. Anterior dissection from this point reaches the cribriform plate and olfactory fibers, which should not be trespassed upon in order to preserve olfaction.

The transplanum approach is indicated for lesions involving the posterior aspect of the anterior skull base (intra- or extradural) at the level of the planum sphenoidale. The suprasellar region is reached through resection of the tuberculum sellae. Craniopharyngiomas and tuberculum sellae meningiomas are examples of lesions that can be resected through a transplanum/transtuberculum approach.

The critical anatomic landmark is the medial optic carotid recess, which has to be removed in order to allow adequate exposure of the suprasellar compartment. Once it is accessed, the dural opening can occur from one internal carotid artery (ICA) to the other with direct safe access to the medial aspect of the carotid cave and optic canals. The most important vital structures related to this module are the optic nerves with the respective ophthalmic arteries, ICAs and the anterior cerebral arteries (A1, Heubner's, anterior communicating and perforators).

An intraoperative view after resection of a tuberculum sellae meningioma through a transplanum approach is shown in Fig. 17.3.

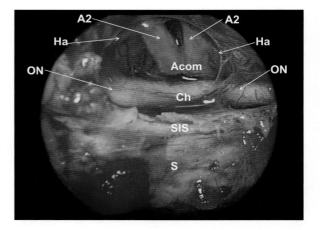

Fig. 17.3 Intraoperative view after resection of a tuberculum sellae meningioma through an expanded endonasal transplanum approach using a zero-degree endoscope. Note the exposure and preservation of the optic chiasm (*Ch*), optic nerves (*ON*), Heubner's arteries (*Ha*), the anterior communicating artery (*Acom*), and the anterior cerebral arteries (*A2*). The superior intercavernous sinus (*SIS*) was preserved as well as the dura of the sella (*S*)

Transsellar Approach

In the transsellar approach [41] the face of the sella as well as its floor are drilled exposing the "four blues", which refer to the bilateral cavernous sinuses and the superior and inferior intercavernous sinuses. Frequently the bone anterior to the ICAs is removed to allow further retraction on the medial wall of the cavernous sinus to permit exposure of the posterolateral contents of the sella turcica. Wide exposure provides adequate space for intrasellar dissections. The transsellar approach can be used in association with the transplanum and transclival (upper third) approaches, particularly to access intradural extrasellar disease.

The most common indication for this approach is a pituitary adenoma. Purely intrasellar craniopharyngiomas and Rathke's cleft cysts are also commonly encountered. Tuberculum sellae or diaphragmatic meningiomas can be resected with a combination of transsellar and transtuberculum approaches, particularly when there is an important intrasellar component of the tumor.

A resection of the tuberculum sellae is essential during the exposure of pituitary macroadenomas with a tall suprasellar component to allow tumor 'waist' decompression and allow further diaphragma herniation.

The most important critical structures related to this module are the cavernous sinuses containing both ICAs and the cranial nerves limiting the area laterally. The chiasm is located in the suprasellar compartment and can be affected in large sellar lesions with suprasellar extension such as large macroadenomas.

An intraoperative view during an endoscopic endonasal transsellar approach after resection of a macroadenoma is shown in Fig. 17.4.

Transclival Approach

The transclival approach [40] can be performed segmentally (upper, middle or lower thirds) or with complete removal of the clivus (panclivectomy). The upper third is related to the dorsum sellae in the midline and the posterior clinoids in the paramedian region. The sellar posterior wall can be removed intradurally via a transsellar approach, particularly where the tumor has created the corridor or after a pituitary transposition and ligation of the posterior intercavernous sinus. The retrosellar bone can also be resected extradurally via a subsellar corridor after removal of the sellar bone and superior retraction of the sellar dura [44]. After transposition, the retrodorsum dura containing the basilar

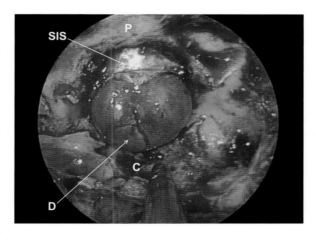

Fig. 17.4 Intraoperative view during an endoscopic endonasal transsellar approach after resection of a macroadenoma. Note that the tuberculum sellae was removed exposing the superior intercavernous sinus (*SIS*) to allow total tumor resection and complete herniation of the diaphragma sellae (*D*). The planum sphenoidale (*P*) and the clival recess (*C*) are seen in the midline

plexus is exposed. Since tumors can move cranial nerves medially, we do not perform extensive dural coagulation at this level to avoid damage to cranial nerves III and VI superolaterally close to the posterior clinoids and inferolaterally at the level of the floor of the sella, respectively. Dural opening with basilar plexus control provides access to the basilar artery and interpeduncular cistern.

A transclival approach is frequently utilized for resection of extradural and intradural diseases as such as chordomas and chondrosarcomas. It is also used to access purely intradural pathologies anterior to the brainstem such as meningiomas and craniopharyngiomas.

The middle clivus can be directly accessed at the posterior aspect of the sphenoid sinus and its resection is limited laterally by both ICAs ascending in the paraclival areas. If the bone drilling continues inferiorly, the lower third of the clivus is restricted laterally by the fossa of Rosenmuller and the torus tubarius. A panclivectomy can extend all the way from the dorsum sellae and posterior clinoids down to the basion at the foramen magnum.

The most vital structures for this module are the brainstem, cranial nerves II, III and VI, basilar and vertebral arteries, superior cerebellar arteries, posterior cerebral arteries and respective perforators.

An intraoperative view after resection of a craniopharyngioma through an endonasal transclival approach is shown in Fig. 17.5.

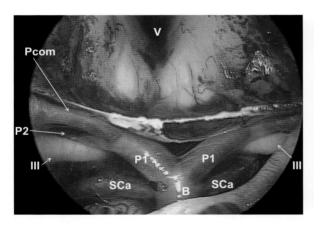

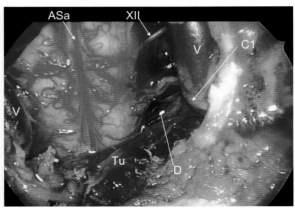

Fig. 17.5 Intraoperative view after resection of a craniopharyngioma through an expanded endonasal transclival approach with pituitary transposition and removal of the dorsum sellae using a 45-degree endoscope. Note the total resection of the lesion and partial visualization of the third ventricle (*V*). The basilar artery (*B*) was dissected from the tumor as well as the posterior cerebral arteries (*P1*, *P2*), posterior communicating arteries (*Pcom*), the third cranial nerves (*III*) and the superior cerebellar arteries (*SCa*) bilaterally

Fig. 17.6 Intraoperative view during an expanded endonasal transodontoid approach for resection of a foramen magnum meningioma (*Tu*) using a zero-degree endoscope. Note that the spinal cord is exposed as well as the anterior spinal artery (*ASa*). Both vertebral arteries (*V*) are exposed and preserved. The dentate ligament (*D*) is seen in the left side with the ventral root of C1 (*C1*). A portion of cranial nerve XII (*XII*) is visualized on the left side as it assumes a lateral position in relation to the left vertebral artery

Transodontoid Approach

The transodontoid approach [45] is a lower extension of the transclival approach. However, if it is performed independently, a sphenoid opening is not required. It is defined by the removal of the odontoid process of the axis (second vertebra). The lower third of the clivus is exposed as well as the anterior arch of C1 after dissection of the nasopharyngeal mucosa and the rectus capitis anterior muscles. The arch of C1 is drilled and the odontoid process is exposed and drilled out. Depending on the case, a posterior cervical fusion might be necessary. If one of the allar ligaments and occipital condyle–C1 articular facet capsules are preserved, stability can be maintained.

The approach was originally described by our group in 2005 as a means to access the extradural craniocervical junction but we have subsequently used it for intradural pathology [45]. This approach can be used for resection of the odontoid process in degenerative/inflammatory diseases and in congenital compressive disorders or to allow exposure of the ventral medulla and upper cervical spinal cord. Foramen magnum meningiomas are examples of intradural lesions that can be treated using this approach.

The most vital neurovascular structures for this module are the vertebral arteries, posterior inferior cerebellar arteries, brainstem and lower cranial nerves. If a decision is made to perform a medial condylectomy, then attention to the XII cranial nerves is critical at the "10 o'clock" and "2 o'clock" positions. The ICAs have to be considered at risk as well because occasionally they can be positioned close to the midline in their parapharyngeal segment under the mucosa. Preoperative CT angiography should always be performed to rule out this potential for a disastrous situation.

An intraoperative view during an endonasal transodontoid approach for resection of a foramen magnum meningioma is shown in Fig. 17.6.

17.3.2 Coronal (Paramedian) Planes (Lateral to Carotid Arteries)

The coronal plane approaches are studied in three different depths. The anterior coronal plane has an intimate relation with the anterior fossa and orbits, the middle coronal plane with the middle fossa and temporal lobe, and the posterior coronal plane with the posterior fossa.

The middle and posterior paramedian modules are divided based on the morphology of the ICAs. In order to allow dissection in the middle and posterior planes, a transpterygoid approach is performed. The vidian nerve and artery are key landmarks for all lateral expanded approaches since the vidian canal leads to the lacerum segment of the ICA.

Transpterygoid approach

All the modules in the midcoronal and posterior coronal plane start with a transpterygoid approach. Initially a maxillary antrostomy is performed exposing the posterior wall of the maxillary sinus. The sphenopalatine artery is identified and its branches are coagulated and ligated. The posterior wall of the maxillary sinus is removed and the soft contents of the sphenopalatine fossa are retracted laterally. The vidian foramen and foramen rotundum are identified posteriorly in the sphenoid bone. Superiorly in this exposure are found the superior and inferior orbital fissures and the orbital apex. The lateral sphenoid recess can be completely exposed once the pterygoid 'wedge' and the base of the sphenoid plates are drilled. This exposure allows direct access to Meckel's cave and the medial temporal fossa where spontaneous CSF leaks are commonly encountered.

17.3.2.1 Anterior Coronal Plane (Anterior Fossa)

Transorbital Approach

This module requires a wide resection of the anterior and posterior ethmoidal air cells in order to expose the lateral wall of the sinonasal cavity. A transorbital approach is defined by the removal of the lamina papyracea or the medial optic canals. It can be performed unilaterally or bilaterally as dictated by the pathology. At the point the ethmoid cells are removed, the surgical field is limited laterally by the lamina papyracea and the orbital apex at depth. After resection of the bone, the periorbita is exposed. These approaches can be divided into intraconal and extraconal. For transorbital intraconal approaches, the periorbita is opened and the medial and inferior rectus muscles are exposed. In general, there is a good window in between these two muscles to allow intraconal dissection dictated by the intrinsic pathology. Subconjunctival localization and mobilization of the eye muscles are extremely helpful during endonasal endoscopic procedures.

A transorbital endoscopic endonasal approach is indicated for resection of sinonasal lesions that are invading the posterior medial wall of the orbit (such as sinonasal malignances), for decompression of the optic nerves in the presence of unresectable intraconal

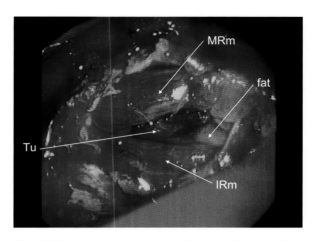

Fig. 17.7 Intraoperative view during dissection of an intraorbital meningioma through an expanded endonasal transorbital intraconal approach with a 45-degree endoscope. Note the window for intraconal dissection between the inferior rectus muscle (*IRm*) and the medial rectus muscle (*MRm*). The intraorbital fat is seen anteriorly and the meningioma (*Tu*) posteriorly

pathologies or for accessing intraconal diseases with the goal of resection such as schwannomas, cavernomas and meningiomas. The most important vital structures related to this module are the optic nerves, the anterior and posterior ethmoidal arteries and the ophthalmic artery with its central retinal branch.

An intraoperative view during dissection of an intraorbital meningioma through an endonasal transorbital intraconal approach is shown in Fig. 17.7.

17.3.2.2 Midcoronal Plane (Middle Fossa)

Petrous Apex (Zone 1)

The petrous apex approach (zone 1 [39]) is fundamentally a lateral extension of the middle third transclival approach. Chondrosarcomas and cholesterol granulomas are typical pathologies in this location. This module is especially useful when lesions expand the petrous apex medially. When the disease is located behind the ICA without medial expansion or remodeling, this medial–lateral corridor should not be used to avoid damage to the ICA. Isolated disease located behind the petrous ICA ('retropetrous') is more safely accessed through an infrapetrous (below the ICA) approach (zone 2; see section 17.3.2.3 Posterior Coronal Plane). The most pertinent structures are the ICAs and the VIth cranial nerve at Dorello's canal.

Suprapetrous Approach (Zone 3)

Suprapetrous refers to above the course of the horizontal ICA).

This module (zone 3 [39]) is indicated to access lesions located in Meckel's cave through the quadrangular space [31]. This space is outlined by the horizontal petrous ICA inferiorly, the ascending vertical cavernous/paraclival ICA medially, the VIth cranial nerve superiorly in the cavernous sinus and the maxillary division of the trigeminal nerve (V2) laterally. In order to get to this region, a transpterygoid approach is performed and the vidian nerve is followed posteriorly up to the level of the lacerum segment of the carotid artery. Once the ICA is identified, it can be skeletonized if needed,

depending on the pathology. The bone of the medial temporal fossa is drilled and the periosteum exposed and opened at the quadrangular space described above.

Pathologies commonly encountered in this region are invasive adenoid cystic carcinomas, juvenile nasal angiofibromas, meningiomas, schwannomas and invasive pituitary adenomas.

The key structures related to this module are the boundaries of the space: ICA, VIth cranial nerve and trigeminal nerve. It is wise to stay below the level of V2 to avoid damage to the VIth cranial nerve.

Image guidance during an expanded endonasal suprapetrous approach for resection of a trigeminal schwannoma located in Meckel's cave is shown in Fig. 17.8.

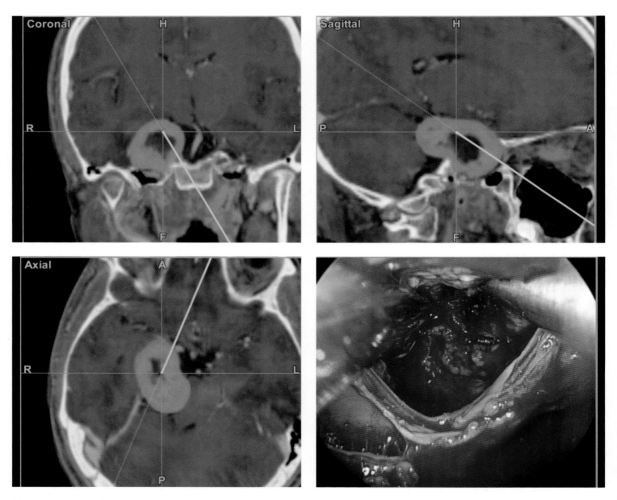

Fig. 17.8 Image guidance during an expanded endonasal suprapetrous approach (zone 3) for resection of a trigeminal schwannoma located in Meckel's cave. Note the trajectory of the blue line (probe)

Supralateral Cavernous Sinus Approach (Zone 4)

Zone 4 [39] refers to the cavernous sinus and is approached lateral to the ICA. It is rarely indicated and most commonly applied in patients who already have cranial nerve deficits (III, IV, VI) such as in apoplectic or functional pituitary adenomas that invade the cavernous sinus causing a cavernous sinus syndrome. It is anatomically defined by the area lateral to the sella turcica where the cavernous carotid siphon is located. The structures at risk during this approach are cranial nerves III, IV, V and VI, and the ICA with its sympathetic fibers.

It is important to mention that we often enter the cavernous sinus just lateral to its medial wall mainly during pituitary surgery with cavernous sinus invasion, which is a lateral extension of a medial transsellar approach. We call that portion of the cavernous sinus the "medial cavernous sinus", since it is located medial or just posterior to the ICA. The medial compartment is a relatively safe area for dissection since all of the cranial nerves are lateral to the cavernous ICA. The inferior hypophyseal artery runs at that level and can be a source of brisk arterial bleeding if not identified and controlled.

Infratemporal Approach (Zone 5)

As one travels from medial to lateral sequentially, the pterygopalatine, infratemporal and temporal fossa are encountered (zone 5 [39]), and these are defined by their relationships to the medial and lateral pterygoid plates. As one progresses from the pterygopalatine fossa, the dissection can be pursued laterally until the lateral pterygoid plate is identified. The lateral pterygoid plate can be drilled rostrally until it is flush with the middle cranial fossa and foramen ovale allowing a corridor even more lateral into the infratemporal fossa. The lateral pterygoid plate is a landmark for identification of the mandibular nerve (V3) immediately posterior.

Pathologies encountered in this region are invasive carcinomas, CSF leaks, encephaloceles, schwannomas and skull-base meningiomas.

The relevant structures in this module are the contents of the pterygomaxillary fissure, such as the internal maxillary artery with its branches, the vidian nerve, the trigeminal nerve (V2 and V3) branches and the superior orbital fissure superiorly.

Image guidance during an endonasal infratemporal approach for resection of a recurrent chordoma is shown in Fig. 17.9.

17.3.2.3 Posterior Coronal Plane (Posterior Fossa)

Infrapetrous Approach (Zone 2)

This region focuses on the petroclival synchondrosis.

The bone under the petrous segment ICA can be removed until the underlying dura of the posterior fossa and venous plexus is identified. The approach (zone 2 [39]) is defined by resections at the petroclival junction. The middle fossa represents the superolateral boundary with the petrous ICA. If required, the dura mater posterior to the drilled petrous bone can be opened to provide access to the paramedian section of the prepontine cistern. for example to expand the corridor to approach a petroclival meningioma. Chondrosarcomas and chordomas are the most common pathologies in this region. Cholesterol granulomas of the petrous apex can be evacuated through this approach particularly when they do not protrude medially into the clival recess.

The vital structures related to this module are the constituents of the inner ear with nerves VII and VIII laterally, the petrous ICA superiorly and the hypoglossal nerve inferolaterally.

Condylar/Hypoglossal Canal Approach

This approach (zone 6 [39]) is an inferior extension of zone 2. It can be approached in combination with an inferior third transclival approach as a lateral extension. However, a zone 6 transcondylar approach is only considered when a partial condylectomy is performed. It is commonly necessary when proximal control of the vertebral artery is important.

The eustachian tube is an important landmark to safely determine the position of the ICA in its parapharyngeal segment where it penetrates the carotid canal in the petrous bone. The fossa of Rosenmüller is followed laterally. The medial aspect of the occipital condyle is encountered lateral to the foramen magnum and followed laterally. The hypoglossal canal is localized rostrolateral to the condyle and should be navigated carefully. This represents the lateral limit of this module. A portion of the condyle can be drilled providing that there is no transgression of the occipital–C1 joint thereby maintaining stability. The dura can be opened behind the drilled condyle and the vertebral artery identified.

Pathologies encountered in this region are invasive carcinomas, paragangliomas, schwannomas and skull-base meningiomas.

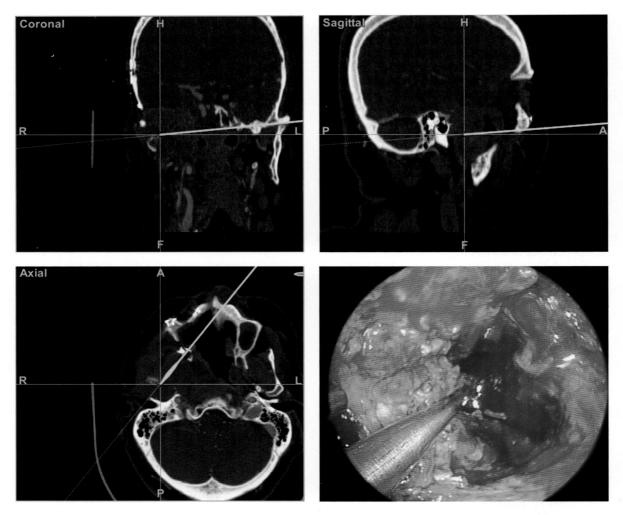

Fig. 17.9 Image guidance during an expanded endonasal infratemporal approach for resection of a recurrent chordoma. Note the trajectory of the blue line (probe)

The relevant structures in this region are the internal maxillary artery, the ICA (parapharyngeal and petrous segments), the trigeminal nerve above and anteriorly, and the XIIth cranial nerve exiting the hypoglossal canal inferiorly and laterally. The lateral limit of zone 6 is the ascending parapharyngeal ICA and the hypoglossal canal.

Jugular Foramen (Zone 7)

Zone 7 is defined by the need for lateral exposure and dissection in close relationship to the parapharyngeal ICA. Zone 7 is a lateral extension of zone 6. The most important landmark for this approach is the eustachian tube, which is sacrificed in order to allow access to the ICA and jugular foramen. The eustachian tube runs parallel and anterior to the petrous ICA and it enters the petrous bone just medial to the ascending parapharyngeal ICA before it enters the petrous canal. Following the eustachian tube laterally allows direct identification of the ICA. Once the ICA is localized, the jugular foramen is located immediately lateral and posterior. Cranial nerves IX, X and XI are located in between the jugular vein and the ICA. This region often requires an endoscopic Denker's (i.e. wide medial) and anterior maxillectomy.

Pathologies encountered in this region are invasive carcinomas, paragangliomas, schwannomas and skull-base meningiomas.

The jugular foramen with jugular vein and lower cranial nerves (IX, X, XI) are the most relevant structures in this module, plus all structures listed in zone 6.

17.4 Reconstruction Technique

Following the principles of reconstruction in open skull-base surgery, we use vascularized tissue to rebuild the skull-base defect. Hadad et al. developed a nasoseptal flap supplied by the posterior nasoseptal arteries, which are branches of the sphenopalatine artery [42]. We have subsequently modified this flap and have shown its ability to reach the entire ventral skull base [43]. This nasoseptal mucosal flap is our preferred reconstruction

technique [43]. The flap is harvested initially during the surgery or as a rescue flap at the end of the procedure in cases in which a CSF leak may not be generated during dissection. In general, it is harvested on the side that requires less lateral exposure, contralateral to the lesion [43]. During the reconstruction, the flap needs to be in contact with the denuded bone for appropriate defect closure, so all the sinus mucosa is extirpated.

Besides the nasoseptal mucosal flap, we use an inlay subdural graft of collagen matrix. Rarely, in cases in which the nasoseptal flap does not cover the entire defect, an additional onlay fascial graft and/or abdominal free fat is used. It is imperative to avoid leaving any foreign body or nonvascularized tissue between the flap and the surrounding edges of the defect.

When a nasoseptal flap is not available, then vascularized tissue can be obtained from other sources. Excellent alternatives are in the nasal cavity, such as an

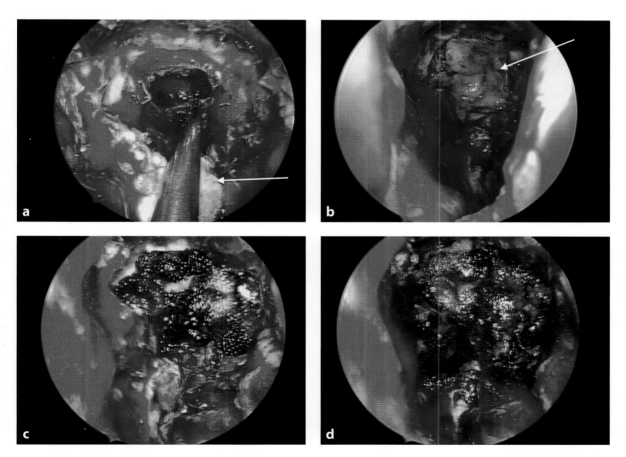

Fig. 17.10 Intraoperative sequence views of skull base reconstruction. **a** The skull-base defect. **b** The nasoseptal flap covering the defect. **c** Surgicel on top of the nasoseptal flap. **d** Duraseal was deposited on the Surgicel. *White arrows* (**a**, **b**) nasoseptal flap

inferior turbinate flap, optimized for clival defects, or middle turbinate flaps for small anterior fossa defects [46]. In situations where a vascularized flap is not available in the nasal cavity, such as after multiple surgeries or radical resections, then healthy vascularized tissue can be elevated externally and rotated into the nasal cavity to cover the defect. Examples of extranasal flaps that can be rotated into the nasal cavity are: (1) the transpterygoid temporoparietal fascia flap based on the superficial temporal artery [47], and (2) a pericranial flap vascularized by the supraorbital artery elevated endoscopically and transferred to the nasal cavity through an opening in the nasal bone.

Biological glue helps to fix the flap in place (but should not be overused) and nasal sponge packing or the balloon of a 12F Foley catheter is inserted to press the Hadad-Bassagasteguy flap against the defect. Inflation of the Foley balloon should be under endoscopic observation, as over-inflation may result in compression of intracranial structures or may compromise the flap vascular pedicle. Silicone splints, left in place for 21 days, protect the denuded septum.

An intraoperative sequence views of skull base reconstruction are shown in Fig. 17.10.

17.5 Conclusion

In our opinion, the two main sources of morbidity in skull-base surgery are the vasculature and the cranial nerves. The selection of approach is determined by the position of the ICAs, circle of Willis, and the cranial nerves. A thorough understanding of and confidence with cerebrovascular surgery is critical for the skull-base surgeon, regardless of the approach being used. The basic guiding principle when choosing an approach is to avoid crossing the plane of these structures, which are then kept on the perimeter of the lesion. In particular, the plane of cranial nerves which are much less tolerant of manipulation.

In accessing lesions of the skull base, the circle of Willis can be approached via medial/ventral corridors (endoscopy) or conventional lateral corridors. Our guiding principle in selecting the appropriate corridor is the need to transgress the plane of cranial nerves and small perforators. Endoscopy does not offer the solution to every surgically treated disease. Therefore, endoscopic approaches are not a substitute but a complement to traditional transcranial and microscopic approaches, and thus it is critical that skull-base surgeons be versed in all techniques to be able to offer the best alternative to their patients.

In summary, the principles we wish to emphasize are:
1. Exposure should be bimanual.
2. Resection should follow the principles of microsurgery.
3. Reconstruction should ideally be vascularized.
4. Selection of the approach should:
   a. Be based on corridors that avoid crossing the plane of cranial nerves and small perforators.
   b. Take account of the surgeon's experience.
   c. Take account of the patient's comorbidities.
   d. Take account of the patient's age.

The endoscope is a tool for visualization while a microsurgical technique is being applied. Outcomes are determined by the judgment with which it is selected and the technique with which it is applied.

References

1. Doglietto F, Prevedello DM, Jane JA Jr et al (2005) Brief history of endoscopic transsphenoidal surgery – from Philipp Bozzini to the First World Congress of Endoscopic Skull Base Surgery. Neurosurg Focus 19:E3
2. Weir N (2000) History of medicine: otorhinolaryngology. Postgrad Med J 76:65–69
3. Messerklinger W (1972) Nasal endoscopy: demonstration, localization and differential diagnosis of nasal liquorrhea (in German). HNO 20:268–270
4. Kennedy DW (1985) Functional endoscopic sinus surgery. Technique. Arch Otolaryngol 111:643–649
5. Kennedy DW, Zinreich SJ, Rosenbaum AE, Johns ME (1985) Functional endoscopic sinus surgery. Theory and diagnostic evaluation. Arch Otolaryngol 111:576–582
6. Stammberger H (1986) Nasal and paranasal sinus endoscopy. A diagnostic and surgical approach to recurrent sinusitis. Endoscopy 18:213–218
7. Draf W (1983) Endoscopy of the paranasal sinuses. Springer, Berlin Heidelberg
8. Griffith HB (1977) Endoneurosurgery: endoscopic intracranial surgery. Proc R Soc Lond B Biol Sci 195:261–268
9. Cappabianca P, de Divitiis E (2004) Endoscopy and transsphenoidal surgery. Neurosurgery 54:1043–1048
10. Maroon JC (2005) Skull base surgery: past, present, and future trends. Neurosurg Focus 19:E1
11. Liu JK, Das K, Weiss MH et al (2001) The history and evolution of transsphenoidal surgery. J Neurosurg 95:1083–1096
12. Apuzzo ML, Heifetz MD, Weiss MH, Kurze T (1977) Neurosurgical endoscopy using the side-viewing telescope. J Neurosurg 46:398–400

13. Bushe KA, Halves E (1978) Modified technique in transsphenoidal operations of pituitary adenomas. Technical note (author's transl) (in German). Acta Neurochir (Wien) 41:163–175

14. Halves E, Bushe KA (1979) Transsphenoidal operation on craniopharyngiomas with extrasellar extensions. The advantage of the operating endoscope [proceedings]. Acta Neurochir Suppl (Wien) 28:362

15. Dusick JR, Esposito F, Kelly DF et al (2005) The extended direct endonasal transsphenoidal approach for nonadenomatous suprasellar tumors. J Neurosurg 102:832–841

16. Couldwell WT, Weiss MH, Rabb C et al (2004) Variations on the standard transsphenoidal approach to the sellar region, with emphasis on the extended approaches and parasellar approaches: surgical experience in 105 cases. Neurosurgery 55:539–547

17. Frank G, Pasquini E, Mazzatenta D (2001) Extended transsphenoidal approach. J Neurosurg 95:917–918

18. Catapano D, Sloffer CA, Frank G et al (2006) Comparison between the microscope and endoscope in the direct endonasal extended transsphenoidal approach: anatomical study. J Neurosurg 104:419–425

19. Frank G, Pasquini E, Doglietto F et al (2006) The endoscopic extended transsphenoidal approach for craniopharyngiomas. Neurosurgery 59:ONS75– ONS83

20. de Divitiis E, Cappabianca P (2002) Microscopic and endoscopic transsphenoidal surgery. Neurosurgery 51:1527–1529

21. Jankowski R, Auque J, Simon C et al (1992) Endoscopic pituitary tumor surgery. Laryngoscope 102:198–202

22. Sethi DS, Pillay PK (1995) Endoscopic management of lesions of the sella turcica. J Laryngol Otol 109:956–962

23. Carrau RL, Jho HD, Ko Y (1996) Transnasal-transsphenoidal endoscopic surgery of the pituitary gland. Laryngoscope 106:914–918

24. Jho HD, Carrau RL (1997) Endoscopic endonasal transsphenoidal surgery: experience with 50 patients. J Neurosurg 87:44–51

25. Litynski GS (1999) Endoscopic surgery: the history, the pioneers. World J Surg 23:745–753

26. Cappabianca P, Alfieri A, Colao A et al (2000) Endoscopic endonasal transsphenoidal surgery in recurrent and residual pituitary adenomas: technical note. Minim Invasive Neurosurg 43:38–43

27. Cappabianca P, Frank G, Pasquini E et al (2003) Extended endoscopic endonasal transsphenoidal approaches to the suprasellar region, planum sphenoidale and clivus. In: de Divitis E, Cappabianca P (eds) Endoscopic endonasal transsphenoidal surgery. Springer, Vienna New York, pp 176–187

28. Cavallo LM, Briganti F, Cappabianca P et al (2004) Hemorrhagic vascular complications of endoscopic transsphenoidal surgery. Minim Invasive Neurosurg 47:145–150

29. Cavallo LM, Cappabianca P, Galzio R et al (2005) Endoscopic transnasal approach to the cavernous sinus versus transcranial route: anatomic study. Neurosurgery 56:379–389

30. Cavallo LM, Messina A, Cappabianca P et al (2005) Endoscopic endonasal surgery of the midline skull base: anatomical study and clinical considerations. Neurosurg Focus 19:E2

31. Cavallo LM, Messina A, Gardner P et al (2005) Extended endoscopic endonasal approach to the pterygopalatine fossa: anatomical study and clinical considerations. Neurosurg Focus 19:E5

32. Cappabianca P, Alfieri A, Thermes S et al (1999) Instruments for endoscopic endonasal transsphenoidal surgery. Neurosurgery 45:392–395

33. Cappabianca P, Cavallo LM, Mariniello G et al (2001) Easy sellar reconstruction in endoscopic endonasal transsphenoidal surgery with polyester-silicone dural substitute and fibrin glue: technical note. Neurosurgery 49:473–475

34. Cappabianca P, Cavallo LM, Valente V et al (2004) Sellar repair with fibrin sealant and collagen fleece after endoscopic endonasal transsphenoidal surgery. Surg Neurol 62:227–233

35. Cappabianca P, de Divitiis E (2007) Back to the Egyptians: neurosurgery via the nose. A five-thousand year history and the recent contribution of the endoscope. Neurosurg Rev 30:1–7

36. de Divitiis E (2006) Endoscopic transsphenoidal surgery: stone-in-the-pond effect. Neurosurgery 59:512–520

37. Prevedello DM, Doglietto F, Jane JA Jr et al (2007) History of endoscopic skull base surgery: its evolution and current reality. J Neurosurg 107:206–213

38. Prevedello DM, Thomas A, Gardner P et al (2007) Endoscopic endonasal resection of a synchronous pituitary adenoma and a tuberculum sellae meningioma: technical case report. Neurosurgery 60:E401

39. Kassam AB, Gardner P, Snyderman C et al (2005) Expanded endonasal approach: fully endoscopic, completely transnasal approach to the middle third of the clivus, petrous bone, middle cranial fossa, and infratemporal fossa. Neurosurg Focus 19:E6

40. Kassam A, Snyderman CH, Mintz A et al (2005) Expanded endonasal approach: the rostrocaudal axis. Part II. Posterior clinoids to the foramen magnum. Neurosurg Focus 19:E4

41. Kassam A, Snyderman CH, Mintz A et al (2005) Expanded endonasal approach: the rostrocaudal axis. Part I. Crista galli to the sella turcica. Neurosurg Focus 19:E3

42. Hadad G, Bassagasteguy L, Carrau RL et al (2006) A novel reconstructive technique after endoscopic expanded endonasal approaches: vascular pedicle nasoseptal flap. Laryngoscope 116:1882–1886

43. Kassam A, Thomas A, Carrau RL et al (2008) Endoscopic reconstruction of the skull base using a pedicled nasoseptal flap. Neurosurgery 63:ONS44–ONS52

44. Kassam AB, Prevedello DM, Thomas A et al (2008) Endoscopic endonasal pituitary transposition for transdorsum sellae approach to the interpeduncular cistern. Neurosurgery 62:57–72

45. Kassam AB, Snyderman C, Gardner P et al (2005) The expanded endonasal approach: a fully endoscopic transnasal approach and resection of the odontoid process: technical case report. Neurosurgery 57:E213

46. Fortes FS, Carrau RL, Snyderman CH et al (2007) The posterior pedicle inferior turbinate flap: a new vascularized flap for skull base reconstruction. Laryngoscope 117: 1329–1332

47. Fortes FS, Carrau RL, Snyderman CH et al (2007) Transpterygoid transposition of a temporoparietal fascia flap: a new method for skull base reconstruction after endoscopic expanded endonasal approaches. Laryngoscope 117:970–976

Introduction

Maxillofacial Surgery: Evolution and Approaches

Luigi Califano

Historical Notes

Skull-base surgery is a very exciting and relatively recent medical discipline that still represents a challenge for the surgeon who is involved in this field.

The history of skull-base surgery is brief, but many pioneers have contributed to its development. Donald reports that the first approaches to the skull base were performed by Francesco Durante (1844–1934) who successfully removed an olfactory groove meningioma in a 35-year-old woman who presented with a loss of smell, proptosis and loss of memory [1].

Historically, most of maxillofacial approaches derive from pituitary gland surgery. Giordano was the first surgeon to describe an extracranial corridor to the sphenoid sinus and intracranial contents [2]. In 1907 the first purely transnasal excision to remove the pituitary gland via the transphenoidal approach was described by Schloffer [3] and, in 1910, Von Eiselsberg performed a transfacial approach to the sphenoid sinus [4]. Subsequently, Cushing in 1914 attempted a sublabial approach to the pituitary fossa preserving the turbinates and nasal function following Killian's suggestion of using a submucosal dissection of the nasal septum [5]. In the same period, Oscar Hirsch, an otolaryngologist, developed the transnasal route combining it with a midline sublabial approach [6].

The first anterior craniofacial resection for a tumor was performed by Dandy in 1941 who, while removing an orbital lesion via an anterior craniofacial approach,

entered the ethmoid complex achieving a better visualization [7].

The work performed by Ketcham et al. in 1963 regarding the combined intracranial–transfacial approach to the paranasal sinuses represent a milestone for the future development of the transfacial approaches in skull-base surgery [8, 9].

More recently, regarding craniofacial surgery for the treatment of skull-base lesions, plastic surgeons, such as Paul Tessier, and maxillofacial surgeons, such as Joram Raveh, recommended that, to reach the central skull base, retraction of the brain parenchyma should be avoided, thus also avoiding related complications [10, 11]. Later, the introduction of the operative microscope contributed tremendously to the improvement of surgical techniques, minimizing brain retraction and improving the functional and esthetic results.

Finally, the transoral approach to the clivus and upper cervical spine was developed by Scoville and Sherman in 1951 [12] and, later, Crockard refined and standardized this approach [13], while median labio-mandibular glossotomy was introduced by Conley in 1970 [14].

Introduction to Maxillofacial Approaches

Often the disease (neoplastic, inflammatory, vascular, traumatic, or congenital) affects the structures on both sides of the base of the skull. Surgery in this region is unique due to its complexity, often requiring the coordinated cooperation and the mutual expertise of at least two surgical disciplines (i.e. neurosurgery and maxillo-

L. Califano (✉)
Dept of Head and Neck Surgery
Università degli Studi di Napoli Federico II, Naples, Italy

facial surgery), since the segmental nature of the craniofacial skeleton lends itself to schematic anatomic compartmentalization of neoplasms involving this region. The development of computed tomography, magnetic resonance imaging, and, more recently, positron emission tomography and image-guided surgery systems (neuronavigation) has allowed an increase in the indications, improvement in the results and a reduction in the complications, thus permitting the evolution and refinement of the surgical techniques. Transfacial approaches are useful as an overall framework for the disassembly of the face for exposure of the cranial base.

Indeed, by using these techniques, multiple segments of the craniofacial skeleton and soft tissue may be disassembled to expose deep-seated tumors, and then reassembled with quite good functional and esthetic results, enabling the surgeon to resect these tumors more efficiently under direct vision and magnification. Transfacial approaches provide a wider exposure of a difficult region and allow resection of almost all anterior skull-base tumors, having in mind the team concept where the essential figures are the craniofacial surgeon and the neurosurgeon.

The transnasal, transseptal, transfacial, transoral, and transmaxillary (Le Fort I maxillotomy) approaches are usually considered alternative routes to the skull base; they often provide adequate tumor removal with minimal morbidity. Although better esthetic results can be achieved with some of these approaches, all of them have pros and cons that are highlighted in the following chapters, each one focusing on a particular subgroup.

The transfacial approaches to the skull base may be roughly divided into midfacial routes, low-facial routes and lateral routes.

Among the midfacial routes, we can include the following:
- Lateronasal approaches:
  – Denker
  – Weber-Ferguson
  – Midfacial degloving
- Transorbital
  – Lynch
  – Medial orbitotomy
  – Lateral orbitotomy
  – Transconjuntival
  – Subciliary
- Transnasal
  – Microscopic
  – Endoscopic
- Transmaxillary
  – Le Fort I maxillotomy with or without palatal split

Among the low-facial routes, we can include the following:
- Transoral
- Transmandibular

Among the lateral routes, we can include the following:
- Approach to the infratemporal fossa
- Approach to the pterygopalatine fossa

Besides the various types of approach to the skull base, it is extremely important to analyze the reconstructive techniques and methods, which greatly contribute to the functional and esthetic results.

The maxillofacial segment of this atlas is focused on the main approaches used to expose the skull base:

Midfacial approaches Such approaches, using transfacial swing osteotomies and based on the principle of disassembly of vascularized midfacial composite units, allow a wide exposure of the anterior and central areas of the skull base and related anatomical regions, such as the nasopharynx or the paranasal sinuses. They are usually completed by esthetic and functional reconstruction.

Transmandibular approaches Such routes can be useful for the surgical management of lesions involving the middle and posterior cranial base, its underlying volumes, and the first cervical vertebrae. The transmandibular approach allows a wider exposure of the middle compartment of the skull base from the foramen magnum up to the sella turcica on the midline, and laterally exposing the infratemporal fossa, petrous bone and parapharyngeal space with its neurovascular contents, compared to other skull-base approaches, i.e. transethmoidal, transoral, transoral–transpalatal.

Orbital approaches Such approaches are frequently indicated for orbital decompression for thyroid orbitopathy, excision of cysts or masses, repair of fractures and reconstruction of defects, abscess drainage, optic nerve decompression, and removal of a foreign body.

Transoral approach The transoral approach provides a direct midline surgical corridor to the midline to expose the craniovertebral junction and ventral foramen magnum. It is indicated principally for extradural lesions such as chordomas, chondrosarcomas and rheumatoid or degenerative pannus. This approach can be extended to increase the exposure via the transmaxillary route without or with palatal split, transpalatal route and median labiomandibular glossotomy.

Reconstructive techniques Accurate planning of reconstruction after most of the approaches described is mandatory. The key point is to separate the endocranial contents from the pharynx and external environment by means of well-vascularized tissue. This chapter gives an overview of the most used and useful reconstructive techniques, with respective indications, complications, advantages and limitations.

References

1. Guidetti B (1983) Francesco Durante. June 29, 1844 to October 2, 1934. Surg Neurol 20:1–3

2. Artico M, Pastore FS, Fraioli B, Giuffre R (1998) The contribution of Davide Giordano (1864-1954) to pituitary surgery: the transglabellar-nasal approach. Neurosurgery 42:909–911

3. Schloffer H (1907) Erfolgreiche Operationen eines Hypophysentumors auf nasalem Wege. Wien Klin Wochenschr 20:621–624

4. Von Eiselsberg A (1910) My experience about operation upon the hypophysis. Trans Am Surg Assoc 28:55

5. Cushing H (1909) Partial hypophysectomy for acromegaly: with remarks on the function of the hypophysis. Ann Surg 50:1002–1017

6. Hamlin H (1981) Oskar Hirsch. Surg Neurol 16:391–393

7. Dandy W (1941) Orbital tumor: results following the transcranial operative attack. OskarPiest, New York

8. Ketcham A, Hoyle R, Van Buren J et al (1966) Complications of intracranial facial resection for tumors of the paranasal sinuses. Am J Surg 12:591–596

9. Ketcham A, Wilkins R, Van Buren J, Smith R (1963) A combined intracranial facial approach to the paranasal sinuses. Am J Surg 106:698–703

10. Raveh J (1983) Das einzeitge vorgehan bei der widerherstellung von frontobasal-mittelgesichtsfrakturen modifikationen und behandlungsmodalitaten. Chirurgie 54:677–686

11. Tessier P, Guiot G, Rougerie J (1967) Cranio-naso-orbitofacial osteotomies. Hypertelorism. Ann Chir Plast 12:103–118

12. Scoville W, Sherman I (1951) Ptalybasia: report of 10 cases with comments on familial tendency, a special diagnostic sign and the end result of operation. Ann Surg 133:496–502

13. Crockard H (1993) Transoral approach to intra/extradural tumors. In: Sekhar L, Janecka I (eds) Surgery of cranial base tumors. Raven Press, New York, pp 225–234

14. Conley J (1970) Concepts in head and neck surgery. Grune & Stratton, New York

Enrico Sesenna, Tito Poli and Alice S. Magri

18.1 Introduction

The orbits represent key structures in the organization of the middle third of the face.

Seven bones form the bony orbital framework: maxilla, zygoma, ethmoid, sphenoid, palatine, frontal and lacrimal (Fig. 18.1). The bony orbit is a pyramid-shaped, conical structure with a total volume of approximately 30 cm³ (7 cm³ corresponding to the globe) completely occupied by soft tissues (eyeball, extraocular muscles, vessels, nerves, lacrimal gland, fat, etc.). To simplify assessment of the orbit, this region is organized into three anatomic compartments: the extraconal space, the intraconal space, and the globe. The orbit is a potential source of a wide range of diseases due to its structural complexity. Because of the anterior anatomic obstacle created by the bony orbital rim and the antero-posterior narrowing of the orbital cavity, the choice of an adequate surgical access to the orbit requires a comprehensive evaluation of the case (clinical, radiological, pathological) and scrupulous adhesion to some basic operative principles: a bloodless operative field, adequate exposure and visualization, optimal instrumentation, safe atraumatic manipulation of the tissues and exposure through nonpathologically involved planes.

A detailed review of the literature reveals no substantial change or innovation in the surgical approaches to the orbit during the last century, but rather a more rational use of well-described procedures mainly related to the topographic characteristics of the disease.

T. Poli (✉)
Maxillofacial Surgery Section, Head and Neck Dept
University Hospital of Parma, Italy

18.2 Surgical Anatomy

The orbit consists of seven bones that form a four-sided pyramid evolving into a three-sided one proceeding from the external rim to the apex. Anteriorly the bony orbit is delimited by a wide rim that Whitnall described as a spiral with its two ends overlapping medially on either side of the lacrimal fossa. The superior orbital rim is constituted by the frontal bone, the lateral rim by the zygoma, the medial rim by the frontal process of the maxilla joined with the maxillary process of the frontal bone, and the inferior rim by the maxilla medially and

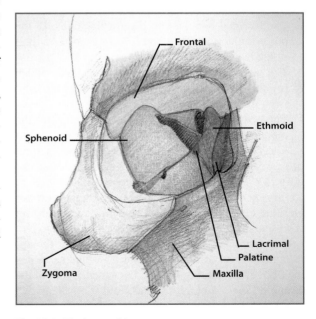

Fig. 18.1 The bony orbit

P. Cappabianca et al. (eds.), *Cranial, Craniofacial and Skull Base Surgery*.
© Springer-Verlag Italia 2010

the zygoma laterally. The orbital roof consists of the thin orbital plate of the frontal bone that separates the orbit from the frontal sinuses anteriorly and the anterior cranial fossa posteriorly. The posterior 1.5 cm of the orbital roof is formed by the lesser wing of the sphenoid bone as the roof tapers backwards and downwards toward the orbital apex into the anterior clinoid process. The optic nerve enters the orbit through the optic foramen located in the posterior orbital roof. More anteriorly the lacrimal gland fossa is located in the lateral part and the trochlear fossa in the medial part of the orbital roof.

The lateral orbital wall is formed by the zygoma anteriorly and the greater wing of the sphenoid bone posteriorly. The thickness of the lateral wall changes widely moving from the rim (the strongest part), through the middle third (the thinnest part) and finally to the sphenozygomatic suture posteriorly (where the thickness rises again). The Whitnall's tubercle is 1.2 cm to 1.5 cm posterior to the lateral orbital rim, and it marks the attachment of the lateral canthal tendon which should be reattached if freed during surgery. The posterior extent of the lateral wall is defined by the superior orbital fissure, which separates the lesser and greater wings of the sphenoid bone, and the inferior orbital fissure created by the gap between the maxilla and the greater wing of the sphenoid bone.

The medial orbital walls are approximately parallel to each other and to the midsagittal plane. From anterior to posterior, the medial orbital wall is formed by:
1. The frontal process of the maxilla, which is a thick bone segment that forms the medial orbital rim.
2. The lacrimal bone, a thin plate which contains the posterior lacrimal crest and forms the posterior half of the lacrimal sac fossa.
3. The lamina papyracea of the ethmoid bone, which is a thin plate (0.2–0.4 mm) that separates the orbit from the ethmoid air cells.
4. The body of the sphenoid bone, that completes the medial wall to the apex.

The frontoethmoid suture marks the superior limit of the medial orbital wall. It contains the anterior and posterior ethmoidal foramina approximately 20 to 25 mm and 32 to 35 mm posterior to the anterior lacrimal crest, respectively. These foramina transmit corresponding arteries, and should be identified to prevent hemorrhage and also because they mark the approximate level of the cribriform plate that separates the floor of the anterior cranial fossa and the roof of the ethmoid sinus. A cerebrospinal fluid (CSF) leak can occur if the medial orbital wall is penetrated superior to these foramina.

The orbital floor is the shortest orbital wall, formed mainly by the orbital plate of the maxilla overlying the maxillary sinus. The anterolateral segment is formed by the zygomatic bone and the posterior segment by the palatine bone. The floor forms a triangular wedge from the maxillary-ethmoid buttress to the inferior orbital fissure horizontally, and the orbital rim to the posterior wall of the maxillary sinus; so it does not reach the orbital apex. The infraorbital groove, transmitting the infraorbital nerve and artery, starts from the inferior orbital fissure and runs forward in the maxilla, becoming the infraorbital canal anteriorly and ending as the infraorbital foramen 6 to 10 mm inferior to the inferior orbital rim. The floor is thin and medial to the infraorbital canal, and surgery on the orbital floor requires special attention to prevent injury.

The orbital contents consist of: eyeball, extraocular muscles, vessels, nerves, lacrimal gland, fat, etc. In particular, the four rectus muscles define the so-called "muscle cone" dividing the orbit into extraconal and intraconal compartments.

The eyelids contain the orbital septum (which represents the anterior soft tissue boundary of the orbit) and the protractor–retractor muscular system (that allows opening and closing of the lids, and provides the blink reflex responsible for protection of the cornea and for pumping tears through the lacrimal excretory system).

The orbital septum, covered by a thin layer of skin, subcuticular tissue and preseptal orbicularis, originates from the orbital rim at the arcus marginalis and inserts onto the eyelid retractors. In both eyelids, there is an analogous triangular space between the eyelid retractor and septum that contains orbital fat. The upper eyelid retractor is represented by the levator muscle, whose aponeurosis passes downward from Whitnall's ligament about 15 to 20 mm to insert onto the tarsal face and to the pretarsal eyelid skin. The lower eyelid retractor is the capsulopalpebral fascia, which originates from and is powered by the inferior rectus muscle and which incorporates the fascial fibers of Lockwood's ligament. After surrounding the inferior oblique muscle, the capsulopalpebral fascia continues forward to insert onto the lower eyelid tarsus and pretarsal skin.

The posterior lamella of the eyelids consists of smooth tarsal muscles (more developed in the upper eyelid as Müller's muscle, which originates from the posterior surface of the levator aponeurosis in the region of Whitnall's ligament and inserts onto the superior tarsal border), conjunctiva, and the tarsal plates, which are fibrous condensations that provide a skeleton for the eyelid margin and contain the meibomian glands (Fig. 18.2).

The orbicularis muscle is divided into pretarsal, preseptal and orbital portions. The muscle fibers form a C-shaped loop and function as the eyelid sphincter. The orbital portion of the orbicularis inserts medially along the superior and inferior orbital rims. The pretarsal and preseptal portions insert with a complex arrangement at the medial canthal tendon by dividing into interdigitating deep and superficial heads. The preseptal muscle divides in a superficial head, which inserts into the anterior limb of the medial canthal tendon, and in a deep head, which inserts onto the fascia of the lacrimal sac. The pretarsal muscle sends anterior slips to the anterior medial canthal tendon and posterior slips (the pars lacrimalis or Horner's muscle) that converge posterior to the lacrimal sac, enclosing the posterior wall of the lacrimal sac and inserting onto the posterior lacrimal crest. The lacrimal sac lies in the lacrimal fossa between the two limbs of the medial canthal tendon.

The lateral canthal tendon is created by the confluence of the upper and lower tarsal tendons and inserts on the lateral orbital tubercle of Whitnall. More anteriorly the lateral canthal tendon receives a contribution from the lateral pretarsal and preseptal orbicularis oculi muscle. The deep portion of the lateral canthal tendon forms the lateral part of the orbital septum.

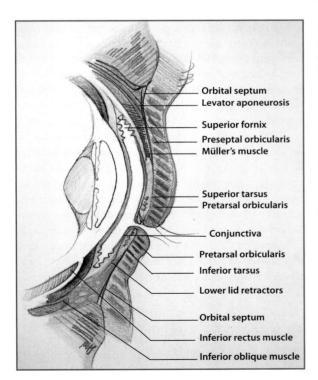

Fig. 18.2 Cross-sectional anatomy of the eyelids and anterior orbit

The lacrimal system is composed of a secretory and an excretory component. The secretory portion is composed mainly of the lacrimal gland (orbital and palpebral portions divided by the levator aponeurosis) that lies in the shallow lacrimal fossa of the anterolateral orbital roof, and the excretory portion comprises the superior and inferior puncta and canaliculi, the lacrimal sac, and the nasolacrimal duct which drains tears into the nasal fossa beneath the inferior turbinate.

18.3 Clinical Aspects

According to Rootman and Durity [1] the anatomic changes caused by a disease in the orbit can be divided into four basic categories of clinical manifestation: inflammatory signs, mass effect, infiltration, and vascular changes. These categories are not necessarily independent, but provide a working framework for characterization of a particular orbital problem.

A mass effect consists of displacement with or without signs of involvement of sensory or neuromuscular structures. Displacement of orbital structures can indicate the localization of the disease and help in defining its nature.

Inflammation is characterized by, and can be suspected by, signs and symptoms of pain, warmth, loss of function, and a mass effect. The degree to which one categorizes the process as either acute or chronic is related to the severity of the signs and symptoms as well as the rapidity of onset.

Infiltrative changes are usually associated with evidence of bone destruction, muscle entrapment, etc., which may lead to effects on ocular movement and neurosensory function (e.g., diplopia, muscle restriction, visual loss, pain or paresthesia).

Alterations in the shape, size, and structural integrity of vessels may imply an underlying vascular process. The major features suggesting vascular changes are venous dilatation, tissue exudation, hemorrhage, infarction, and structural alterations of vascular components.

Statistically the most common manifestation related to neoplasia is a mass effect while the second one, which is usually associated with a malignant process, is infiltration.

Patients affected by orbital diseases must be investigated with a thorough history and physical analysis, which would define the structural and functional changes as well as the location of orbital lesions. The steps of investigation are comprehensive and comprise a careful clinical examination, ocular and visual function assessment, orbital imaging, systemic survey, and pathological study.

The objective assessment of the eye and adnexal structures should include an evaluation of the color and texture of the adnexal tissues and surface of the eye, an observation of any disparity in the anatomic relationship of the eye and covering eyelids, and palpation of the orbital rim and soft tissue components of the anterior orbit [2]. Protrusion (any combination of proptosis and displacement) of the eye, mono- or bilateral, is the most frequent manifestation of Graves' orbitopathy or an orbital tumor; on the contrary, enophthalmos is sometimes secondary to a retraction effect of an infiltrative, sclerosing malignant tumor. Dynamic proptosis is usually associated with a carotid–cavernous sinus fistula of traumatic origin or with a bony dysplasia of the orbit present in neurofibromatosis. Palpation of an orbit with a protruding or displaced eye is of diagnostic value essentially in cases of a tumor located along the orbital rim, in the lacrimal gland fossa, and in adnexal structures.

The next step is the assessment of ocular function and motility, which is helpful in diagnosis and essential in judging the "before and after" of therapy. Ocular function may be affected in several ways by an orbital mass such as malposition of the eye secondary to increased orbital pressure, anatomic contact of tumor and eye, infiltration by tumor of nerves and muscles connected to the eye, and direct or indirect compromise of the blood supply to the eye and appendages by the tumor.

Finally, ocular and psychophysical investigations should include visual field assessment, oculomotor examination, psychophysical studies, such as color vision and contrast sensitivity, and electrophysiological investigations (visual evoked response, VER).

18.4 Orbital Imaging

Orbital imaging has undergone an extraordinary evolution over the last 30–40 years and nowadays provides detailed information. It is not only able to display the exact localization but also to suggest features of inflammatory, mass, infiltrative, and vascular changes. These radiographic data, combined with clinical and ophthalmological investigation results, allows increasing specificity in terms of defining the position, nature, and clinical course of lesions. In particular they can reveal fundamental information regarding evidence of infiltration, capsular definition, tissue characteristics, and

the relationship to the vascular and nervous systems, which will aid in determining both the need for surgery and the type of approach. In addition, changes with time on follow-up can aid in diagnosis and assessment of a treatment modality.

In modern imaging routines radiographic methods are of limited use, but can outline dense tumors such as osteomas and the bony changes associated with both expansive and destructive lesions and fractures.

Nowadays the gold standard in orbital imaging investigation remains accurate high-resolution computed tomography (CT) with or without administration of contrast agent. The CT scan can define the margin of lesions (smooth, nodular, or infiltrative) and demonstrate contrast enhancement in inflammatory, vascular, and some solid tumors. Density differentiation may help in defining fat and calcium, and delineate adjacent soft tissues. The location of the lesions as well as their extension into either the nasosinusal cavities or intracranial spaces can also be studied with both soft tissue and bone dedicated settings.

Magnetic resonance imaging (MRI) may give additional information regarding the structural nature of orbital lesions and is particularly useful in the study of optic nerve masses when the normal nerve structures can be defined separately from adjacent tumor masses, thus differentiating between intrinsic and extrinsic optic nerve tumors. In addition, this modality is useful in demonstrating some vascular lesions and delineating the anatomy of and relationship to intracranial structures in lesions that have extended beyond the orbit into adjacent cavities. Finally, gadolinium-enhanced fat-suppressed MRI is the first choice imaging modality in patients affected by Graves' orbitopathy.

Vascular studies, both arterial and venous, are useful only for selected aspects of orbital tumors. Magnified and subtracted views of the arterial supply can aid in defining preoperatively the location and character of the blood supply of tumors. Some vascular tumors can be treated with preoperative embolization and occlusion. Venography is rarely used now except for specific indications in case of orbital varices. Echography can provide useful information on location, size, shape, tissue characteristics, and vascular features of many lesions.

18.5 Pathological Diagnosis

In order to provide a framework for understanding surgical indications and approaches to the orbit, orbital disorders can be classified into six major categories (Graves' disease, neoplasia, structural disorders, inflammatory processes, vascular lesions, degenerative diseases) [1, 3]. These diseases can occur either independently or together, in or around the orbit, and all enter into the differential diagnosis of "orbital tumors" insofar as they produce mass and functional effects based on displacement or infiltration of healthy structures.

Pathological assessment of biopsied tissue has become increasingly sophisticated and it is important to emphasize that the appropriate management and processing of these tissues should be clearly outlined in advance of surgery to maximize the diagnostic yield. Orbital masses with a clear benign clinical behavior and benign imaging (well-defined boundaries/borders, etc.) can be approached without any pathological preoperative assessment. On the other hand, masses showing an infiltrative pattern on imaging and/or a malignant clinical course need open biopsy or a fine-needle aspiration biopsy (FNAB). This is the case for malignant tumors, and also for inflammatory processes (inflammatory pseudotumor) and systemic diseases not requiring surgery (lymphomas).

Orbital lesions can be biopsied not only with open surgical procedures but also with B-scan ultrasound- or CT-guided FNAB, especially for lesions involving the optic nerve. The basic tenet of FNAB is to establish a histological diagnosis of an orbital tumor in an office setting, which may spare the patient the morbidity of an orbitotomy. To this end, Kennerdell [4] standardized the technique, tried to ensure its safety, noted the complications, and assessed the accuracy and efficacy of the procedure. The accuracy of the procedure has, however, been the subject of ongoing discussion in the literature, considering both the pros and cons: inadequacy of the quantity and quality of the tissue aspirate has been noted; false-negative and false-positive diagnoses have been recorded; and the interpretive skill of the cytopathologist has been questioned.

18.6 Indications for Surgical Intervention

The approach and timing of surgical intervention depends on the nature of the disease as defined by preoperative investigation. Statistically the main/more-frequent indications for intervention are: orbital decompression for thyroid orbitopathy, excision of a cyst or mass, repair of fractures and reconstruction of de-fects, abscess drainage, optic nerve decompression, and removal of a foreign body [1].

In particular orbital masses can be divided into two broad categories in terms of the indications for surgery:
1. Well-defined, limited, circumscribed, slow-growing, or nonprogressive lesions whether they are cystic, neoplastic or structural not causing functional deficit, can usually be monitored. In such cases surgical intervention is based on the size, location, rate of progression, or functional impairment produced by the lesion and is usually radical.
2. Progressive, poorly defined, or infiltrative lesions that cause functional deficits or entrapment of orbital structures generally require FNAB or incisional biopsy prior to definitive management. The surgical intervention is then based on the specific histopathological diagnosis.

Neurogenic tumors require special surgical considerations. The indication for excision of an optic nerve glioma or meningioma is limited to lesions showing growth during follow up toward the optic chiasm which are associated with blindness, severe pain and proptosis. Only rare exophytic and anterior optic nerve meningiomas (nerve sheath meningiomas) can be resected sparing the optic nerve. Finally, sphenoid wing meningiomas are usually resected via craniofacial approaches, reserving such complex surgical procedures to patients with large lesions that cause progressive, functional deficit and/or severe proptosis.

18.7 Surgical Approaches to the Orbit

The progressive refinements in imaging modalities (CT, MRI) and the anatomic studies of Koornneef [5, 6], which have disclosed the definite structural organization and constant pattern of the intraorbital connective tissue system, have led to the codification of so-called "topographic orbital surgery" which provides a more rational selection of surgical technique. In particular, in the above-mentioned studies, Koornneef did not find any anatomic evidence for the existence of a common muscle sheath behind the globe, as suggested by radiologists, subdividing the orbit into central and peripheral surgical spaces. Based on this study, the terms "intraconal" and "extraconal" are merely radiological definitions, as confirmed, for example, by the biological behavior of tumors that, regardless of their origin within the orbit, extend freely through the two spaces.

The available surgical techniques are classically divided into anterior or soft-tissue approaches, orbital marginotomies or osseous approaches, and craniofacial approaches.

Surgical access to the orbital skeleton and periorbital structures through the eyelids and anterior orbit can be accomplished using a wide range of cutaneous incisions. Historically, these incisions were developed mainly from the surgical treatment of orbitozygomatic fractures and blepharochalasis [7]. The choice of incision is mainly influenced by the surgeon's personal experience. Classical cutaneous approaches to the orbital skeleton and periorbital structures are illustrated in Fig. 18.3.

Access to the orbital region is quite difficult because the orbital skeleton and in particular the bony rim often limit surgical maneuvers in a narrow anatomic space. For this reason in 1889 Krönlein [8], in order to expose and remove an intraorbital dermoid cyst, proposed mobilization of the lateral orbital wall. This basic concept was then extended to other orbital walls so that now orbital or cranioorbital bone segments may be temporarily removed and replaced in their original position without any morphological sequelae. Orbital marginotomies available for surgical treatment of orbital diseases are classified into four distinct procedures according to the spatial organization of the bony walls: inferior, lateral, superior and medial [9] (Fig. 18.4).

Of the surgical approaches to the orbit, 8% to 10% are performed combining an orbital marginotomy with a neurosurgical approach, the so-called craniofacial or combined approaches [10].

The superior approach to the orbit, via either a transfrontal or a frontotemporalorbitozygomatic approach, is usually chosen for the resection of apical or combined apical/intracranial lesions (gliomas, meningiomas) or malignances requiring en bloc orbitectomy.

Finally, the surgical treatment of specific diseases involves the selection of dedicated procedures, such as transethmoidosphenoidal decompression of the intracanalicular part of the optic nerve in cases of posttraumatic neuropathy [11, 12], optic nerve sheath decompression via lateral or medial orbitotomy in cases of papilledema related to idiopathic intracranial hypertension [13], and two- or three-wall orbital decompression [14, 15] and/or Olivari's technique (orbital fat lipectomy) in cases of Graves' orbitopathy [16].

Based on various series in the literature, the majority of orbital procedures can be carried out through an anterior incision with or without osseous orbitotomy (with variations in the amount and location of bone removal depending on the size and location of the orbital lesion; Figs. 18.5 and 18.6).

In our personal experience, lateral orbitotomy is the gold standard in the surgical treatment of benign orbital diseases (benign orbital tumors, Graves' orbitopathy, papilledema related to intracranial hypertension, etc.) and it is preferred for about 60% of orbital surgical pathologies.

18.7.1 Lateral Orbitotomy

First described by Krönlein in 1889 [8], the lateral orbitotomy is nowadays the workhorse in the surgical treatment of benign orbital diseases. This approach involves the temporary mobilization of the lateral rim, which can be either left pedicled to the fascia and temporalis muscle, or completely removed. This versatile surgical approach provides adequate access to the orbital region which is anatomically encased in the bony framework and so quite difficult to visualize (due to the narrow surgical field), and permits easy removal of the overwhelming majority of orbital lesions (intra- or extraconal, located in the superior, inferior or lateral compartment of the orbit).

The skin incisions selected for lateral orbitotomy depend upon the surgeon's personal experience. In most cases we prefer an incision (lateral canthotomy) that starts horizontally from the external canthus, proceeds laterally for about 2–3 cm toward the ear and extends down to the temporalis fascia. The external canthotomy

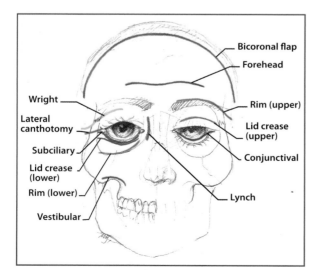

Fig. 18.3 The anterior approaches to the orbit

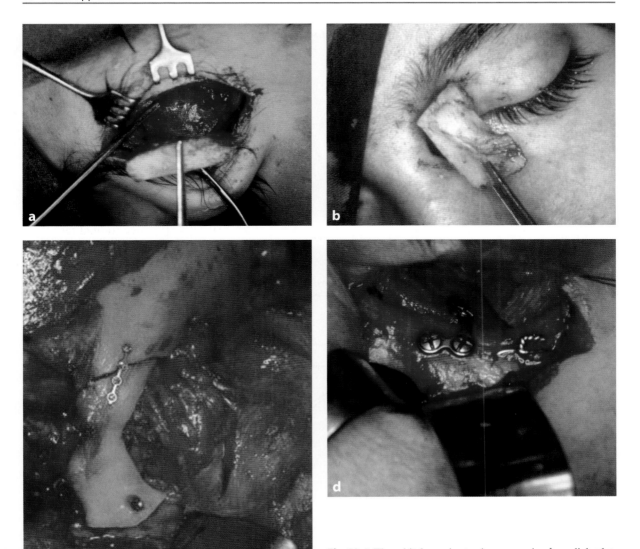

Fig. 18.4 The orbital marginotomies: **a** superior, **b** medial, **c** lateral, **d** inferior

is then carried out for a short way through the conjunctiva with scissors so that the lower and upper skin flaps can be dissected. The ligament, together with the septum orbitale, is freed from the lateral orbital margin and the dissection is extended up to the superior and down to the inferior orbital rims. At this point the periosteum can be incised exposing the lateral margin of the orbit and marking the site of the bone cuts. Before performing the osteotomies, the temporalis muscle must be detached and retracted posteriorly. Good esthetic results following this incision (an almost invisible scar) depend on its well-hidden drawing in a cutaneous fold [17, 18].

A less-common incision is the superolateral or "lazy S" which starts from the lower tip of the eyebrow and runs down along the lateral orbital rim to the zygomatic arch, extending along the superior margin of the arch approximately 2–3 cm backwards [19]. The incision is deepened and the subcuticular tissues are dissected to the level of the temporal fascia, where they are then separated by blunt dissection to minimize damage to critical overlying tissues. This subcuticular dissection is carried forward over the orbital margin. The next step involves fascial and periosteal incisions that include a superior relaxing incision along the zygomatic arch allowing mo-

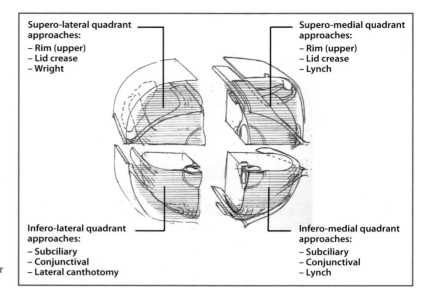

Fig. 18.5 Topographic surgery: anterior orbit

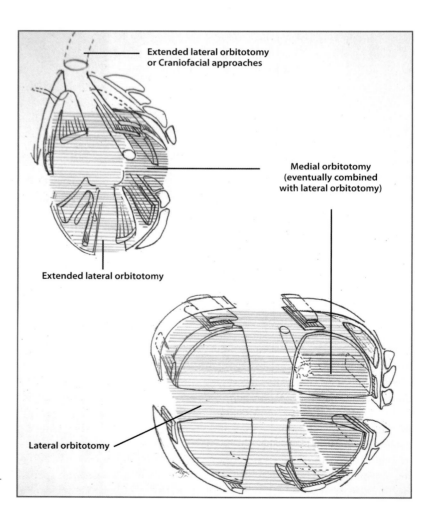

Fig. 18.6 Topographic surgery: midapical orbit and optic canal

bilization of the temporalis muscle. At this point the periosteum is elevated to the anterior orbital rim and posteriorly the temporalis muscle is detached. The major disadvantage of the superolateral incision is the prominent scar created beneath the brow, which results in a minimally shaded facial area. In conclusion, the superolateral incision leaves more visible scarring than the former incision, although it provides a wider operating field.

An incision along the hairline in the temporal area (coronal or hemicoronal) has been used for three-wall decompression in Graves' exophthalmos, to correct craniofacial malformations in cases of craniofacial trauma or malignancy, in cosmetic surgery of the face and sometimes for deeply located orbital tumors. In the coronal approach the incision begins inferiorly in the preauricular crease for adequate exposure of the zygomatic arch. The incision then proceeds superiorly above the root of the helix to approximately 3 to 4 cm behind the hairline. In male patients, the incision should be adapted to temporal recession, and in children it should be traced well away from the hairline to avoid migration of the scar with growth. If a hemicoronal incision is planned, the incision curves forward at the midline, while in the coronal approach it proceeds in a symmetric fashion to the contralateral temporal and preauricular region.

The incision is made parallel to the hair follicles through the galea into the loose areolar plane, leaving the periosteum intact. As the incision proceeds laterally and inferiorly, the depth is constant but the underlying plane becomes the deep temporalis fascia. The flap is then dissected inferiorly in the loose areolar plane with special attention to proper elevation of the temporoparietal fascia laterally. A horizontal incision is made 2 to 3 cm above the orbital rim(s) so that a subperiosteal elevation over the superior orbital rim(s) can be accomplished. Medially, the supraorbital neurovascular bundle(s) is (are) released from their respective notches, allowing adequate reflection of the flap and further subperiosteal dissection of the entire nasoethmoid region to expose the medial orbit(s).

Prior to exposing the whole lateral orbital rim and detaching the deep temporal fascia from its insertion along the lateral posterior aspect, it is necessary to enter the proper plane of dissection over the temporalis muscle and zygomatic arch to avoid injury to the upper divisions of the seventh nerve. For this purpose, an incision is made approximately 0.5 to 2.0 cm above the zygomatic arch, and so well inferior to the line of fusion of the two layers of the deep temporalis fascia, the superficial leaf and the inner leaf, that encase a curvilinear fat pad just superficial to the temporalis muscle,

the so called superficial temporal fat pad (the line of fusion corresponds approximately to the level of the superior orbital rim). This incision starts at the zygomatic root in an oblique direction at an angle of approximately 45° toward the lateral orbit through the superficial layer of the deep temporal fascia into the superficial temporal fat pad. Within this fat pad, the superior aspect of the whole zygomatic arch can be exposed, usually starting with dissection of the root of the zygoma, allowing subperiosteal dissection and exposure of the arch. Then dissection of the lateral orbital rim continues in a subperiosteal fashion inferiorly beyond the frontozygomatic suture toward the malar process, allowing at the same time the deep temporal fascia to be detached from its insertion along the lateral posterior aspect. At this point it is possible to connect the arch and lateral orbital rim dissections with complete exposure of the malar region and lateral orbital rim. Using this safe surgical plane first described by Yasargil et al. [20], it is possible to avoid injury to the upper divisions of the seventh nerve.

A coronal approach selected for a lateral orbitotomy allows greater exposure, but it is a more aggressive procedure that should be limited to cases in which even a postcanthotomy scar is to be avoided (for example, in young girls) or in craniofacial resections when the lateral access is performed in order to proceed with an endocranial step (for example, in optic meningiomas which extend intracranially or to the optic canal, or retrobulbar malignant tumors, etc.). In such cases, however, the lateral marginotomy is only a minor part of the whole surgical procedure.

Considering mobilization of the lateral orbital wall, the superior osteotomy is commonly performed 0.5–1 cm above the frontozygomatic suture and slanted 45° toward the orbital floor. The inferior osteotomy is designed parallel to the orbital floor, where the frontozygomatic process is attached to the zygoma itself. Mobilization can be accomplished either by displacing the segment externally (involving a vertical fracture along the lateral orbital wall which extends between the two mentioned horizontal osteotomies) or by lifting/detaching the temporalis muscle and performing the vertical osteotomy directly. For better access to the posterior orbital region, an ostectomy of the lateral orbital wall (corresponding to the greater wing of the sphenoid) can be extended posteriorly and, in selected cases, it is possible to expose the dura of the middle cranial fossa [9, 21] (Figs. 18.7 and 18.8).

The original design of the osteoplastic lateral marginotomy as described by Krönlein was modified in a

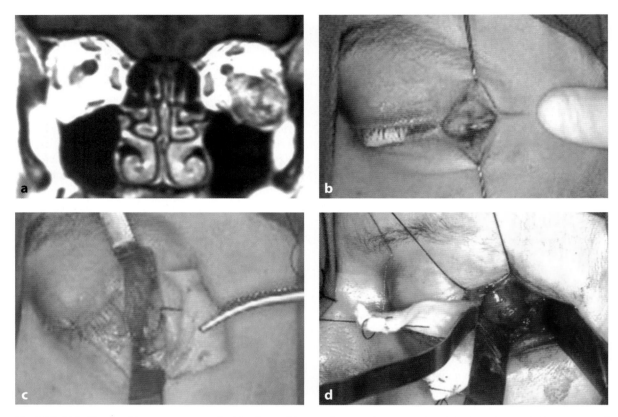

Fig. 18.7 This 45-year-old woman presented with a 2-year history of progressive proptosis, diplopia and upward displacement of the left eye due to a large lesion located into the midapical inferolateral intraconal space (**a**). **b** A lateral orbitotomy was carried out through a lateral canthotomy. **c** After superior, inferior and vertical osteotomies had been performed the whole lateral margin and part of the lateral orbital wall were mobilized. **d** The periorbita was incised and the huge tumor was gently removed

variety of different options mobilizing the lateral orbital rim en bloc with adjacent bony segments such as the body of the zygoma, the greater wing of the sphenoid (as far as the pterion exposing the middle cranial fossa dura), the supraorbital rim and orbital roof, and so on. Furthermore, in craniofacial orbital approaches the lateral marginotomy is almost always combined with frontal, temporal and parietal bony segments to gain access to orbital tumors with intracanalicular or intracranial extension.

Lateral orbitotomy has also been performed in association with medial conjunctival orbitotomy (medial 180° periectomy around the cornea) for the treatment of intraconal medial tumors. Although intraconal medial masses can be resected by microsurgical methods without bony orbitotomy, a lateral marginotomy permits lateral displacement of the globe and consequently better access to the lesion [22].

18.7.2 Inferior Orbitotomy

For lesions located extraconally in the inferior orbit, various approaches are available. A palpebral skin incision is usually adopted, but authors disagree as to where to place it: precisely just below the eyelashes or along a cutaneous fold in the eyelid itself.

A subciliary (blepharoplasty) incision is probably the best option from the aesthetic point of view. The incision is placed approximately 2 mm below and parallel to the lower lid margin beginning medially at the punctum and continuing laterally beyond the lateral canthus in a skin crease. The incision is carried down dividing the pretarsal fibers of the orbicularis muscle, and then the dissection is accomplished under the muscle to expose the septum. The junction between the arcus marginalis and the septum is very useful for determining the plane of entry either through the septum

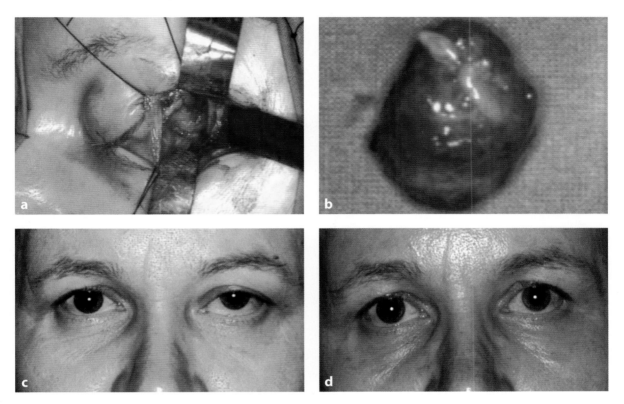

Fig. 18.8 **a**, **b** The surgical field after resection of the tumor (**a**) which proved to be a cavernous hemangioma (**b**). **c**, **d** Comparison of the patient's preoperative (**c**) and postoperative (**d**) views shows an optimal aesthetic result (no scar detectable in the lateral canthal area) associated with a complete functional recovery

into the orbital space or subperiosteally into the floor of the orbit. This access guarantees wide exposure of the inferolateral orbit, but some authors consider unacceptable the potential morbidity (postoperative ectropion and increased scleral show) caused by vertical lid shortening secondary to fibrosis from the dissection [23]. Other authors consider the subciliary incision completely acceptable considering that a musculocutaneous flap would be harvested [24] (Fig. 18.9).

The inferior orbital rim incision is one possible alternative. This incision has undoubtedly evolved from its first description to avoid any lid complications, as well as to provide the shortest route between skin and bone. For these reasons, it is placed several millimeters lower than the blepharoplasty incision at the inferior orbital margin where a minor fold with the cheek indicates the junction of the orbital and palpebral portions of the orbicularis as well as the region where the orbital septum extends upward from the periosteum of the rim. Although this clearly appears to be an advantageous in-

cisional choice, it is no longer considered acceptable because of the risk of an unsightly scar.

The conjunctival approach through the fornix was originally proposed in 1923 by Bourquet (quoted by Manson et al. [24]) and was popularized in the early 1970s by Tenzel, Tessier and Converse [9]. An incision placed in the fornix results in equal exposure of the floor and rim when compared with the other inferior orbital approaches. When combined with a lateral canthotomy incision in the so-called swinging eyelid incision, it provides wide exposure of both the inferior orbit and the zygoma. Despite its early popularity and wide use, an increasing number of reported complications (ectropion, entropion, and tearing of the lid margin), combined with the initial limited familiarity with manipulation of inner lid tissues and lateral canthus, probably explain a more selective use of this incision for fracture repair, malformation correction, tumor removal, orbital decompression, and cosmetic lid surgery.

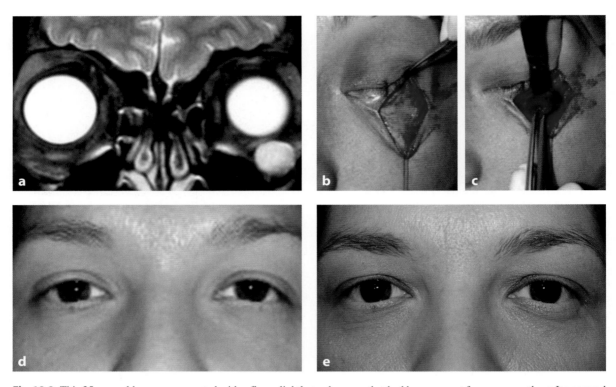

Fig. 18.9 This 25-year-old woman presented with a firm, slightly tender mass that had been present for some months. **a** It appeared to be located inferolaterally and projected just over the orbital rim. **b** Through a subciliary incision placed 2 mm below the ciliary margin blunt dissection under the orbicularis muscle exposed the septum. **c** The septum was opened to enter the orbital space and finally to resect the tumor, which proved to be a cavernous hemangioma. **d, e** Preoperative (**d**) and postoperative (**e**) frontal views. Note in the latter the good aesthetic result with favorable healing of the subciliary scar

Many suggestions have been proposed to decrease the potential complications from the conjunctival incision. The incision should be placed between the lower border of the tarsus and the lowest point of the fornix. If carried to/at a higher level, the necessary vertical dissection within the lid increases the risk of fibrosis and ectropion; if carried to/at a lower level, injury to the inferior oblique muscle is more likely and the dissection must proceed through orbital fat. Considering the preseptal versus retroseptal approach, the identification of the anterior fat capsule, which almost always protrudes into the wound after transection of the inferior lid retractors, allows an anterior dissection (preseptal) down to the level of the rim preventing fat prolapse (which may result in adhesions with the mucosal lining of the lid and consequent vertical lid shortening) and providing better visualization. The conjunctival access has the advantage of leaving no cutaneous scar, with the exception of cases in which a wider exposure (manipulation of the zygoma or lateral orbit, placement of bone

plates, etc.) requires a lateral extension of the canthotomy that leads to facial scarring.

The intraconal inferior compartment is better approached as previously seen with lateral orbitotomies.

In very selected cases we can employ, through the same incisions, the inferior marginotomy that involves the temporary removal of a segment of the inferior orbital rim. This bony fragment is delimited by two distinct osteotomies: one extends laterally from the inferolateral corner of the orbital frame, the second is traced medial to the infraorbital neurovascular bundle. In the original description of Tessier et al. [25], the lateral osteotomy is inclined medially 30° and extends to the inferior orbital fissure, so that the segment also includes a considerable area of the orbital floor. The horizontal osteotomy is conducted on the anterior wall of the maxilla at the level of the infraorbital foramen, thus permitting the complete dissection/freeing of the corresponding neurovascular bundle. This access is particularly suitable for orbital floor fractures with herniation of the orbital contents into the maxillary sinus and for resection of extraconal lesions very deeply located in the inferior orbit.

18.7.3 Superior Orbitotomy

Lesions located extraconally just below the orbital roof can be approached in most instances by an upper eyelid crease, a sub-brow/brow or a coronal incision.

The superior eyelid crease (blepharoplasty) incision is placed in a naturally developing, age-independent skin fold and offers the best aesthetic result among all the superior orbital approaches. A skin-muscle flap may be developed superiorly, medially, and laterally (with an incisional extension following the natural skin fold and curving upward) in a plane deep to the orbicularis muscle and can be raised close to the brow. At this point the periosteum can be divided over the rim for bony exposure and dissection can proceed for access to the deeper superior orbital spaces. The lid crease approach decreases

many of the risks associated with more peripherally placed incisions. Despite wide undermining and raising of the flap, the vascularity of its orbicularis muscle component ensures skin viability and optimal healing.

Through the upper lid crease incision the whole superior orbit can be approached and, if necessary, this access can be extended laterally onto the zygoma for more peripheral aspects. The resulting scar is usually undetectable [7] (Fig. 18.10).

The use of incisions placed over the superior (medial brow) and lateral (lateral brow) orbital rims was first described in fracture repairs. The advantages of these incisions are the speed of execution and the acceptable exposure of the underlying bony anatomy due to the anatomical proximity. Possible disadvantages of these approaches are a poor-quality scar and eyebrow hair loss (due to transection of hair follicles if the incision is not directed completely parallel to the emerging hairs). The risk of supraorbital nerve injury can be reduced by limiting the length of the incision (with consequently more limited access) and by performing a

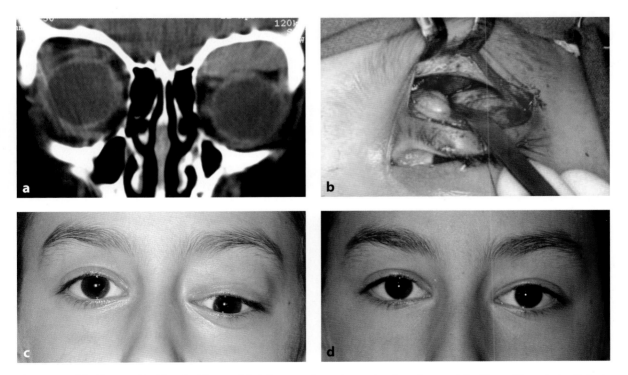

Fig. 18.10 This 12-year-old girl had a history of facial trauma 6 months previously and presented with swelling, ptosis, diplopia and slight tenderness of her upper left eyelid associated with a downward displacement of the globe and progressive limitation of upward gaze, caused by a subperiosteal organized hematoma involving the superior orbit (**a**). **b** Through a direct lid crease incision the mass was easily resected. **c, d** The patient's preoperative (**c**) and postoperative (**d**) views show an optimal aesthetic result which was associated with a complete functional recovery

blunt dissection carried down through the orbicularis muscle and periosteum [7].

The superior rim can be mobilized alone or en bloc with a segment of the orbital roof depending on the indication. In the great majority of patients, the superior marginectomy is limited to the superior rim and so the procedure remains totally extracranial often involving the frontal sinus. Based on high-resolution CT scans, an osteotomy adequate in depth and inclination can be traced avoiding intracranial extension. The temporary mobilization of the superior orbital rim allows easier and safer dissection of the orbital roof. This procedure is indicated for fractures of the orbital roof or in the presence of deeply located extraconal tumors. For superiorly located intraconal tumors lateral orbitotomy provides a more reliable approach.

A superior orbitotomy limited to the orbital rim can be performed through a skin incision placed along the eyebrow or better in the superior lid crease as described above. When a segment of the orbital roof is removed along with the rim, the approach is either intra- and extracranial. The supraorbital frame can be mobilized alone or attached to the frontal bone. The lifted fronto-orbital fragment provides adequate access to the orbital region as well as to the anterior cranial base, with wide exposure and without significant retraction of the brain. This procedure can be selected for the treatment of optic nerve meningiomas located intracranially as well as extracranially, orbitopalpebral neurofibromatosis, benign or malignant tumors and dysplasias of the anterior cranial base. Soft tissue access is through a coronal or hemicoronal incision, because this approach not only provides wide exposure but also offers the advantage of leaving an unnoticeable scar hidden in the hairline [9].

18.7.4 Medial Orbitotomy

Lesions of the medial orbit can be divided into those located extraconally or intraconally. The former are

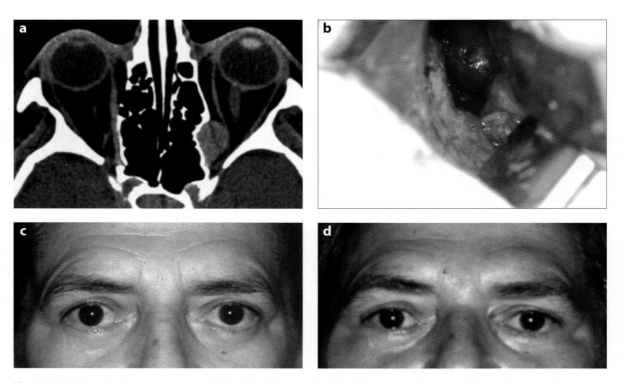

Fig. 18.11 A 50-year-old woman presented with only mild proptosis of the left eye, caused by a deeply located extraconal cavernous hemangioma, occupying the medial apical orbit (**a**). **b** The lesion was approached via a simple Lynch incision with medial canthal detachment, through which an adequate surgical field was obtained; note in the intraoperative view the tumor lying in the far end of the operating field. **c**, **d** The patient's preoperative (**c**) and postoperative (**d**) frontal view; note in the latter the optimal aesthetic result with favorable healing of the epicanthal scar

best approached through a coronal, a Lynch (combined with temporary detachment of the medial canthal tendon), a limited subciliary or a superior eyelid crease (medial crease) incision.

The intraconal medial compartment can be managed through a conjunctival incision (transcaruncular; medial 180° periectomy around the cornea) alone or combined with a lateral orbitotomy with bone removal.

The Lynch incision, a nearly vertical incision placed medial to the canthal ligament, provides excellent exposure of the medial orbit [26]. It is useful for access to extraconal medially located orbital tumors, for repair of medial wall fractures, for decompression of the optic canal, and for treatment of ethmoidal sinus disease. The inferior portion of the incision may also be used as the approach for a dacrocystorhinostomy. Section of the medial canthal tendon provides a wider surgical field and a safer removal of more deeply located masses

(Fig. 18.11), in particular concerning control of possible hemorrhage from the anterior and posterior ethmoidal arteries. Obviously at the end of the procedure, the common tendon of the medial canthus has to be reattached to the medial wall with a direct suture or more frequently with a transnasal canthopexy as described by Markowitz et al. [27]. The Lynch incision results in a minimally noticeable scar because of its prominent location in the midface and because it crosses relaxed skin tension lines that normally run superomedially from the medial canthus to the glabella. Modifications of the original incision design, including Z- and W-plasty, have been suggested to reduce the scar.

The transcaruncular approach, first described by Garcia et al. in 1998 [28] for the repair of medial orbital fractures, consists of a 10 to 15-mm vertical incision through the caruncle and conjunctiva into the condensed fibrous tissue just deep to the caruncle,

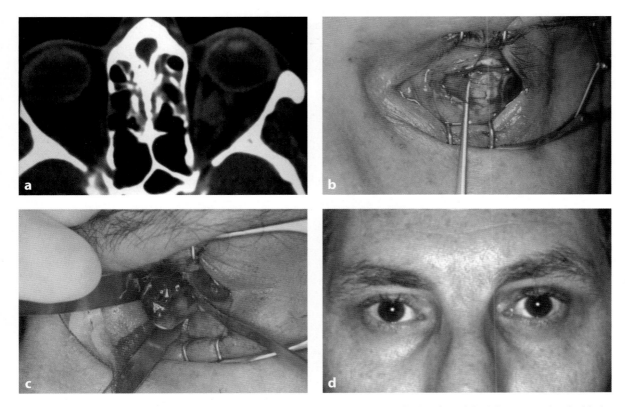

Fig. 18.12 A 45-year-old man presented with mild proptosis and slight limitation of adduction of the left eye associated with the presence of a medially located enhancing mass occupying the mid intraconal orbital space (**a**). **b**, **c** Through a medial conjunctival incision (180° periectomy) and with detachment of the medial rectus muscle (**b**), the tumor was removed uneventfully (**c**) and it proved to be a cavernous hemangioma. **d** The postoperative frontal view shows a good aesthetic result associated with complete functional recovery

avoiding any trauma to the plica semilunaris. An important landmark in the technique is the posterior lacrimal crest. In fact, placing a malleable retractor on the medial orbital wall just posterior to the crest discloses the proposed plane of dissection between the medial part of the orbital septum and Horner's muscle (which inserts at the posterior lacrimal crest) so that the muscle delineates a safe and bloodless plane from the lacrimal sac apparatus. The incision is a relatively new technique that has several advantages over traditional medial approaches: the incision is hidden in the conjunctiva and provides excellent access to the medial orbit, but it does not permit the same access as the cutaneous incisions.

Through the medial 180° periectomy, combined with conjunctival relaxing incisions traced superiorly and inferiorly to the medial rectus muscle, it is possible to dissect and free the muscle from its inner septa, to imbricate it near its insertion site with a 6-0 double-arm Vicryl suture at both borders, and finally to sever it from the insertion site. Once the medial rectus muscle is detached, it is possible to dissect more deeply into the medial intraconal compartment and finally to gently remove masses and eventually perform cryoprobe-assisted procedures (Fig. 18.12). As first described by McCord, if additional exposure is required, a lateral orbitotomy may be carried out so that the globe can be retracted even further laterally for excellent visualization [22] (Figs. 18.13 and 18.14).

The use of the medial half of a standard upper lid crease incision has been described for both removal of superomedial orbital masses and anterior medial orbital wall fracture repair. The stretching of the lid skin and underlying orbicularis muscle permits adequate access

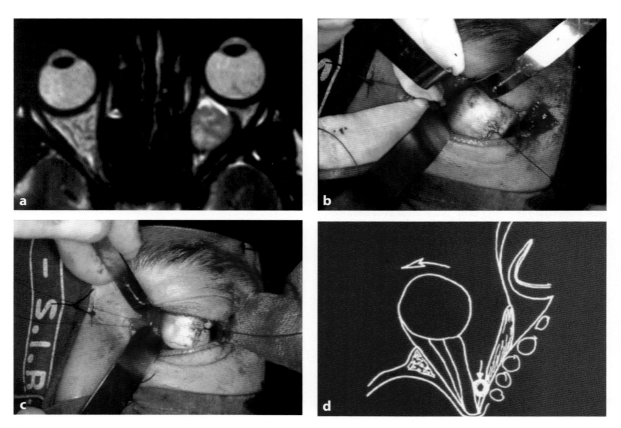

Fig. 18.13 An 35-year-old man presented with significant diplopia, proptosis, and slight limitation of adduction of the left eye associated with the presence of an enhancing mass located in the medial midapical intraconal space (**a**). The lesion was approached via a combined medial conjunctival incision (with detachment of the medial rectus muscle) and a lateral orbitotomy (through a canthotomic incision) to allow distraction of the globe laterally and access to the deep orbital space (**b**) and uneventful removal of the cavernous hemangioma (**c**), using the technique first proposed by McCord et al. (**d**)

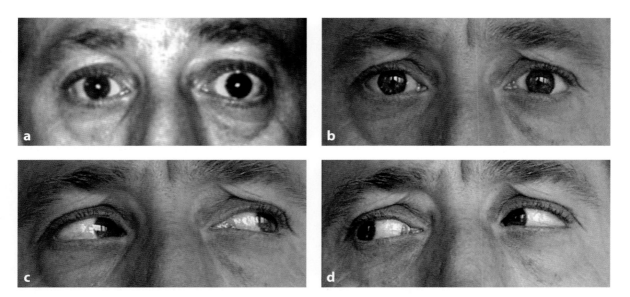

Fig. 18.14 Same patient as in Fig. 18.13. Comparison of the preoperative (**a**) and 4-year postoperative (**b**) frontal views show an extremely satisfying aesthetic result associated with a complete functional recovery of ocular movement (**c, d**)

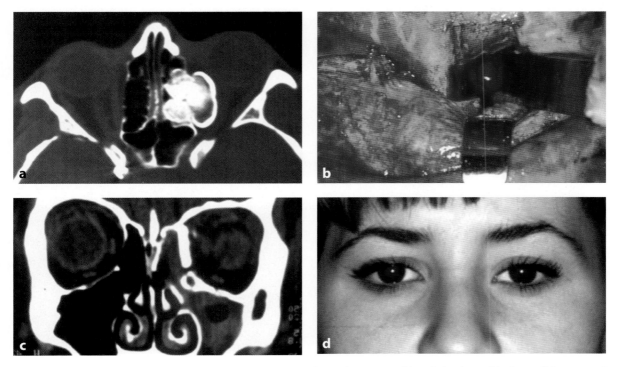

Fig. 18.15 A 25-year-old woman presented with mild proptosis of the left eye, caused by a lesion located in the medial extraconal midapical orbit and arising from the ethmoid (**a**). The tumor was approached through a coronal incision and a higher located medial marginotomy. Due to hypoplasia of the frontal sinus the dura mater of the frontal lobe was exposed and the osseous lesion was cored with a drill and removed piecemeal (**b**). After resection of the osteoma, the medial orbital wall was reconstructed with a split thickness calvarial graft (**c**). At 1-year the patient shows excellent aesthetic and functional results (**d**)

to the medial orbital wall. The trochlea and the superior oblique tendon can be temporarily detached from the orbital wall with limited secondary functional impairment. This approach results in a less-detectable scar than the Lynch incision, but provides narrower access to deep areas.

The temporary removal of the medial orbital rim in the treatment of posttraumatic sequelae was proposed by Sullivan and Kawamoto in 1989 [9]. In the original technique a bone segment extending from the frontomaxillary apophysis anteriorly to the lacrimal bone

posteriorly can be mobilized. Medial marginotomy is mainly selected in cases of either early or delayed posttraumatic deformities of the medial orbital wall, especially in fractures close to the optic foramen. This osteotomy also provides an excellent approach for the excision of benign tumors of the ethmoidal sinuses (osteomas, etc; Fig. 18.15). As a final note on medial marginotomy, the transnasal medial canthopexy can be avoided at the end of the procedure leaving the canthus attached to the bone during osseous segment mobilization.

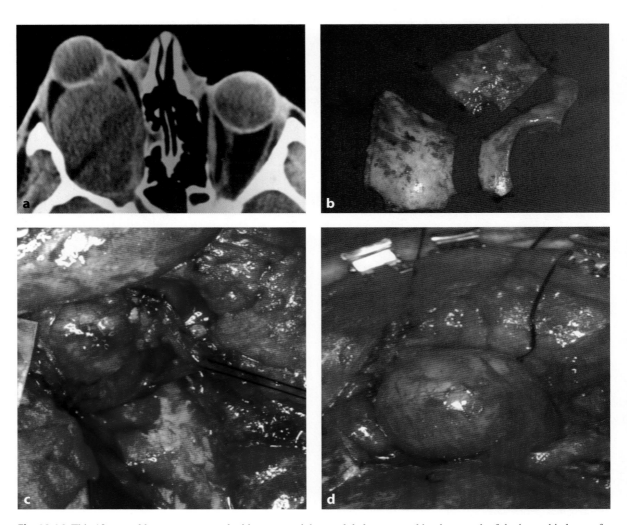

Fig. 18.16 This 18-year-old women presented with a severe right exophthalmos caused by the growth of the intraorbital part of a huge glioma (**a**). A frontotemporozygomatic approach was adopted to gain better control of the inferolateral orbit and the optic canal. **b** The three bone segments removed. **c, d** Intraoperative views: c the tumor was carefully freed from intraorbital structures (the lateral rectus muscle was displaced with a silk filament); d the huge glioma was completely isolated before its resection including the intracanalicular part of the optic nerve

18.7.5 Craniofacial Approaches

As already stressed, the approach directed through the lateral orbital wall is selected for tumors located in the superior, temporal, or inferior compartment of the orbit and those in the lateral part of the apex; on the other hand the medial approach is used for tumors located medial to the optic nerve but not deep in the apex. The limitations of the approaches mentioned above forced the development of craniofacial techniques that have allowed significant advances in access to the orbit and anterior cranial fossa. Dandy was the first to report a transcranial approach to the orbit in 1922 [29], and this was followed by various other reports. The transcranial approach is commonly selected for orbital tumors with intracranial extension, for tumors located medially intraconal in the orbital apex, optic canal, or both areas, and for intracranial tumors with extension into the orbit.

The transcranial surgical approaches to the orbit may be arbitrarily divided into two types: the first involves removal of a frontal or frontotemporal bone flap with preservation of the supraorbital rim, as initially recommended by Dandy; the second approach involves removal of the supraorbital rim with the bone flap. Although first proposed early in the 20th century by McArthur and Frazier for pituitary surgery, the standard frontoorbital craniotomy was popularized and standardized by Jane and associates who modified the original technique to include the orbital roof and the zygomatic process of the frontal bone down to the frontozygomatic suture [30]. When a more complete exposure of the lateral and inferior orbit, as well as the middle cranial fossa, is required, almost the entire zygoma can be removed along with the frontal craniotomy moving the lateral osteotomy at the level of the zygomatic arch. Finally, extensive exposure of the anterior and middle cranial fossae can be achieved using an orbitozygomatic craniotomy as proposed by Sekhar and others [30]. For such applications the procedure is best performed as a two-part craniotomy, the first being a standard frontotemporal craniotomy followed by an orbitozygomatic osteotomy (Figs. 18.16 and 18.17).

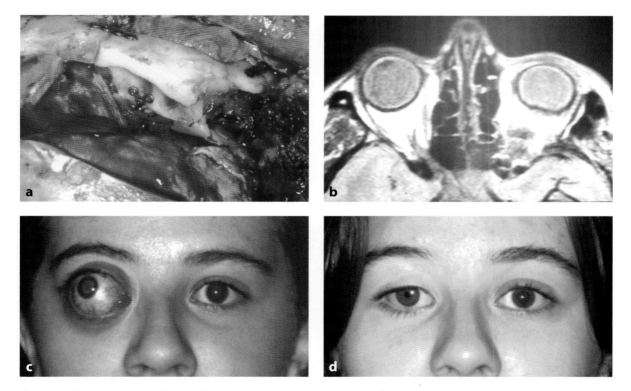

Fig. 18.17 Same patient as in Fig. 18.16. **a** Orbital bony reconstruction with split thickness calvarial grafts. **b** Radiological view of the radical removal of the glioma with preservation of the globe. **c, d** The preoperative (**c**) and postoperative (**d**) frontal views show a satisfying final clinical result at 1 year

Bifrontoorbital craniotomy consists of extending the frontal craniotomy to the opposite side. This allows extensive access to the anterior cranial fossa, while giving additional access to the orbit on one side. Concerning the bifrontal-bizygomatic craniotomy, this complex bilateral approach is almost exclusively reserved for the correction of craniofacial anomalies with craniosynostosis such as Cruzon and Apert syndromes. All these craniofacial approaches to the orbit are accomplished through coronal or hemicoronal incisions.

18.8 "Special" Surgical Approaches

In addition the main surgical approaches discussed above, some specific orbital diseases require treatment using, or represent indications for, specific surgical techniques which are briefly described below.

18.8.1 Optic Canal Decompression in Posttraumatic Optic Neuropathy

Despite considerable controversy persisting about the management of trauma to the nerve in the optic canal, mainly because no controlled data to guide decision making are available to date, anecdotal series suggest possible benefit from megadose corticosteroid treatment (based on data from studies of spinal cord injury) and surgical canal decompression. In patients not responding to megasteroid therapy, a swollen optic nerve within the bony canal should be decompressed to improve the possibility of recovering visual function. The transethmoidal–sphenoidal route via a Lynch incision allows an almost direct view of the optic canal, using the bony landmarks of the posterior orbit to gain access to the region of the optic nerve [11, 12]. Today in experienced hands this procedure can also be performed via an endoscopic route.

18.8.2 Optic Nerve Sheath Decompression in Pseudotumor Cerebri

Pseudotumor cerebri is a condition characterized by the following features: increased intracranial pressure without evidence of an intracranial space-occupying lesion or enlargement of the ventricles; normal CSF

cytology and chemistry (except for a low protein level); headache, blurring of vision, transient loss of vision, diplopia, and swollen optic discs in an otherwise healthy patient; and normal mental status. The major complication of this disorder is visual loss, which occurs in 10–26% of patients and is due to damage to the nerve fibers at the optic disc caused by papilledema. In patients with loss of vision related to pseudotumor cerebri, optic nerve sheath fenestration is an effective route to prompt recovery of vision. As first described by Tse et al. [13], through a lateral orbitotomy approach and using an operating microscope, a rectangular window of dura and arachnoid (measuring approximately 3×5 mm) can be excised from the bulbous portion of the optic nerve to obtain prompt release of CSF.

An alternative approach is the medial one that involves a conjunctival incision, detachment of the rectus muscle and removal of a window of dura from the medial side of the bulbar portion of the optic nerve.

18.8.3 Orbital Wall Decompression in Graves' Ophthalmopathy

Graves' disease is a multisystem disorder of unknown etiology characterized by the clinical triad of infiltrative pretibial dermopathy, thyroid glandular hyperplasia, and ophthalmopathy. Expansion of the bony orbital volume is an effective method of treating moderate to severe exophthalmos. In general, the indications for surgical expansion of the orbit are to relieve exophthalmos (which is accompanied by corneal exposure and disfigurement), or to reduce the increased orbital pressure produced by the swelling of extraocular muscles which results in compressive neuropathy and visual loss.

Several techniques have been proposed over the years reflecting individual surgical specialties [15]:
1. Lateral orbital decompression.
2. Antral-ethmoidal decompression (via the translid, fornix or transantral approach).
3. "Three-wall decompression", in which lateral wall decompression is added to antral–ethmoidal decompression.
4. Kennerdell-Maroon "four-wall decompression", in which the lateral wall portion of three-wall decompression is extended to a large portion of the sphenoid bone in the apex of the orbit and to the lateral half of the orbital roof.

Among these surgical procedures, the most commonly performed is "two- to three-wall decompression" which is eventually combined with a valgus rotation lateral displacement of the zygoma to gain more space, usually performed through a swinging eyelid or a coronal approach [14]. Finally, removal of intraconal fat through a radial incision in the periorbita further decompresses the orbital contents.

18.8.4 Transpalpebral Decompression of Graves' Ophthalmopathy (Olivari's Technique)

This surgical technique is an alternative to previous described orbital decompression procedures in patients with minor to mild Graves' proptosis. Decompression is obtained by removing intraorbital fat through a transpalpebral incision. The average volume of fat that can be resected is 6 cm^3 per orbit. Usually only one orbit is decompressed at a time [16].

18.9 Complications

In general, the potential complications of orbital surgery are classified into four main types [3]: hemorrhage, infection, emphysema, and CSF rhinorrhea.

Hemorrhage

Hemorrhage can occur at any time following orbital surgery, early (related to inadequate intraoperative control of bleeding vessels) or late (usually 4 to 6 days after surgery, due to local factors influencing hemostasis and clot formation with secondary hematoma). It is identified by cardinal symptoms of pain, tense proptosis, ecchymosis, decreased vision and/or afferent pupillary defect. Immediate assessment of optic nerve function is imperative and immediate decompression of the orbit is indicated, which is accomplished by wound opening, lateral canthotomy, and even reoperation and bony decompression.

Infection

Postoperative infection is unusual in well-vascularized tissues of the orbit even in cases which have involved direct exposure of the sinuses or abscess drainage, with the only exception being foreign bodies. Acute postoperative infection is characterized by clinical local symptoms (pain, redness, and swelling) eventually associated with purulent drainage from the wound or through the sinuses, and systemic symptoms. Broad-spectrum antibiotics should be instituted immediately, with revision in the regimen guided by culture results. In case of acute onset of severe intraorbital swelling with rapid deterioration of vision or visual acuity, emergency surgical procedures such as cantholysis and/or canthotomy should be performed as soon as possible to decompress the nerve.

Emphysema

Orbital emphysema can occur after nose blowing or sneezing when a direct connection with the paranasal sinuses has been surgically created. A severe increase in orbital pressure may compromise the neurovascular structures and require urgent decompression, but usually the problem resolves spontaneously with a simple wait and see monitoring of visual function.

CSF rhinorrhea

If possible, a CSF leak is best controlled at the time of surgery. If a CSF leak develops postoperatively or an intraoperative leak is poorly controlled, the patient will develop a standard CSF rhinorrhea and has to be treated with the standard protocol which includes a lumbar drain, head elevation, and immobilization. If control from below is not possible, open craniotomy may be necessary to close the dural defect.

References

1. Rootman J, Durity F (1993) Orbital surgery. In: Sekhar LN, Janeka IP (eds) Surgery of cranial base tumors. Raven Press, New York, pp 769–785
2. Henderson JW (1994) Orbital tumors, 3rd edn. Raven Press, New York
3. Rootman J, Stewart B, Goldberg LA (1995) Orbital surgery: a conceptual approach. Lippincott-Raven, Philadelphia New York
4. Kennerdell JS (1989) Fine-needle aspiration biopsy. Ophthalmol Times 1:13
5. Koornneef L (1977) New insights in the human orbital connective tissue. Arch Ophthalmol 95:1269–1273

6. Koornneef L (1988) Eyelid and orbital fascial attachments and their clinical significance. Eye 2:130–134

7. Eppley BL, Custer PL, Sadove AM (1990) Cutaneous approaches to the orbital skeleton and periorbital structures. J Oral Maxillofac Surg 48:842–854

8. Krönlein RU (1889) Zur Pathologie und operativen Behandlung der Dermoidcysten der Orbita. Beitr Klin Chir 4:149–163

9. Sesenna E, Raffaini M, Tullio A et al (1994) Orbital marginotomies for treatment of orbital and periorbital lesions. Int J Oral Maxillofac Surg 23:76–84

10. Bumpous J, Janecka IP (1995) Transorbital approaches to the cranial base. Clin Plast Surg 22:461–481

11. Steinsapir KD, Goldberg RA (1994) Traumatic optic neuropathy. Surv Ophthalmol 38:487–518

12. Goldberg RA, Steinsapir KD (1996) Extracranial optic canal decompression: indications and technique. Ophthal Plast Reconstr Surg 12:163–170

13. Tse DT, Nerad JA, Anderson RL et al (1988) Optic nerve sheath fenestration in pseudotumor cerebri. A lateral orbitotomy approach. Arch Ophthalmol 106:1458–1462

14. Tessier P (1969) Les exophthalmies: expansion chirurgicale de l'orbite. Ann Chir Plast 12:273–285

15. McCord CD (1985) Current trends in orbital decompression. Ophthalmology 92:21–33

16. Olivari N (1991) Transpalpebral decompression of endocrine ophthalmopathy (Graves' disease) by removal of intraorbital fat: experience with 147 operations over 5 years. Plast Reconstr Surg 87:627–641

17. Swift GW (1935) Malignant exophthalmos and operative approach. West J Surg 43:119–123

18. Berke RN (1954) A modified Krönlein operation. Arch Ophthalmol 51:609–632

19. Wright JE, Stewart WB, Krohel GB (1979) Clinical presentation and management of lacrimal gland tumors. Br J Ophthalmol 63:600–606

20. Yasargil MG, Reichman MV, Kubik S (1987) Preservation of the frontotemporal branch of the facial nerve using the interfascial temporalis flap for pterional craniotomy. J Neurosurg 67:463–466

21. Maroon C, Kennerdell MD (1984) Surgical approaches to the orbit. J Neurosurg 60:1226–1235

22. McCord CD Jr (1978) A combined lateral and medial orbitotomy for exposure of the optic nerve and the orbital apex. Ophthalmic Surg 9:58–66

23. Holtmann B, Wray RC, Little AG (1981) A randomized comparison of four incisions for orbital fractures. Plast Reconstr Surg 67:731–737

24. Manson PN, Ruas E, Ilif N et al (1987) Single eyelid incision for exposure of the zygomatic bone and orbital reconstruction. Plast Reconstr Surg 79:120–126

25. Tessier P, Rougier J, Hervouet F et al (1977) Chirurgie plastique orbito-palpébrale. Masson, Paris

26. Lynch RC (1921) The technique of a radical frontal sinus operation which has given me the best results. Laryngoscope 31:1–5

27. Markowitz BL, Manson PN, Sargent L et al (1991) Management of the medial canthal tendon in nasoethmoid orbital fractures: the importance of the central fragment in classification and treatment. Plast Reconstr Surg 87:843–852

28. Garcia GH, Goldberg RA, Shorr N (1998) The transcaruncular approach in repair of orbital fractures: a retrospective study. J Craniomaxillofac Trauma 4:7–12

29. Dandy WE (1922) Prechiasmal intracranial tumors of the optic nerves. Am J Ophthalmol 5:169–188

30. Haines SJ, Marentette LJ, Wirtschafter JD (1992) Extended fronto-orbital approaches to the anterior cranial base: variation on a theme. Skull Base Surg 2:134–141

Transoral Approaches

Francesco S. De Ponte and Evaristo Belli

19.1 Anatomy

The anatomical structures that should be taken into consideration when referring to the transoral approaches are: the clivus, the foramen magnum, the occipital bone, the atlas, the axis and the joints between some of these structures [1, 2].

19.1.1 Clivus

Embryologically, the clivus consists of two bones: the sphenoid bone and the occipital bone, both of which extend from the foramen magnum to the sphenoid sinus. The clivus is wedge-shaped (38–42 mm long) as it is about 25 mm thick at its rostral end and 3 mm at the foramen magnum. In adults, it is 22 to 26 mm wide and it represents a surgically "safe" area between the carotid arteries rostrally and, caudally, the vertebral arteries along with the lower cranial nerves. The oval-shaped foramen magnum, the atlas and the axis constitute the craniocervical junction (Fig. 19.1).

19.1.2 Foramen Magnum

The foramen magnum is the wide aperture between the squamous and the basilar parts of the occipital bone. At

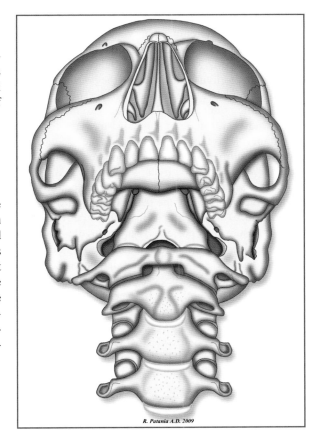

Fig. 19.1 Upper cervical spine and skull base

the sides of the foramen magnum are the condylar parts. The occipital bone, the atlas and the axis are the structures that need to be considered in planning an approach to the foramen magnum.

F.S. De Ponte (✉)
School of Maxillofacial Surgery
University Hospital G. Martino of Messina, Italy

P. Cappabianca et al. (eds.), *Cranial, Craniofacial and Skull Base Surgery*.
© Springer-Verlag Italia 2010

19.1.3 Occipital bone

The occipital bone is an unpaired, median and symmetrical bone situated at the back and lower part of the cranium. It is involved in shaping the basis and the cranial vault. It articulates with the first cervical vertebra. In its lower part is a wide hole (foramen magnum) through which the bulb passes to become the spinal cord.

The portion in front of the foramen magnum is the body or basilar part (the clival part). The portion situated behind the hole is called the squama which resembles a concave leaf in form. A condylar part connects the squamosal and clival parts.

The basilar part articulates forward with the sphenoid and, at about the 15th year of age, it merges with it by synostosis. At the center of its external or extracranial surface is a small protuberance called the pharyngeal tubercle (tuberculum pharyngeum) which is the point of attachment of the superior end of the pharynx. On the intracranial surface is a sagittal shallow depression called the clivus against which the pons varolii and a portion of the medulla oblongata lean. The clivus is a thick quadrangular plate of bone that extends forward and upward at an angle of about 45° from the foramen magnum. It joins the sphenoid bone at the sphenoccipital synchondrosis just below the dorsum sellae. The superior surface of the clivus is concave from side to side and is separated on each side from the petrous part of the temporal bone by the petroclival fissure. On the upper surface of this fissure is the inferior petrosal sinus and the fissure ends posteriorly at the jugular foramen

At the sides of the foramen magnum, the external or extracranial portion of the condylar parts exhibit a smooth sole-shaped surface called the occipital condyle which articulates with the first cervical vertebra or atlas. In front of the condyle is a hole (the anterior condylar foramen). This is the external foramen of a short canal, the hypoglossal canal which is a "passageway" for the hypoglossal nerve exiting the skull. The internal condylar foramen, through which the hypoglossal canal is reached, is situated in the intracranial portion. Behind the condyle is another hole called the condylar foramen or canal into which an effluent vein runs connecting the vertebral venous plexus with the sigmoid sinus. Laterally the condylar parts contribute to delimiting the jugular foramen (or posterior foramen lacerum) with the jugular process.

The jugular foramen is situated lateral and slightly superior to the anterior half of the condyles. It is bordered posteriorly by the jugular process of the occipital bone, and anteriorly and superiorly by the jugular fossa

of the petrous portion of the temporal bone. The foramen sits at the posterior end of the petroclival suture. The jugular foramen is divided into two parts by the intrajugular processes on the opposing edges of the petrous and occipital bones, which either join directly or are connected by a fibrous band. The smaller anteromedial part, the petrous part, transmits the inferior petrosal sinus, and the larger posterolateral part, the sigmoid part, transmits the sigmoid sinus. The intrajugular part, situated along the intrajugular processes, transmits the glossopharyngeal, vagus, and accessory nerves. The enlarged part of the internal jugular vein located within the foramen is referred to as the jugular bulb. The jugular process also serves as the site of attachment of the rectus capitis lateralis muscle behind the jugular foramen.

The squama of the occipital bone, situated behind the occipital foramen, as mentioned above, has an external and an internal surface. The external surface, convex and almost irregular, exhibits on the median line a protuberance called the external occipital protuberance, which is more or less prominent. Two parallel ridges radiate laterally from the protuberance: the highest and upper nuchal lines. A vertical ridge, the external occipital crest, descends from the external occipital protuberance to the midpoint of the posterior margin of the foramen magnum. The inferior nuchal lines run laterally from the midpoint of the crest. The area between the upper and inferior nuchal lines and the area immediately below, are wrinkled and irregular and function as the insertion point for several muscles.

The internal or intracranial surface of the squamous part is concave and has a prominence, the internal occipital protuberance, near its center. The internal surface is divided into four unequal fossae by the sulcus of the superior sagittal sinus that extends upward from the protuberance, by the internal occipital crest, a prominent ridge that descends from the protuberance, and by the paired sulci for the transverse sinuses that extend laterally from the protuberance. The upper two fossae are adapted to the poles of the occipital lobes. The inferior two fossae conform to the contours of the cerebellar hemispheres. The internal occipital crest bifurcates above the foramen magnum to form paired lower limbs, which extend along each side of the posterior margin of the foramen. A depression between the lower limbs, the vermian fossa, is occupied by the inferior part of the vermis. The falx cerebelli is attached along the internal occipital crest.

The superior edge of the squama is jagged. The mastoid process articulates its inferior and lateral parts, while the parietal bone articulates its superior part. The suture between the occipital squama and the parietal bones is called the lambdoid suture.

The inferior occipital margin constitutes the postero-medial contour of the jugular foramen or posterior foramen lacerum.

19.1.4 Atlas

The first cervical vertebra, called the atlas, as it supports the head articulating with the occipital bone. It differs from the other cervical vertebrae in that it has no real vertebral body. It comprises two lateral masses dorsally and ventrally linked together by two arch-shaped laminae respectively constituting the posterior arch and the anterior arch. The two arches and two lateral masses encircle the vertebral foramen.

The anterior arch exhibits at its center on its lower convex surface, a tubercle (anterior tubercle). On the opposite concave face, in front of the vertebral foramen, is an articular facet which articulates with the dens of the axis. The posterior arch is convex backward and has a median posterior tubercle and a groove on the lateral part of its upper-outer surface in which the vertebral artery courses.

Each lateral mass has a superior articular process articulating with the occipital bone condyle with an elliptical facet, an inferior articular process articulating with the articular process of the axis, a transverse process with a wide foramen transversarium, and only one tubercle or two slightly prominent ones at its edge. The vertebral foramen can be divided into two parts: an anterior quadrangular part and a posterior half-elliptical part. These two portions are split by the transverse ligament in the skeleton covered with soft tissue. The first portion houses the dens of the axis; the second houses the spinal cord and its sheaths. Only the latter corresponds to the vertebral foramen of other vertebrae.

19.1.5 Axis

The second cervical vertebra does not differ anatomically from vertebrae in general and from the cervical vertebrae in particular, as the first vertebra does. It exhibits, in fact, all the constituent elements of the vertebrae below: a body, a vertebral foramen, a spinous process, two transverse processes, two articular processes, two laminae and two peduncles. The body of the axis is transversally stretched with a flat posterior part and a prominent anterior part. Its unique feature is that it has on its superior face a vertical prominence called the odontoid process or dens. Actually the dens is the vertebral body of the atlas, detached from it and fused to the axis forming a cylindrical pivot on which the atlas and the upper cranium can rotate. It is 12 to 15 mm high and about 1 cm wide.

From the bottom upwards the vertebra shows: (1) an enlarged portion or base connecting it with the body of the axis; (2) a narrow portion or neck very slightly prominent; (3) a body corresponding to the median portion that has a flattened side where the alar ligaments are attached; and (4) an apex, more or less wrinkled, where numerous ligaments from the occipital bone are attached.

Considering it as a whole, it is possible to detect two faces, anterior and posterior, each of which shows an articular facet: the anterior facet, oval in shape, a little higher than wide, slightly transversally convex and corresponding to the anterior arch of the atlas; and the posterior facet, structurally similar to the anterior facet, running in vivo on the transverse ligament and grooved at the base of its posterior surface where the transverse ligament of the atlas passes.

The body of the axis exhibits an inferior lip-shaped extension, passing on the anterosuperior border of the third cervical vertebra. Its anterior surface shows, at the level of the median line, a ridge split with small hollows that allow the long muscles of the neck to flow. The posteroinferior border of the vertebral body is less prominent and the tectorial membrane and the posterior longitudinal spinal ligament are stuck to it. The peduncles and the laminae are strong and the latter end in a squat bifid spinous process. The vertebral foramen of the axis is sometimes smaller than that of the atlas.

The dens and the body are flanked by a pair of large oval facets that extend laterally from the body onto the adjoining parts of the pedicles and articulate with the inferior facets of the atlas. The superior facets do not form an articular pillar with the inferior facets, but are anterior to the latter.

The transverse processes of the axis are small. Their blunt tips show a single tubercle, the anterior tubercle, situated at or near the junction of the anterior root of the transverse process and the body. Their transverse foramina are superolaterally skewed in order to provide arteries and vertebral nerves with an easier passage into the wider transverse foramina of the atlas. The inferior articular facets are situated at the junction of the pedicles and laminae, and face downward and forward. The spade-shaped vertebral foramen is relatively large.

19.1.6 Atlantoaxial Joints

The articulation of the atlas and axis comprises four synovial joints: two median ones on the front and back of the dens, and paired lateral ones between the opposing articular facets on the lateral masses of the atlas and axis (Fig. 19.2). Each of the median joints situated on the front and back of the dens has its own fibrous capsule and synovial cavity. The atlas and axis are united by the cruciform ligament, the anterior and posterior longitudinal ligaments, and the articular capsules surrounding the joints between the opposing articular facets on the lateral masses. The cruciform ligament has transverse and vertical parts that form a cross behind the dens. The transverse part, called the transverse ligament, is a thick strong band that arches across the ring of the atlas behind the dens and divides the vertebral canal into a larger posterior compartment containing the dura and the spinal cord and a smaller anterior compartment containing the odontoid process.

In front, the atlas and axis are connected by the anterior longitudinal ligament, which is a wide band fixed above to the lower border of the anterior arch of the atlas and below to the front of the body of the axis. The posterior longitudinal ligament is attached below to the posterior surface of the body of the axis, and above to the transverse part of the cruciform ligament and the clivus. Posterior to the spinal canal, the atlas and axis are joined by a broad, thin membrane in series with the ligamentum flavum that is attached above to the lower border of the posterior arch of the atlas, and below to the upper edges of the laminae of the axis. This membrane is pierced laterally by the second cervical nerve.

19.1.7 Atlantooccipital Joints

The atlas and the occipital bone are united by the articular capsules surrounding the atlantooccipital joints and by the anterior and posterior atlantooccipital membranes. The anterior atlantooccipital membrane is attached superiorly to the anterior edge of the foramen magnum, inferiorly to the superior edge of the anterior arch of the atlas, and laterally to the capsule of the atlantooccipital joints.

The posterior atlantooccipital membrane is a thin sheet connected above to the posterior margin of the foramen magnum and below to the upper border of the posterior arch of the atlas. The lateral border of the membrane is free and arches behind the vertebral artery and the first cervical nerve root.

19.1.8 Axis and Occipital Bone

Four fibrous bands, the tectorial membrane, the paired alar ligaments, and the apical ligament, connect the axis and the occipital bone. The tectorial membrane is a cephalic extension of the posterior longitudinal ligament that covers the dens and cruciform ligament. It is attached below to the posterior surface of the body of the axis, above to the upper surface of the occipital bone in front of the foramen magnum, and laterally to the medial sides of the atlantooccipital joints. The alar ligaments are two strong bands that arise on each side of the upper part of the dens and extend obliquely superolaterally to attach to the medial surfaces of the occipital condyles. The apical ligament of the odontoid process extends from the tip of the dens to the anterior

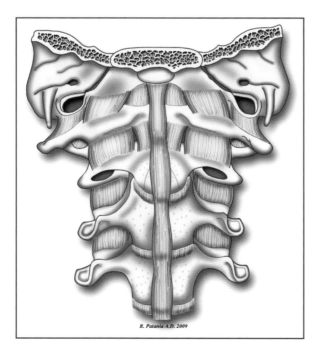

Fig. 19.2 Upper cervical spine joints and ligaments

margin of the foramen magnum and is situated between the anterior atlantooccipital membrane and the superior prolongation of the cruciform ligament.

19.2 Pathology

A huge variety of lesions involve this area including congenital anomalies, traumas, benign and malignant tumors, inflammatory conditions and those of uncertain etiology. They have in common the production of medullary compression or spinal instability [3].

19.2.1 Congenital

Congenital anomalies include basilar impression, odontoid malformations and a group of cranial anomalies of the posterior basicranium. They all compress the brainstem and the superior spinal cord. Basilar impression, even though not frequent, is one of the most usual indications for odontectomy. Sometimes it may be necessary to perform a craniectomy to allow proper decompression of the brainstem. Basilar impression is the "upward compression" or the introflexion of the occipital bone usually convex by the superior cervical tract. This implies involvement of the odontoid process in the surface of the brainstem, as well as introflexion of the occipital bone, adding further compression to this structure. Such lesions can be either congenital and acquired:

- Hajdu-Cheney syndrome or acroosteolysis combined with dolichocephaly, an unusual protuberance of the squamous part of the occipital bone (bathrocephaly) and progressive basilar invagination with specific anomalous facies and anomalies of the extremities, including osteolysis of the terminal phalanges.
- The cloverleaf brain or Klieblättschadel is another rare genetic syndrome, in which thanatophoric dwarfism and multiple anomalies of the extremities are combined with a trilobate cranium. Such calvarial anomalies, with bony protuberances at the same level as the floor of the posterior cranial fossa markedly reduced in height, are associated with basilar impression.
- Sjögren-Larsson syndrome.
- Pyknodysostosis.
- Achondroplastic dwarfism exhibits associated cranial anomalies, one of which may be basilar impression.

The acquired disorders of the cranial bones, such as osteomalacia, osteogenesis imperfecta, cretinism and rachitism, cause bony impairment. This produces a bony malleability that can lead to a progressive occipital introflexion.

The odontoid congenital anomalies are associated with a number of disorders, including Morquio syndrome (IVB type mucopolysaccharidosis), Aarskog syndrome, Dyggve-Melchior-Clausen syndrome, pseudoachondroplasia, cartilage-hair hypoplasia, congenital spondyloepiphyseal dysplasia and spondylometaphyseal dysplasia.

Morquio syndrome exhibits multiple spinal anomalies, including severe kyphoscoliosis and shortened cervical vertebrae. The odontoid can be hypoplastic, lacking or anomalous, and causes a superior medullary compression. In Aarskog syndrome (faciodigitogenital syndrome), the posterior arch may be open and placed in an upper position together with the odontoid into the foramen magnum during cranial extension. Dyggve-Melchior-Clausen syndrome is also associated with dwarfism. There is instability of the atlantoaxial junction that can lead to medullary compression.

19.2.2 Traumatic

The traumatic lesion most frequently needing this kind of approach is fracture of the odontoid. This is not a frequent lesion and it can be considered as a part of a "hangman's fracture", a bilateral fracture of the pars interarticularis with subsequent dislocation of C2 upon C3. If the dens is fractured, the craniocervical junction can be destabilized and the spinal cord can be compressed in an acute way. Fractures of C2 account for 10–20% of all cervical spine traumatic injuries [4] in adults and for 70% in children. The neurological morbidity in patients reaching hospital is extremely low. The real frequency of such fractures and their real mortality are unknown, and are surely underestimated. Indeed, such fractures are probably the cause of immediate death in some polytraumas.

Odontoid process fractures are the most common C2 fractures, representing approximately 60% of fractures at this level [5]. They have been classified into three types depending on the site of the rim of the fracture (Anderson and D'Alonzo classification) [6]:

- Type 1: very rare, involves the tip of the odontoid.
- Type 2: the most frequent (65–80%), exhibits the rim of the fracture at the base of the odontoid.
- Type 3: extends to the body of C2.

They are frequently associated with a certain degree of atlantoaxial dislocation. They are a consequence of forces produced by hyperflexion or hyperextension.

Odontoid type 1 and type 3 fractures are typically effectively treated with rigid external immobilization. The treatment of odontoid type 2 fractures remains controversial because of the high rate of nonunions with external immobilization. Mostly, surgery is indicated for nonunion after conservative treatment and when the dislocation of the dens is >6 mm [4]. The surgical treatment can be performed posteriorly with fixation of C1–C2, anteriorly with insertion of a screw into the dens or via a transoral route.

19.2.3 Inflammatory

Rheumatoid arthritis (RA) [7] is a chronic inflammatory disorder with unknown etiology. Even though it is a multisystemic disorder, RA is fundamentally a severe form of chronic synovitis which leads to the destruction and ankylosis of the affected articulations. The clinical course is variable and is not easy to predict in the individual patient. In most cases it is a persistent disease with alternate periods of major and minor activity. The peripheral joints are usually severely affected, before symptoms occur in the superior cervical cord.

From an anatomopathological point of view arthritis starts with an nonspecific inflammatory thickening of the synovial membrane. As the disease advances specific alterations occur such as proliferative synovitis or synovial pannus characterized by marked thickening of the synovial membrane, stratification of synovial cells and deep infiltration of inflammatory cells. Such an exuberant inflammatory infiltrate will fill the whole joint space and the released mediators progressively damage the cartilage. The pannus then invades the damaged cartilage and subsequently the subchondral bone, with subsequent demineralization and reabsorption.

Though any vertebral segment can be affected, the distribution of the lesions is anything but homogeneous. The cervical tract is most frequently involved while the thoracic and lumbar tracts are rarely involved. Since the area most frequently involved by cervical RA is the synovial membrane of the dens, impairment of the cruciform and alar ligaments and reabsorption of the odontoid process will typically occur. The joints between the occipital condyles and the lateral masses of C1 and between those of C1 and C2 are affected by RA and the process is characterized by bony erosion and impairment of the attachment points of the joint capsules and alar ligaments.

All the above-mentioned lesions lead to instability which is exhibited in different forms [8]:

- Anterior atlantoaxial subluxation characterized by anterior sliding of C1 in relation to C2; this occurs in the presence of cruciform ligament degeneration and/or a marked erosion of the dens.
- Posterior atlantoaxial subluxation characterized by posterior sliding of C1 in relation to C2; such a situation can become more severe because of erosion of the occipital condyles.

Sometimes penetration of the dens of the atlas into the foramen magnum is associated to anterior subluxation. Such a situation is known as vertical atlantoaxial subluxation or basilar impression. It arises as a result of reabsorption of the lateral masses of C1 with the subsequent migration of C2 upwards; it can worsen due to erosion of the occipital condyles.

19.2.4 Neoplastic

Various tumors can start at the level of the craniocervical junction. They may be benign or malignant, and the malignant lesions may be primary or secondary. The most common epithelial lesion is the squamous cell carcinoma and the most common bony lesion is the chordoma, even though the latter is not frequent. Squamous cell carcinomas are usually rhinopharyngeal or oropharyngeal. The robust pharyngobasilar fascia provides a barrier to tumor penetration. Tumors of rhinopharyngeal origin have a greater propensity to spread into the bone of the clivus than oropharyngeal tumors have to spread into the cervical column.

Chordomas [9] should be considered as low-grade malignant tumors. However, their behavior is more malignant because they are difficult to remove totally, they have a high recurrence rate, and they can metastasize. They are slow growing, locally aggressive and osseodestructive. They arise from the notochordal remnants extending from the clivus to the sacrum (which normally differentiates into the nucleus pulposus of the intervertebral disks).

The most frequent sites are: sacrococcygeal (50%), sphenooccipital and clival (35%), and vertebral (15%). The reason for such major occurrence is the presence of a large amount of notochordal cell remnants in sacrococcygeal and basioccipital sites. The average age at presentation is 40 years. Because of the slow rate of growth chordomas appear quite large at presentation. Histologically physaliphorous cells (vacuolated cells that probably represent cytoplasmic mucus vacuoles seen ultrastructurally) are distinctive. Macroscopically they are grayish, lobulated masses without a distinct capsule, and they contain varying amount of calcification. Irregular bone destruction is evident on CT scans. The consistency of the tumors may vary from soft and gelatinous to hard. They are extradural in origin and tend to displace the dura. It is usually possible to establish a plane of dissection around the tumor and the neurovascular structures; however, such a plane cannot be developed in the bone because of tumor infiltration. Malignant transformation into fibrosarcoma or malignant fibrous histiocytoma is rare.

Chondrosarcomas and chondromas should be considered in the differential diagnosis. Chondrosarcomas [9] are slow-growing, malignant neoplasms. They are believed to originate in the primitive mesenchymal cell rests in the cartilaginous matrix at the skull base. They are rarer than chordomas, tend to have a better prognosis, are less aggressive, and their recurrence rate is lower.

The most frequently occurring tumors of the spinal column are metastatic and the spine is the most common site for skeletal metastases [10]. Secondary spinal tumors most often arise from carcinomas of the breast, prostate and lung.

Neurological symptoms occur when the tumor compresses the brainstem or extends through the foramen magnum.

19.2.5 Clinical Presentation

Lesions of the clivus can be occasional findings on a routine CT scan or radiograph of the head, with few or lacking clinical manifestations. Odontoid lesions and atlantooccipital or atlantoaxial disease are typically symptomatic [3].

Lesions of the clivus can simply occur with posterior cervical pain or occipital cephalea claimed at the anamnesis. The involvement of the canal of the hypoglossal nerve can produce paresis or paralysis of cranial nerve XII, causing speech impediment and oral dysphagia. Such symptoms often tend to be transitory, since the patient rapidly adjusts to unilateral lingual paralysis. Extension of the lesion at the level of the jugular foramen causes impairment of cranial nerves IX, X and XI (jugular foramen syndrome). Such a well-known constellation of symptoms, consisting of weakness of shoulder movements, secondary to paralysis of the sternocleidomastoid and trapezius muscle, hoarse voice, food aspiration, pharyngeal dysphagia caused by vagus nerve paralysis and additional paralysis of the glossopharyngeal nerve, can be severely debilitating.

The presence of a mass in the rhinopharynx can cause a swelling sensation in the throat and an auditory deficit in conduction.

Malignant lesions of the mucous membrane, such as rhinopharyngeal carcinoma, are usually ulcerating and the bleeding, even though it is seldom profuse, is a recurrent symptom. Posterior extension of clival tumors can cause brainstem compression. The early symptomatology may only be a suboccipital pain and a minor dysesthesia in the arms. As the compression of the inferior portion of the clivus becomes greater, the patient may report weakness of the upper limbs and balance disorders, as well as paresis of cranial nerve XI. If compression has reached the medial and superior portion of the clivus, symptoms may include: a deficit of cranial nerve VI, dizziness, ataxia, syncopal episodes, and hydrocephalus.

The basilar impression syndrome causes brainstem compression and can indicate a cerebromedullary syndrome with ataxia, dizziness, oscillopsia and vertical nystagmus. The inferior cranial nerves may also be involved. Compression of the pons can produce sudden cardiorespiratory arrest. Compression in the atlantoaxial area can cause lower limb paralysis, upper limb paresthesia, hyposthenia and quadriparesis.

Odontoid fractures, especially with posterior luxation, can cause cardiorespiratory arrest and sudden death. There may be severe pain in the posterior surface of neck, which increases in intensity with coughing or leaning forwards, upper limb paresthesia and hyposthenia, lower limb hyposthenia or paralysis or quadriparesis.

19.3 Radiological Assessment

Radiological investigations are extremely important both in the diagnosis phase and in surgical intervention planning, as it is easy to deduce. Modalities include:
- Conventional radiology (including dynamic projections in flexion-extension and open mouth projection).
- CT.
- MRI.
- Angio-MRI.

A simple cross-table lateral is usually the first image of the cervical spine to be obtained following trauma. A swimmer's view may be required, as it is necessary to image from the skull base to the top of the T1 vertebral body. An open-mouth odontoid view should be obtained to assess the C1–C2 vertebrae and articulations and is particularly valuable for assessment of the odontoid process. The anteroposterior view may be useful to identify injuries with a rotatory component.

In the oncological patient, plain radiographic imaging of the spine allow assessment of: qualitative bony alterations (e.g. lytic, blastic, or sclerotic abnormalities); site of involvement (e.g. posterior elements, pedicles, or vertebral body); ancillary findings (e.g. paraspinal soft-tissue shadow, vertebral collapse, pathological fracture dislocation, or malalignment).

The lateral radiograph of the cranium allows the odontoid edge position to be emphasized in relation to the basicranium. Chamberlain's line [11] connects the dorsal margin of the foramen magnum with the posterior edge of the hard palate. The extremity of the odontoid process should be below this line. Since the dorsal margin cannot be so easily detected, McGregor defined another line connecting the posterior margin of the hard palate to the most caudal point of the occiput (no more than 4–5 mm of dens should be above this line) [12]. Fischgold's lines are also useful measures and are reproducible radiographically using an anteroposterior projection. Fischgold's digastric line joins the digastric notches. The normal distance from this line to the middle of the atlantooccipital joint is 10 mm (this distance is reduced in basilar impression) [13]. No part of the odontoid should be above this line. Fischgold's bimastoid line joins the tips of the mastoid processes. The odontoid tip averages 2 mm above this line (range 3 mm below to 10 mm above) and the line should cross the atlantooccipital joint [14].

With current MRI technology these measures are less important than they were since compression of soft tissues can be demonstrated with high precision.

CT in the assessment of the trauma patient is particularly useful for analyzing the occipitocervical and the cervicothoracic junctions. Areas identified as possible pathology on plain radiographs should be further investigated with CT imaging with fine sections through the suspicious areas. In the oncological patient CT scans are useful to demonstrate the distribution of spinal tumors, the displacement of the spinal cord and nerve roots, the degree of bony destruction, and paraspinal extension of the lesion in the horizontal plane. CT could be effective in distinguishing between benign spinal degenerative disease and neoplastic lesions [15, 16].

MRI is an extremely useful tool in the assessment of the patient with a cervical spine injury and may identify injuries, such as disk herniations, not seen on plain radiographs or CT scans. MRI has become the imaging modality of choice for spinal tumors, including metastases [17, 18]. The MRI scan helps in defining the relationships between pathology and the brainstem, the cervical cord and vertebral arteries. Gradient-echo sequences and images after contrast agent administration allow the assessment of soft-tissue pathologies and the integrity of the C1–C2 ligament complex, important factors in surgical planning.

The angio-MRI or angiography is necessary in the surgery of tumors with possible embolization, and is also useful in some congenital or acquired abnormalities.

The evaluation of radiological images of the craniocervical junction is an essential step in selecting the best approach and in evaluating for the presence of instability at the level of the craniovertebral junction. As discussed in section 19.4 Surgical Considerations, it is very important to distinguish between an intradural lesion and an extradural lesion and to evaluate the lateral extension of the lesion.

Tracing on an MRI image an imaginary sagittal plane between the hard palate and the craniocervical junction permits, in the preoperative phase, the superior extension of the exposure to be estimated. The possibility of choosing a transsphenoidal approach is to be considered for lesions above such a line. A solely transoral approach could be enough when the lesion is below the plane of the hard palate. As an alternative, a Le Fort I maxillectomy, with or without splitting the palate, can be considered for lesions extending both above and below the plane of the hard palate. If the lesion extends inferiorly over the body of C2 a transmandibular approach will provide a better exposure.

19.4 Surgical Considerations

The transoral approach [3, 19–24] to the basicranium allows exposure alongside the midline of the third inferior of the clivus, the craniovertebral junction and the C1/C2 complex.

The primary advantage of such a surgical approach is direct extradural approach without surgical tensile forces upon the encephalus. Though exposure alongside the midline allows access to intradural structures

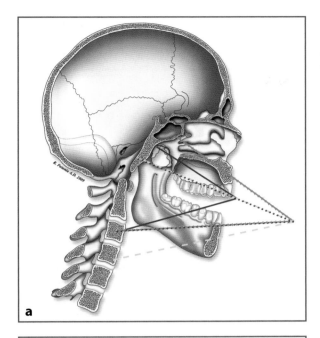

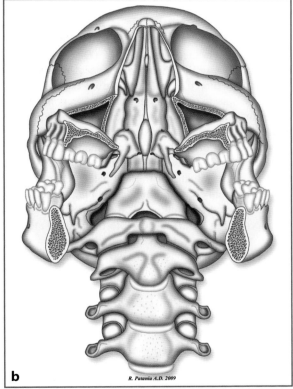

Fig. 19.3 a Transoral approaches (*blue dotted line* transmaxillary palatal split approach, *green dotted line* transpalatal approach, *red dotted line* transmandibular approach, *yellow dotted line* standard transoral approach). **b** Skull base and upper cervical spine frontal view after palatal and mandibular splitting

such as the caudal portion of the pons, spinal cord, cervicomedullary junction, and vertebrobasilar artery complex, a transoral approach for the treatment of intradural lesions appears not to be the most suitable intervention due to contamination of the surgical field. A watertight dural closure is difficult to obtain using such an approach and the probable fluid fistula would put the patient at risk of meningitis.

The limits of a transoral approach are laterally the mandible and tonsillar pillars, and superiorly and inferiorly the third inferior of the clivus and the medioinferior portion of the C2 body. Some clinical conditions such as RA can result in a reduction in the extension of the exposure because of a decreased ability to open the mouth. Therefore it is necessary to perform accurate radiological investigations before planning the intervention. First it is necessary to consider the possibility of approaching the lesion by an exposure of the basicranium alongside the midline and distinguishing between an intradural lesion and an extradural one. In the case of an extradural lesion, such an intervention should be considered only when the lesion does not extend laterally. In order to obtain an adequate surgical field, mouth needs to be open at least 2.5–3 cm between the incisor teeth of the two dental arches. An extended transoral approach [3, 19–21] (by maxillectomy, palate splitting [25], mandibulectomy [26–28] and glossectomy [26–28]) undoubtedly allows a wider exposure which is useful for lesions of larger dimensions (Fig. 19.3), but it is also associated with greater morbidity.

In the preoperative phase radiography of the cervical spine will reveal the presence of instability at the level of the craniovertebral junction. Stabilization of the cervical spine (occipitocervical or atlantoaxial) may be necessary if a lesion has already destabilized the atlantooccipital or atlantoaxial articulation, or if the removal of a lesion has resulted in instability.

19.5 Surgical Technique

19.5.1 Patient Preparation

Before covering the patient with a surgical drape, setting the brilliance amplifier will provide useful information for intraoperative orientation. The patient is placed in a supine position. The head can be rested on a surgical donut-shaped cushion or fixed rigidly. In the former case the head needs to be held still during the intervention. The patient's head will be hyperextended so as to provide the best view of the craniovertebral region. The extent of opening of the mandible, the size of the oral cavity and the isthmus of the fauces should be assessed. In patients suffering from RA involvement of the temporomandibular joint is common, and in such cases surgical mobilization of the joint or the use of an extended approach (labiomandibular glossotomy) may be necessary. A tracheostomy must be performed in patients suffering from respiratory complications related to bulbar dysfunction and in patients needing an extended approach involving labiomandibular glossotomy. Considerations in favor of such a procedure are the possibility to:

- Obtain a wider surgical field.
- Avoid a probable source of bacterial contamination (endotracheal tube).
- Prevent damage related to aspiration and dysphagia that frequently occur in the postoperative period.
- Provide airway protection in the first days after the intervention.

The endotracheal tube, passing through the oral cavity, is usually set under the tongue retractor and this increases tongue compression and the probability of postoperative swelling. It is advisable to perform a tracheotomy because of the occurrence of postoperative edema of the tongue together with stenosis of the airways.

The eyes are protected by the use of Frost knots or, in short interventions, by corneal protectors. Sterile skin preparation should include besides the head and neck region, any region that is likely to be used for tissue harvest (e.g. the thigh for fascia lata). Thorough oral hygiene in the days preceding a surgical intervention is important. All gum or tooth infections must be cleared before the intervention. Sterile preparation includes washing with a disinfectant solution.

Exposure of the surgical field is guaranteed by placement of a retractor (such as a Dingman, Crockard or Spetzler-Sonntag retractor) which allows retraction of the tongue and cheeks and keeps the oral fissure open. For orotracheal intubation it the tube can be placed under the tongue retractor ensuring that excessive compression of the tongue is avoided (Fig. 19.4). Moreover the tip of the tongue should not be too compressed against the tooth arch. A few minutes after placing the retractor it will be possible to obtain the widest opening allowing further tool release, while the perioral and mandibular muscles carry on loosening and stretching. The surgeon will be at the patient's head and will use a surgical microscope which is very useful for working in such a narrow and hard-to-illuminate surgical field.

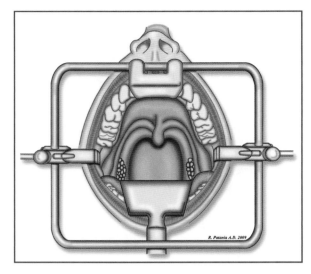

Fig. 19.4 Surgical field after retractor placement

19.5.2 Surgical Procedure

The posterior part of the pharynx is infiltrated with 0.5% lidocaine with epinephrine at 1/200,000. If necessary, the soft palate and the hard palate are also infiltrated. Touching the tubercle of C1 the midline is found, but it should be born in mind that this point of anatomical reference may be lacking or anatomically altered in patients with a tumors located at this level. When the procedure involves the inferior clivus and foramen magnum it is necessary to split the soft palate, and at times, the hard palate. In other situations, the soft palate and uvula are retracted superiorly with a malleable blade retractor or catheters are passed via the nasal passages into the nasopharynx (Fig. 19.5). To elevate the soft palate, the catheters are secured to its edges, and it is then withdrawn into the high nasopharynx (a palatal incision is avoided when possible because it can cause nasal regurgitation, dysphagia, and a nasal tone to the voice).

The soft palate incision starts at the base of the uvula and, continuing between the hard palate and soft palate, ends laterally at 3–5 mm from the tooth root. The incision runs around the anterior margin of the hard palate, just behind the incisive foramen, contralaterally and downwards, and up to the first molar of the opposite side (Fig. 19.6). The mucoperiosteal flap of the hard palate is then dissected at the junction between the hard palate and soft palate. The principal palatal neurovascular bundle is isolated at the side of the incision and sectioned after tying it with a suture thread. The insertions of the

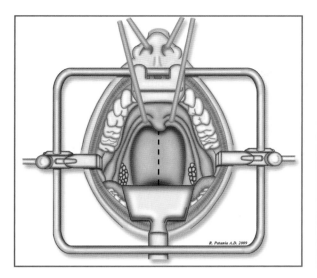

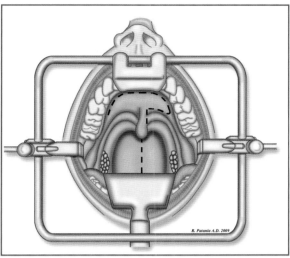

Fig. 19.5 Surgical field after retractor placement and soft palate and uvula retraction superiorly using catheters passed via the nasal passages into the nasopharynx

Fig. 19.6 Incision line for the pharyngeal wall, soft palate and hard palate

soft palatal muscles into the hard palate are dissected. This is performed contralaterally via the submucosa.

The posterior pharyngeal wall is longitudinally incised alongside the midline in correspondence to the lesion that will later be resected. An electroscalpel can be used for this incision. The incision is carried progressively through the mucosa, the midline raphe between the pharyngeal muscles, and the anterior longitudinal ligament down to the bone using a regular monopolar cautery tip. The lateral retractors help to ex-

pose the tissues as the incision is deepened. Then the tip of a regular monopolar cautery, bent to a near right angle, is used in a sweeping motion to detach the ligaments from the bone in a subperiosteal fashion. This technique greatly reduces bleeding from these well-vascularized tissues. The longus colli and the longus capitis muscles are mobilized laterally and held in place with tooth-bladed lateral pharyngeal retractors to expose the inferior clivus, C1 arch, and C2 vertebral body (Fig. 19.7).

Fig. 19.7 **a** Exposure obtained by a pharyngeal wall incision. **b** Exposure obtained by a pharyngeal wall incision combined with a soft and hard palate incision

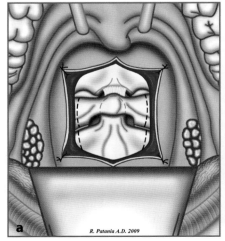

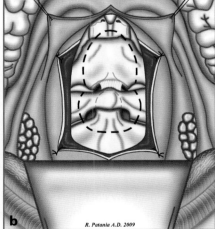

Detailed descriptions of odontoidectomy, tumor removal, extended procedures, and closure of the wound can be found in the respective sections.

19.5.3 Removal of C1 Arch and Odontoidectomy

When is removal of the dens necessary?
- When a fracture and irreducible subluxation of the dens cause an anterior compression of the spinal cord.
- When an anterior compression of the cervicomedullary junction arises from a rheumatoid pannus or a tumor.
- When decompression must be performed in basilar impression.

First soft tissues are freed using an electroscalpel and a periosteal elevator before the anterior arch of C1 and the odontoid process of C2 are removed. Then, by means of a high-speed drill, the arch of C1 is cut on each side of the odontoid process and the underlying odontoid process exposed by removing the arch of C1 using rongeurs. After distinctly defining the edges of the odontoid process the alar and apical ligaments are detached sharply with curved curettes. The base of the dens is partially transected with a cutting burr. The osteotomy is completed by removing the posterior cortex with a small Kerrison rongeur or diamond burr. At this point the dens is removed en bloc.

The transverse ligament is identified. Sometimes removal of the pannus might first involve removal of the transverse ligament, tectorial membrane, and any other residual ligaments. To decompress the underlying craniovertebral junction dura mater, a proper resection of the compressive pathology is performed and, if necessary, the inferior clivus is removed using a high-speed drill and rongeurs.

19.5.4 Tumor Removal

Sometimes opening the posterior pharyngeal mucosa may reveal a tumor that has caused misshaping of the anatomy of the craniovertebral junction. In such cases removal of the tumor, in a piece-meal fashion, is indicated. Any ligaments involved by tumor should also be removed.

Odontoidectomy could be indicated for a neoplastic mass extending more deeply, being mindful to detach the apical and alar ligaments first, in order to avoid upward tip retraction.

Posterior stabilization is advisable if tumoral erosion of the atlantooccipital joints or disruption of the arch of C1 or of the odontoid process has occurred. If the tumor has involved the occipital condyle, care must be taken not to injure the hypoglossal nerves (passing through the hypoglossal canal) while drilling it. If the tumor has involved the dura mater, care must be taken not to injure the basilar artery, perforators and brainstem. If an intraoperative cerebrospinal fluid leak occurs, the dura mater should be reconstructed with autologous or allograft fascia lata, fat and fibrin glue in several layers. At the end of such a procedure temporary lumbar drainage should be performed. If the tumor has not involved the dura mater the extent of decompression can be evaluated intraoperatively by injecting contrast material into the epidural space and viewing it fluoroscopically.

19.5.5 Closure

Proper wound closure is not an easy task. Two conditions have to be recognized:
1. If the dura mater is intact the wound is closed in two layers. First, the muscle layer is approximated in a horizontal mattress using 3-0 vicryl sutures. Then, the mucosal layer is approximated using simple interrupted 3-0 vicryl sutures.
2. If the dura mater has been lacerated by the tumor or the surgical approach, it is necessary to reconstruct the cranial base followed by placement of a temporary lumbar drain in order to prevent a cerebrospinal fluid leak. The dural defect can be reconstructed by grafting a piece of fascia lata, previously harvested from the thigh. Then the muscle layer and mucosa can be closed as previously described.

19.5.6 Posterior Stabilization

It is advisable to perform a posterior stabilization immediately after transoral resection since it allows both restoration of normal alignment which is often disrupted by the pathological process and its subsequent stabilization. If the patient is in good alignment initially, the stabilization could be performed before the transoral approach. The surgery itself contributes to weakening of the craniovertebral junction, which in many cases, is already impaired by the underlying pathology. The key structure for stabilization in the atlantoaxial region is the odontoid process of C2, which is held within the anterior ring of C1 by the very strong transverse ligament. Resecting the anterior arch of C1 or performing a transoral odontoidectomy will therefore disrupt this complex leading to a significant increase in the amount of translational and rotational motion making the spine very unstable.

An occipitocervical stabilization is usually required when a basilar invagination is found preoperatively.

For posterior stabilization, the patient is repositioned in the prone position with the head placed in three-point fixation. A cervical collar is used to increase the stability during careful turning of the patient. Then, the craniovertebral junction is placed in anatomic alignment under fluoroscopic visualization for subsequent stabilization. The motion segments requiring stabilization are definitively determined during surgery because it is not easy to determine whether there is atlantooccipital instability if atlantoaxial instability is also present. After exposing the spine, a towel clamp or Kocher clamp is placed on the posterior arch of C1, and force is carefully applied under fluoroscopic visualization. The atlantooccipital joint is unstable if C1 translates in the anteroposterior plane by more than 1 mm. If this is the case the fusion construct is extended to the occipital bone to perform an occipitocervical fusion. If no translation of C1 in relation to the occipital bone occurs, only C1/C2 stabilization is usually performed with transarticular screws or a direct C1 lateral mass screw and C2 pars screw construct (Harms' technique). If the fixing of C1 and C2 cannot be directly performed it is necessary to extend the construct to achieve an instrumented occipitocervical stabilization. Nevertheless, in most cases a short segment fusion is achieved thanks to the versatility of modern instrumentation systems.

19.6 Extended Transoral Approaches

The extended transoral approach is usually required when lesions extend beyond the exposure limits of a standard transoral approach. The need for an extended approach can be determined preoperatively from radiographic images, as described above. Extended approaches involve additional incisions and facial osteotomies to mobilize structures that may obstruct the

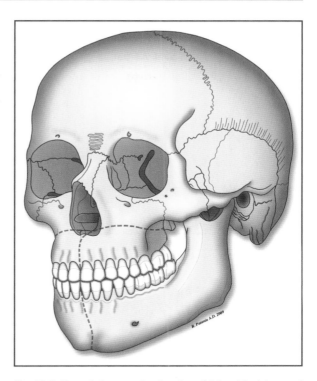

Fig. 19.8 Extended approaches involve additional incisions and facial osteotomies to mobilize structures that may obstruct the line of sight to the lesion

surgeon's line of sight to the lesion (Fig. 19.8). Accurate reconstruction of maxillofacial osteotomies is essential to achieve excellent cosmesis and avoid malocclusion. The options for gaining more superior exposure of the upper and middle clivus and sphenoid sinus are the transmaxillary (Le Fort I maxillotomy) approach, transmaxillary palatal split (extended "open-door" maxillotomy) approach, or the transpalatal approach. To gain more inferior exposure from C2 to C4, a median labiomandibular glossotomy (transmandibular split) can be used.

19.6.1 Transmaxillary Approach (Le Fort I Maxillotomy)

The transmaxillary approach involves a Le Fort I maxillotomy through a gingival fornix incision that allows inferior mobilization of the maxilla and hard palate, much like a trap door [22, 29, 30]. The lateral limits of the exposure are the carotid arteries (Fig. 19.9).

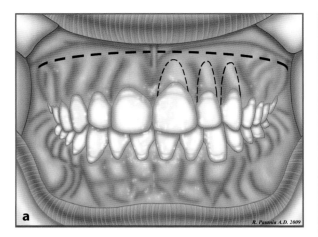

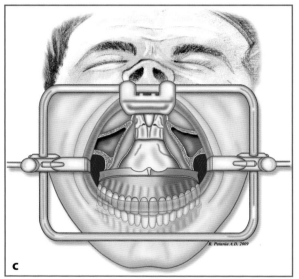

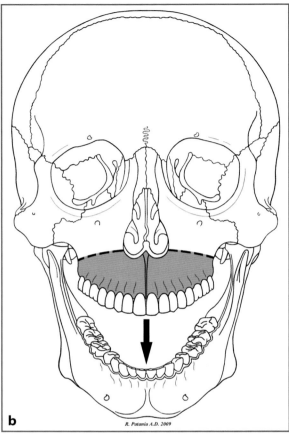

Fig. 19.9 a Gingival fornix incision in the transmaxillary approach. **b** Downward displacement of the maxilla. **c** Exposure obtained by the transmaxillary approach

19.6.1.1 Indications

This maneuver provides more upward viewing to the sphenoid sinus and upper and middle clivus and also provides a wider panoramic exposure of the posterior nasooropharynx. Inferior displacement of the hard palate, however, obstructs inferior viewing of the inferior portions of the body of C2, which is the major limitation of this approach. This approach is appropriate for midline extradural lesions that are wider and involve the sphenoid sinus, clivus, and odontoid process.

The Le Fort I maxillotomy has advantages over the extended transsphenoidal approach in that it provides wider exposure as well as more inferior viewing past the plane of the hard palate.

19.6.1.2 Surgical Technique

A gingival fornix incision is made along the upper alveolar margin extending from one maxillary tuberosity to the other. The gingival mucosa is elevated subperiosteally to expose the anterior maxilla up to the level of the infraorbital nerve. Once the piriform aperture has been identified, the nasal mucosa is elevated from the nasal floor and the nasal septum up to the level of the inferior nasal turbinates. The pterygomaxillary fissures on both sides must be exposed prior to the osteotomy.

The intended Le Fort I osteotomy is marked on the maxilla with a sterile pen. It is important to perform preplating with titanium plates and screws to ensure an exact fit when the maxilla is returned to its anatomic position during closure. This technique reduces the risk of postoperative malocclusion. The titanium miniplates and screws are secured over both sides of the intended Le Fort I osteotomy line. They are then removed and carefully labeled for subsequent replacement during closure. Using an oscillating saw, bilateral Le Fort I osteotomies are made, staying above the roots of the teeth to avoid dental injury.

Another osteotomy is made to separate the bony nasal septum from the hard palate. Using a curved osteotome, the maxillary tuberosities are disarticulated from the pterygomaxillary fissures bilaterally. Then the hard palate is down-fractured and mobilized inferiorly into the oral cavity. The remainder of the operation is similar to the transoral approach described above. At the time of closure, the maxilla is replaced and fixed with the preregistered titanium plates and screws. The gingival mucosa is reapproximated with interrupted 2-0 absorbable sutures.

19.6.2 Transmaxillary Palatal Split Approach (Extended Maxillotomy)

This modified approach is referred to as the transmaxillary palatal split approach, or extended "open-door" maxillotomy, and is essentially a Le Fort I osteotomy enhanced with an additional split of the hard and soft palate. The lateral limits of this exposure are the cavernous carotid arteries, the occipital condyles, and the lateral masses of the C1–C2 complex (Fig. 19.10).

19.6.2.1 Indications

This approach provides rostral exposure of the sphenoid sinus and upper and middle clivus while maintaining the inferior exposure provided by a standard transoral approach. This is particularly useful for extensive lesions that involve the sphenoid sinus and clivus down to the body of C2.

The splitting of the hard and soft palate and subsequent mobilization of the hemimaxillae laterally permits a wider exposure of the inferior limits. Each hemimaxilla has its own blood supply and innervation from its respective palatine artery and nerve.

The major disadvantages of this approach are an extended operating time and the complexity of reconstruction and wound closure.

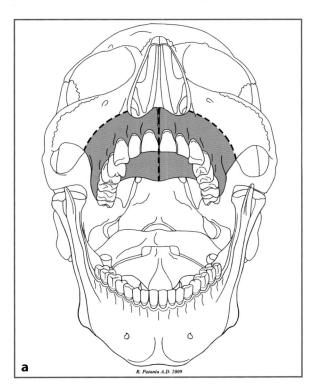

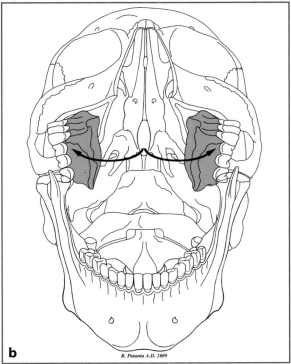

Fig. 19.10 a Incision lines in the transmaxillary palatal split approach. **b** Palatal splitting in the transmaxillary palatal split approach

19.6.2.2 Surgical Technique

A Le Fort I osteotomy is initially performed as described above. The mucosa over the hard palate is incised slightly off the midline, continuing posteriorly through the soft palate, staying on one side of the uvula. Using an oscillating saw, the hard palate is split in the midline starting between the front incisors. The osteotomy traverses around the anterior nasal spine and continues posteriorly in the sagittal plane. Each hemimaxilla is rotated outward and retracted laterally into the cheek. A midline incision is made in the posterior pharyngeal wall and the surgical resection is continued as described previously (Fig. 19.11). At the time of closure, each hemimaxilla is restored to its anatomic location and fixed with preregistered titanium plates and screws. The mucosa is reapproximated over the hard palate and the sublabial incisions with interrupted absorbable sutures. The soft palate is closed in three layers with interrupted absorbable sutures.

19.6.3 Transpalatal Approach

The transpalatal approach provides increased rostral exposure of the upper and middle clivus through a standard transoral approach by excising the hard palate.

19.6.3.1 Indications

This approach is useful for tumors of the craniovertebral junction that extend superiorly beyond the plane of the hard palate. It allows minimal facial disassembly.

19.6.3.2 Surgical Technique

To disarticulate the hard palate, exposure is obtained above and below the hard palate through the nasal floor and oral cavity, respectively. Initially, a gingival fornix incision is made and the gingival mucosa elevated subperiosteally to expose the piriform aperture. Submucosal dissection is performed to expose the nasal floor and nasal septum, similar to a sublabial transsphenoidal approach. A midline incision is made through the mucosa of the inferior surface of the hard palate that continues through the soft palate, staying on one side of the uvula. The mucosa is elevated subperiosteally to the alveolar margin around the greater palatine foramen, and the levator muscle detached from the posterior mar-

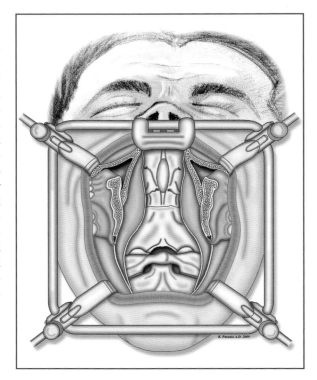

Fig. 19.11 Exposure obtained by the transmaxillary palatal split approach

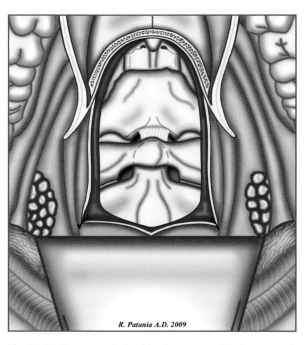

Fig. 19.12 Exposure obtained by the transmandibular approach

gins of the hard palate. An oscillating saw is used to cut around the margin of the palate near the alveolar edge, staying medial to the greater palatine foramen. Through the sublabial exposure, the hard palate is disarticulated from the nasal septum and lateral nasal walls with an osteotome. The bony hard palate is removed from the oral cavity, thereby exposing the nasal septum, sphenoid sinus, and upper clivus (Fig. 19.12). The posterior pharynx is incised and tumor removal proceeds as described previously. At the time of closure, titanium microplates and screws are used to fix the hard palate back into its anatomical position. Take care not to place screws into the tooth roots. The soft tissues of the soft palate and the palatal mucosa are reapproximated with interrupted absorbable sutures, and the sublabial incision is also closed with interrupted absorbable sutures.

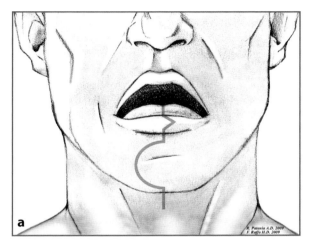

19.6.4 Transmandibular Approach (Median Labiomandibular Glossotomy)

The median labiomandibular glossotomy involves a lower lip and chin incision followed by a midline split of the mandible and tongue (Fig. 19.13).

Fig. 19.13 a Skin incision lines in the transmandibular approach. **b** Mandibular incision line in the transmandibular approach. **c** Exposure obtained by the transmandibular approach. **d** Closure after the transmandibular approach

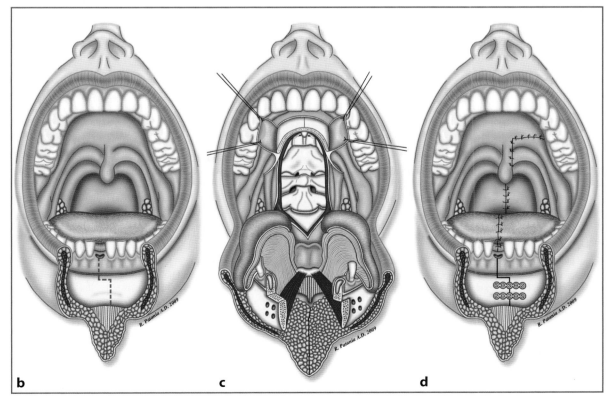

b   c   d

19.6.4.1 Indications

This approach is useful to access craniovertebral junction tumors and other lesions that extend inferiorly beyond C2 to about the C4 level if they are not accessible through a standard transoral approach.

19.6.4.2 Surgical Technique

It is advisable to perform a tracheostomy before performing this extended approach. A vertical curvilinear incision is made in the lower lip, starting in the midline and curving around the skin crease of the chin, then continuing inferiorly in the midline to the hyoid bone. The soft tissues and mucosa are elevated from the mandible laterally. Titanium plates and screws are contoured to the mandible and preregistered for later replacement. Using an oscillating saw, the mandible is split in the midline between the two lower incisors. Removal of the teeth is not required in performing this osteotomy. The tongue is incised with monopolar cautery along the median raphe, a relatively avascular plane, posteriorly toward the median glossoepiglottic fold. Because the incision is in the midline, the innervation from the hypoglossal nerves to their respective halves of the tongue is preserved, as is the vascular supply to the tongue. The halves of the mandible and tongue are retracted laterally. The floor of the mouth is split between the submaxillary ducts, and the incision extended inferiorly to the level of the hyoid bone. The posterior pharyngeal wall is incised in the midline, exposing the middle-to-inferior clivus down to the C3 and C4 vertebral bodies. Tumor removal and closure proceed as described above. The mandible is restored to its anatomic position and reapproximated with the preregistered titanium plates and screws. The tongue is reapproximated with interrupted absorbable sutures. The lip and skin incisions are reapproximated with 3-0 nylon sutures.

19.7.5 Complications

There are intra- and postoperative complications:

- Intraoperative: vascular damage, cerebrospinal fluid leakage, edema of soft tissues (tongue and lips), cranial nerve paralysis.
- Postoperative: local infection and dehiscence of the wound, cerebrospinal fluid leakage and meningitis, hematoma formation, velopalatine dysfunction, dysphagia and nasal regurgitation, dental malocclusion after resection of the mandible or jaw, pain and rigidity of the mandible, craniocervical junction instability, mandibular luxation.

Acknowledgment: The authors thank Andrea Braconi, Noemi Mazzone, Guido Rendine and Fabio Romano for their precious collaboration.

References

1. Testut L, Latarjet A (eds) (1972) Trattato di anatomia umana, 5th edn. Utet, Torino
2. Rhoton AL Jr (2000) The foramen magnum. Neurosurgery 47:S155–S193
3. Donald PJ (ed) (2001) Chirurgia del basicranio. Antonio Delfino Editore, Rome
4. Hadley M, Dickman C, Browner C, Sonntag V (1989) Acute axis fractures: a review of 229 cases. J Neurosurg 71:642–647
5. Hadley MN, Browner C, Sonntag VK (1985) Axis fractures: a comprehensive review of management and treatment in 107 cases. Neurosurgery 17:281–290
6. Anderson LD, D'Alonzo RT (1974) Fractures of the odontoid process of the axis. J Bone Joint Surg 56A:1663–1674
7. Lipsky PE (2004) Rheumatoid arthritis. In: Kasper DL, Braunwald E, Hauser S, Longo D, Jameson JL, Fauci AS (eds) Harrison's principles of internal medicine,16th edn. McGraw-Hill, New York
8. Rana NA, Hancock DO, Taylor AR (1973) Atlanto-axial subluxation in rheumatoid arthritis. J Bone Joint Surg 55B:458–470
9. Sen CN, Sekhar LN, Schramm VL et al (1989) Chordomas and chondrosarcomas of the cranial base. Neurosurgery 25:931–941
10. Willis RA (ed) (1973) The spread of tumors in the human body, 3rd edn. Butterworth, London
11. Chamberlain WE (1939) Basilar impression (platybasia); bizarre developmental anomaly of occipital bone and upper cervical spine with striking and misleading neurologic manifestations. Yale J Biol Med 11:487–496
12. McGregor J (1948) The significance of certain measurements of the skull in the diagnosis of basilar impression. Br J Radiol 21:171–181
13. Hinck VC, Hopkins CE, Savara BS (1961) Diagnostic criteria of basilar impression. Radiology 76:572–585
14. Fischgold H, Metzger J (1952) Etude radiotomographique de l'impression basilaire. Rev Rhum Mal Osteoartic 19:261–264
15. O'Rourke T, George CB, Redmond J et al (1986) Spinal computed tomography and computed tomographic metriza-

mide myelography in the early diagnosis of metastatic disease. J Clin Oncol 4:576–583

16. Redmond J, Spring DB, Munderloh SH et al (1984) Spinal computed tomography scanning in the evaluation of metastatic disease. Cancer 54:253–258

17. Jaeckle KA (1991) Neuroimaging for central nervous system tumors. Semin Oncol 18:150–157

18. Sze G (1991) Magnetic resonance imaging in the evaluation of spinal tumors. Cancer 67:1229–1241

19. Fessler RG, Sekhar L (2007) Neurochirurgia. Colonna vertebrale e nervi periferici. Testo e atlante. Verduci Editore, Rome

20. Liu JK, Couldwell WT, Apfelbaum RI (2008) Transoral approach and extended modifications for lesions of the ventral foramen magnum and craniovertebral junction. Skull Base 18:151–166

21. Menezes AH, Gregory DF (2005) Transoral approach to the ventral craniocervical border. Oper Tech Neurosurg 8:150–157

22. Ammirati M, Bernardo A (1998) Analytical evaluation of complex anterior approaches to the cranial base: an anatomic study. Neurosurgery 43:1398–1407

23. Crockard HA (1985) The transoral approach to the base of the brain and upper cervical cord. Ann R Coll Surg Engl 67: 321–325

24. Dickman CA, Locantro J, Fessler RG (1992) The influence of transoral odontoid resection on stability of the craniovertebral junction. J Neurosurg 77:525–530

25. Williams WG, Lo LJ, Chen YR (1998) The Le Fort I-palatal split approach for skull base tumors: efficacy, complications, and outcome. Plast Reconstr Surg 102:2310–2319

26. Arbit E, Patterson RH Jr (1981) Combined transoral and median labiomandibular glossotomy approach to the upper cervical spine. Neurosurgery 8:672–674

27. Delgado TE, Garrido E, Harwick RD (1981) Labiomandibular, transoral approach to chordomas in the clivus and upper cervical spine. Neurosurgery 8:675–679

28. Moore LJ, Schwartz HC (1985) Median labiomandibular glossotomy for access to the cervical spine. J Oral Maxillofac Surg 43:909–912

29. Sasaki CT, Lowlicht RA, Astrachan DI et al (1990) Le Fort I osteotomy approach to the skull base. Laryngoscope 100: 1073–1076

30. Uttley D, Moore A, Archer DJ (1989) Surgical management of midline skull-base tumors: a new approach. J Neurosurg 71:705–710

Midfacial Approaches

20

Luigi Califano, Pasquale Piombino, Felice Esposito
and Giorgio Iaconetta

20.1 History

The first rudimentary transfacial approaches were performed in ancient Greece to cure warriors and wrestlers. Aesculapius and Hippocrates reported treatment of people suffering from trauma to the head and face. During the Renaissance period, the practice of anatomy on cadavers led to the meticulous description of the anatomy of the face and its cavities. At the end of the 18th century, Dionis described some techniques to perform maxillofacial resections and, during the 19th century, in relation to the wars that involved all of Europe, interest in this surgery came back again. It was only in the second half of the last century that the modern concepts involved in the performance of maxillofacial surgery were developed. These include an interest in treating tumors involving the paranasal sinuses and skull base extending within the cranium, the opportunity to use prostheses after extensive surgery, and the respect of the different tissue layers during surgery in order to achieve an adequate and optimal esthetic reconstruction of the face. In the 1980s, Curioni introduced the concept of the box in oncological surgery.

20.2 Indications

Transfacial approaches are used to treat tumors sited within the ethmoid cells, within the maxillary sinuses,

in the central skull base and clivus, and within the pterygopalatine and subtemporal fossa. Furthermore, nasopharyngeal tumors, and tumors invading the orbit and anterior skull base, require a subtotal or total ethmoidomaxillectomy using different techniques [1–6].

20.3 Investigations

Radiological investigations are extremely useful in diagnosis and surgical planning. The modalities used include plain radiography, computed tomography, angiography, and magnetic resonance imaging.

20.3.1 Radiography

The role of plain radiography has declined in popularity following the introduction of more recent techniques. The value of plain radiography is in determining the stability at the occipitoatlantoaxial joints. The lateral views in extension and in flexion can give useful information regarding the extent and level of alterations. The angles and the distances between bone landmarks can indicate significant discrepancies from normal.

20.3.2 Computed Tomography

This investigation, before and after the administration of contrast agent, can predict the boundaries, nature, consistency, and relationship with the near structures of tumoral lesions. Possible edema and necrosis and the

L. Califano (✉)
Dept of Head and Neck Surgery
Università degli Studi di Napoli Federico II, Naples, Italy

P. Cappabianca et al. (eds.), *Cranial, Craniofacial and Skull Base Surgery*.
© Springer-Verlag Italia 2010

extent of invasion can be accurately assessed as well. Thin slices and high resolution bone windows (1 mm) are tremendously important for detection of such lesions. Three-dimensional reconstructions also play an important role in preoperative surgical planning.

20.3.3 Angiography

Sometimes it is important to assess the precise tumoral vascular supply and to study the displacement, distortion or occlusion of the main vessels. Also, preoperative angiography gives the opportunity to perform endovascular embolization if the tumor is extensively vascularized, thus helping to reduce intraoperative blood loss. Angiography can be performed not only in its traditional form but also, more recently, as angio-CT and angio-MR.

20.3.4 Magnetic Resonance Imaging

MRI gives high-quality images, with clear demarcation between normal and pathological soft tissues, allowing the operation to be performed more safely. This examination can be associated with high-resolution CT to study the soft and hard tissues simultaneously, thus giving the navigation system information that is extremely important in decreasing the risk of error.

The operative field is adequately prepped with antiseptic solution from the forehead to the upper half of the neck. The oral cavity is also cleaned with antiseptic solution after a pharyngeal pack has been inserted. In relation to the extension of the surgical approach and the areas involved by the tumor lesion, the opportunity to prepare the carotid artery to the neck should be considered if any manipulation of this artery may be needed during surgery.

The precise planning of the skin incision is extremely important considering its functional and cosmetic implications. The most used incision is the Weber-Ferguson incision (Fig. 20.1). The incision is drawn using a skin marker and before the incision is performed, a solution of epinephrine is injected within the soft tissues in order to reduce bleeding. The classic Weber-Ferguson incision starts 1 cm above and medial to the medial canthus, curving inferiorly along the lateral border of the nose, following the nasofacial sulcus, to reach the alar groove.

The curve has to be as obtuse as possible to be sure that the skin has an adequate blood supply to avoid necrosis. The incision then continues inferiorly, curving in the direction of the midline, turning downward at right angles and extending along the philtrum to divide the upper lip up to the vermilion. The incision over the vermilion of the upper lip has a "zig-zag" line in order to avoid subsequent contraction and upward retraction of the lip. The incision continues over the gum to reach the groove between the two central incisors. The palatal

20.4 Surgical Technique

20.4.1 Skin Incision and Soft Tissue Dissection

Surgery is carried out under general anesthesia with the patient in the supine position with the head slightly elevated and not fixed to any device. In order to keep the nasal and oral cavities free, tracheostomy is usually required, but in many cases, after intubation, we pass the tube through the floor of the oral cavity so it exits in the submandibular region, being careful to position it on the opposite side from the maxillectomy and lateral to the tongue. A temporary tarsorrhaphy is performed on the eyelid of the operative side if orbital exenteration is not required, and the other eye is simply covered by protective tape.

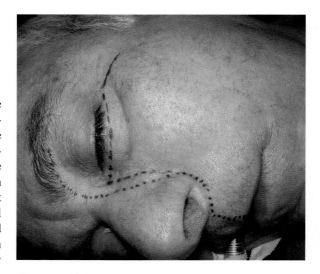

Fig. 20.1 Skin incision

incision is sited on the lingual aspect of the upper alveolus, between the central incisors, and curves along the inner border of the upper alveolus 0.5 cm from the mucosa, toward the operative side, reaching the third molar area and then turning laterally toward the oral mucosa behind the maxillary tuberosity. The gingival attachment of the vestibular surface is resected by knife as far as the third molar. The attachment of the soft palate to the hard palate has to be detached and divided to enter the posterior nasal cavity. This incision allows a skin flap to be reflected providing a wide exposure of the paralateronasal and maxillary regions (Fig. 20.2).

Over the years different variations of skin incision have been suggested. We mostly use the Tabb incision which is an upper prolongation of the previously described incision, following the ciliary margin of the upper eyelid, eventually prolonged into the temporal region. The Schuknecht incision is useful if orbital exenteration is required. If more exposure of the deep midface and maxilla is needed, we perform the Moure incision, along the upper border of the orbital cavity, or the modified Moure with infraorbital incision to reach the lateral canthus and in some cases extending more laterally to the zygomatic arch.

The incision along the eyelid has to be 3 mm away from and parallel to the eyelashes in order to avoid edema if too close, or ectropion if too far from the eyelashes, complications that evolve into esthetic and functional problems for the patient. The soft-tissue layers and muscles are then incised and elevated until the periosteal layer is reached, taking care to avoid excessive stretching of the orbicularis muscle. This is then incised following the section line of the skin and is dissected with a smooth dissector.

The soft tissue dissection should be limited to exposure of the bony surface enough to perform the osteotomies; excessive retraction may lead to scar formation after an inadequate reconstruction at the end of surgery. Attention has to be paid to preserving the arteries and veins while accurate hemostasis of the soft tissues has to be performed. The lacrimal sac is elevated from its lodge while the periosteum at this level is left in position. The periosteum is superiorly dissected to expose the frontoethmoidal suture taking great care to preserve the ethmoidal arteries which represent the upper limit of the resection.

Obviously, the techniques of incision we use have to be tailored according to the approach for each specific lesion treated; for example, if an ethmoidectomy only has to be performed, it is unnecessary to split the superior lip.

The soft tissues of the nasal pyramid are laterally reflected toward the contralateral eye and the median nasal suture is exposed; the nasal fibrocartilage is hence dissected from the bony margin and the orbital contents are gently dissected and lateralized in order to elevate the periorbit from the bony structures of the lamina papyracea (Fig. 20.3). The soft tissues are covered by wetted gauze to avoid accidental trauma during the osteotomies and their drying.

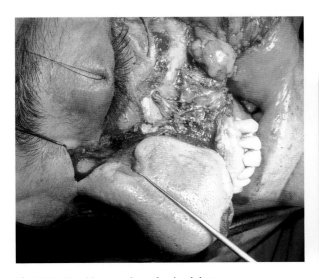

Fig. 20.2 Nasal bone and nasolacrimal duct

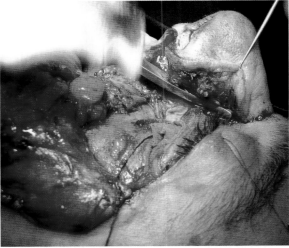

Fig. 20.3 Nasal bone osteotomy

20.4.2 *Osteotomies*

After skeletonization of the maxilla, there are two main approaches: ethmoidectomy with medial maxillectomy, and total ethmoidomaxillectomy.

20.4.2.1 Ethmoidectomy and Medial Maxillectomy

If this approach is required, the superior lip has to be left intact because the hard palate is not resected. The ipsilateral nasal bone is disconnected at the level of the maxillary suture and the orbit contents are lateralized to enlarge the surgical corridor. The nasofrontal suture is disconnected with a straight osteotome. The anterior wall of the maxilla is opened with a drill and a total of three osteotomies are performed. The first is necessary to mobilize the entire lateral nasal wall and is performed transecting the bone that limits the piriform incisures laterally.

The second osteotomy is carried out in correspondence with the frontoethmoidal suture 2–3 mm below the ethmoidal arteries, gently displacing the periorbit laterally, keeping in mind that the optic nerve is quite close. The third osteotomy is carried out on the orbital floor, very close to the lacrimal bone, disconnecting the maxilla from the zygomatic bone. After these osteotomies have been performed, the maxilla is still in place because the soft tissue connections have still to be resected. By gently using osteotomes and levers, and also scissors, the maxilla is progressively elevated and removed. After having obtained accurate hemostasis, the bony irregular margins are resected and smoothed in order to avoid scar formation. At this point the surgical corridor is widely open in all directions and the sphenoid sinus and upper third clivus are the deepest structures. This approach is generally indicated to treat tumors located within the ethmoid and nose with involvement also of the orbit

20.4.2.3 Total Ethmoidomaxillectomy

This approach (Figs. 20.4 to 20.6) allows the surgical corridor to be tremendously enlarged compared to the previous one since it consists of removing the entire ethmoid and maxilla to extend the opening within the orbit, pterygopalatine fossa and anterior skull base, and is particularly indicated for tumors extending in these areas. The nasal bone is disconnected from the maxillonasal suture, for example the nasofrontal suture by

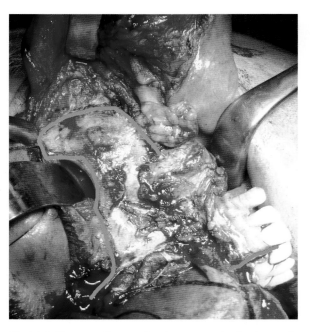

Fig. 20.4 The green lines outline the osteotomies for the maxillectomy

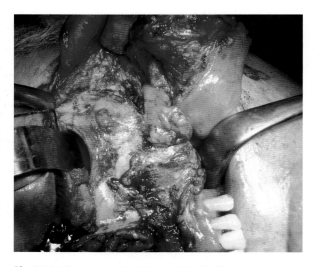

Fig. 20.5 The osteotomies delineated in Fig. 20.4 are being performed. Different osteotomes can be used, together with the ocillating saw, or drills, etc

using a straight osteotome 10 mm in width. An osteotomy is performed at the level of the frontoethmoidal suture 2–3 mm below the ethmoidal arteries, stopping before the optic nerve is encountered. An oscillating saw is generally used. A second osteotomy is

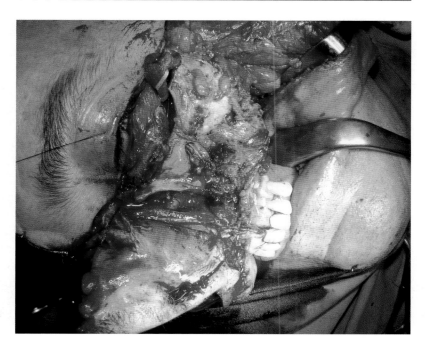

Fig. 20.6 The left maxilla has been freed and is ready to be removed

carried out along the inferior orbital floor, close to the lacrimal bone, extending laterally and inferiorly to disconnect the maxillozygomatic suture. The third osteotomy concerns the hard palate. After separating the soft palate from the posterior border of the hard palate through a transoral approach, a straight osteotome or a Gigli saw can be used. This is inserted in the nasal fossa in the middle of the central incisors, and is passed through the previously performed uranostaphiline incision. The hard palate is then resected on the midline. A fourth osteotomy is performed positioning a curved osteotome between the maxillary tuberosity and the pterygoid plates. This maneuver has to be very gentle in order to avoid fractures to the sphenoid bone and lesions of the dura, which can result in cerebrospinal fluid leakage.

With a strong instrument we start mobilizing the bone, resecting using scissors all soft-tissue connections from the pterygoid muscles and soft palate. Often the venous pterygoid plexus is bleeding at this stage of the approach and bipolar coagulation and/or the use of hemostatic tools is required.

After removal of the ethmoid-maxillary bony complex, the nasopharynx and the central skull base are exposed. Attention has to be paid to protecting the carotid artery and the maxillary artery, which often has to be clamped and ligated.

20.5 Tumor Resection

The surgeon, before performing the approach, has to have the procedure clearly in mind. If the tumor extends within the maxilla and surrounding structures, Curioni's oncological "box" concept is the best choice for the patient. This consists of total removal of the maxilla, ethmoid, orbit, and invaded soft tissues (Fig. 20.7). Of course, the extent of destruction is related to the histology of the lesion. For greater enlargement of the surgical corridor, the posterior part of the nasal septum, the vomer and septal cartilage are removed, which also widely exposes the nasopharynx and the paranasopharyngeal space. The wide exposure achieved after total removal of the maxilla or after the maxilla is swung laterally, allows total removal of tumors such as schwannomas and angiofibromas, and lymph nodes, under direct vision. We consider the use of the endoscope extremely useful; we have used this tool in every procedure and found it necessary for total tumor removal.

20.6 Reconstruction

If the maxilla has been swung laterally and pedunculated as an osteocutaneous flap, it can be repositioned

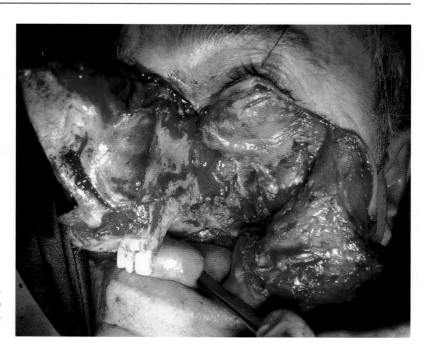

Fig. 20.7 The surgical field after removal of the maxilla together with the tumor, according to Curioni's oncological box concept

and fixed and stabilized using titanium miniplates, as also can the nasal bone. An inferior antrostomy is performed to drain the sinus, and the mucosa of the inferior turbinate can be placed as a free flap within the operative field covering the nasopharynx. Also, after extensive bone removal from the skull base, tissue transplantation is required. We usually transplant the temporal muscle when a total maxillectomy has been carried out in order to fill the enormous residual space. A question-mark skin incision is carried out in the temporal region as described in other chapters of this book. The temporal muscle is then disconnected from its attachment to the temporal fossa, and reflected after channelization of the teguments between its lodge and the zygoma leaving intact the vascular pedicle. The edge of the muscle is then fixed around the half hard palate using holes that have been previously prepared in the bone, to separate the nasal fossa from the oral cavity. The use of the rectus abdomini muscle is also reported in the literature.

When the orbit floor has been removed its reconstruction is mandatory to avoid a blow-out of the bulb, using hard enough materials. We usually use titanium mesh, but also septal cartilage, or ceramic or dural substitutes can be used. The lacrimal sac is identified and a dacryocystorhinostomy with marsupialization is performed, if needed. The medial canthal ligament is identified and

sutured to the periosteum. Synthetic prostheses have recently been introduced and we are convinced that in the near future they will be more extensively used.

20.7 Closure

The wide cavity is filled with a long gauze with Vaseline and antibiotics, the extremity of the gauze being fixed to a suture thread in order to avoid losing it within the nasal cavity. The anterior nasal cavity is packed with Merocel. Drains from the temporal fossa, when the temporal muscle is transplanted, are positioned for a couple of days. The nasal packing is removed after five or six days. The wounds are closed with interrupted sutures in layers. An occlusive bandage on the ipsilateral eye should be left in place.

20.8 Postoperative Care

The surgical wound is dressed daily. The ocular bandage is removed after two days and a medicated cream is used in the conjunctival sac. The nasal packing is partially removed three days later, and totally on the sixth day. The patient should avoid blowing the nose. The suture is removed seven or eight days after surgery.

20.9 Complications

The most likely complication is hemorrhage usually due to bleeding from the maxillary artery. If this occurs, the patient is taken back to the operating room and this artery is ligated. Another possible complication is cerebrospinal fluid leakage. A lumbar drain can be placed for four or five days and, if the leak is not resolved, a reoperation for leak repair should be considered. Bacterial infections are treated by antibiotics, and a bone sequester, should it occur, should be surgically removed. The incidence of infection can be reduced by frequent irrigation and cleansing during the operation. Trismus is avoided by active and passive stretching exercises.

References

1. Arriaga MA, Janecka IP (1989) Surgical exposure of the nasopharynx: anatomic basis for a transfacial approach. Surg Forum 40:547–549
2. Casson PR, Bonnano PC, Converse JM (1974) The midface degloving procedure. Plast Reconstr Surgery 53:102–113
3. Hernández Altemir F (1986) Transfacial access to the retromaxillary area. J Maxillofac Surg 14:165–170
4. James D, Crockard HA (1991) Surgical access to the base of skull and upper cervical spine by extended maxillotomy. Neurosurgery 29:411–416
5. Janecka IP, Sen CN, Sekhar LN, Arriaga MA (1990) Facial translocation: a new approach to the cranial base. Otolaryngol Head Neck Surg 103:413–419
6. Price JC, Holliday MJ, Kennedy DW et al (1988) The versatile midface degloving approach. Laryngoscope 98:291–295

Midfacial Translocation Approach

21

Julio Acero-Sanz and Carlos Navarro-Vila

21.1 Introduction

The skull base is an anatomic region that separates the facial viscerocranium from the neurocranium. Pathological processes affecting this region can arise within the skull base or extend there by direct growth from neighboring territories. Metastases of distant origin can also affect this area. Pathological entities affecting the skull basis may include dysplasia, benign or malignant tumors, congenital deformities or inflammatory processes [1]. Operative treatment of these pathological processes is a challenging issue, since the cranial base and related regions are a complex anatomical area with structures that are critical for life and important functions. As has been discussed in other chapters of this book, during the last two decades advances in anesthesia, imaging techniques, surgical technology and reconstructive procedures including rigid fixation, bone grafting and microvascular techniques, have made possible the surgical treatment of many entities affecting this region. Development of different surgical approaches to the skull base including midfacial translocation has been essential to allow adequate access to this territory.

21.2 Anatomical Basis

The base of the skull can be divided by the internal carotid artery into a central compartment and two lateral

compartments (right and left), which are further subdivided into anterior, middle and posterior segments (Fig. 21.1). The central region contains the anterior cranial fossa, clivus, body of the sphenoid and the upper cervical spine. The central anterior cranial fossa includes the cribiform plate, planum sphenoidale, orbital roof and greater wing of the sphenoid bone. The lateral compartment has an anterior segment which extends from the anterior middle cranial fossa to the anterior

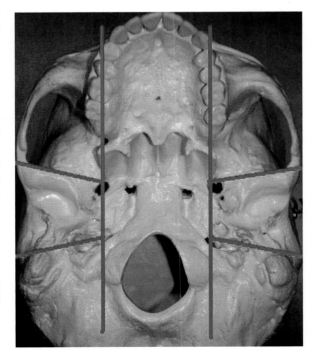

Fig. 21.1 Compartments of the cranial base: central and lateral (anterior, middle and posterior segments)

J. Acero-Sanz (✉)
Complutense University and Dept of Oral and Maxillofacial Surgery, G. Marañon University Hospital, Madrid, Spain

P. Cappabianca et al. (eds.), *Cranial, Craniofacial and Skull Base Surgery.*
© Springer-Verlag Italia 2010

edge of the petrous temporal bone. This segment includes part of the greater wing of the sphenoid bone as well as the inferior surface of the petrous temporal bone, related to the infratemporal and retromaxillary areas [2, 3]. Another classification considers the central skull base as a part of the middle skull base, located in the midline posterior to the anterior fossa corresponding to the region of the brainstem and the pituitary gland.

Intracranial structures related to this region are the ventral surface of the brainstem, basilar artery, intracranial optic nerve, optic chiasm and the medial aspect of the cavernous sinus, lateral to the sphenoid sinus and sella. The most frequent tumors affecting this area are pituitary adenoma, juvenile angiofibroma, chordomas and craniopharyngioma, although many different pathological entities can affect this region. Lesions located anterior to the neuroaxis should be approached through an anterior access whilst the anterior segment of the lateral compartment requires a lateral or a combined anterolateral approach.

21.3 Basic Principles

According to Janecka and Tiedemann [1], there are several principles that are applicable to cranial base surgery, such as a proper sequential logic to the procedure and an adequate exposure while minimizing brain retraction. Surgical access to skull-base lesions aims to allow complete tumor removal if possible and correction of the defect with acceptable morbidity. Defect reconstruction must lead to the best functional and esthetic result including restoration of critical barriers [4]. Management by a multidisciplinary team is essential in order to achieve the goals of treatment.

Following these basic principles, various surgical approaches have been developed to access the different parts of the skull base. Craniofacial approaches combine an intracranial and a transmaxillary or transfacial approach. Techniques such as the frontocranial or subfrontal–subcranial approach, the intraoral transmaxillary approaches or the infratemporal fossa approach have been described in other parts of this book. Endoscopically assisted approaches are also being increasingly used for selected cases [5]. Transfacial swing osteotomies are valuable approaches to the skull base, providing a wide exposure to facilitate tumor resection especially in the anterior and central areas of this region [6]. A midfacial translocation approach is based in the principle of the displacement or disassembling of vas-

cularized midfacial composite units allowing wide access to the cranial basis and deep facial regions and safe reconstruction once the midfacial units are reassembled [1, 4]. This technique was popularized by Curioni [7] and Hernandez-Altemir, who reported in detail the techniques of unilateral and bilateral maxillocheek flap to approach the retromaxillary area (Fig. 21.2) [8], although Krause and Heymann [9] in 1915 referred to its description by Von Langenbeck for the excision of tumors located in the nasopharyngeal area (Fig. 21.3).

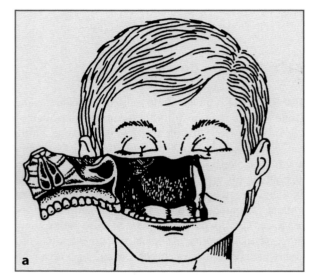

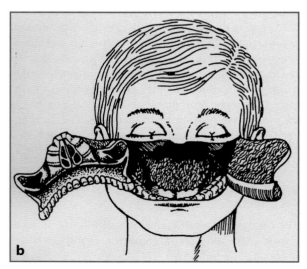

Fig. 21.2 a Unilateral technique as designed by Hernandez-Altemir (courtesy of the author). **b** Bilateral technique. The upper maxilla and the nasal and ethmoidal structures are pedicled to the cheek flap

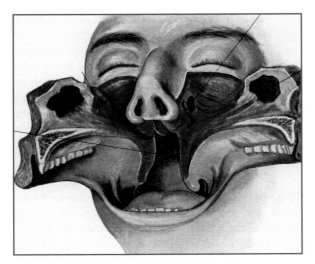

Fig. 21.3 Bilateral maxillocheek flap described by Krause for the excision of tumors located in the nasopharyngeal area (from original drawing published by Krause, 1915 [9])

Janecka and Tiedemann [1] systematized the advantages of the transfacial approaches, which are related to anatomical and embryological features:

1. Separation of the facial units in the midline or paramedian region across the lines of fusion between embryonic facial processes is associated with low morbidity and facilitates extensive approaches to the skull-base regions through the division and reassembly of the facial units. The blood supply to the facial units is ensured by the external carotid artery system, which is in a lateral to medial direction.
2. Use of the facial cavities (oronasal cavity, nasopharynx, paranasal sinuses) as surgical highways through the skull base.
3. The extracranial approaches offer less morbidity and greater tolerance to postoperative surgical swelling than the intracranial techniques.
4. Once the normal anatomy is reestablished through the repositioning of the facial units, reconstruction of facial esthetics, isolation of the neurocranium, and the functional result will be successful in experienced hands.

21.4 Indications

Before a surgical approach to a lesion in the anterior skull base is performed, it is important to carry out careful preoperative planning, including adequate imaging (CT scanning and MRI), angiography in selected cases and, if possible, histological diagnosis. These methods, which are discussed in detail in other chapters, will provide information on the location and extension of the lesion, its anatomical relationships with vital structures such as the carotid and vertebral arteries system, the dura and brain and cranial nerves (V2, V3, XII), and its histological features, leading to the selection of an adequate surgical approach. The selection of the surgical access will be based on the suspected histology, and location and extension of the lesion, including the extent of dural or intradural involvement.

Anterior transfacial approaches are an excellent alternative for extensive tumors affecting the central skull base and related anatomical regions. Any part of the orbit, maxilla or mandible can be mobilized, thus providing excellent exposure which facilitates three-dimensional tumor removal. The midfacial swing osteotomy is used mainly in the treatment of tumors involving the lower two-thirds of the clivus, being more effective in these cases than a maxillotomy. Techniques such as the transnasal, transsphenoidal and transoral approaches have some limitations and are more suitable for the treatment of small tumors [6]. Le Fort I downfracture is a highly cosmetic approach and offers good access to tumors affecting the nasopharynx and central skull base with low morbidity, but it is a poor approach for very extensive lesions or malignant tumors affecting these territories. In these cases, the maxillonasal cheek flap is more versatile, since it provides wide access and can be combined with other approaches such as an intracranial approach if necessary. A partial maxillary resection can be included if indicated. In addition to the treatment of tumors of the skull base, the facial translocation technique can be useful in the treatment of tumors of the paranasal sinuses, nasopharynx, pterigomaxillary and infratemporal fossa and orbit [6, 8]. The orbital swing can be performed in order to approach large orbital tumors lying inferior to the optic nerve and posterior to the globe.

21.5 Surgical Technique

All patients are given a course of broad-spectrum antibiotics in the perioperative period which is continued for 48 to 72 hours postoperatively, or until the spinal drain is removed. Anticonvulsant therapy is added if there is a neurosurgical indication. An active infection in the oronasopharynx area will delay surgery until it is successfully treated.

21.5.1 Patient positioning

Supine on the operating table with the head secured in a headrest, and occasionally with rigid head fixation, is the most common surgical position for this type of approach. An alternative position for a limited midline tumor approached transorally is the right lateral position. Preparation of the oral cavity, face and neck is completed with antiseptic solution and correct draping, also including possible distant donor sites for reconstruction flaps.

21.5.2 Anesthetic Technique

Oral–endotracheal intubation must be the first option for airway management. In some cases we could need to perform a preliminary tracheostomy or a submental endotracheal intubation [10]. Fixing the endotracheal tube to the mandible molars with a wire provides supplementary stability to the anesthetic framework. All patients will have arterial as well as central venous pressure lines. Elective hypotension is not always used. When dural transgression is anticipated a spinal drain may be inserted.

21.5.3 Operative Techniques

As discussed above, the facial translocation approach is based on modular disassembly of the craniofacial structures as units along the principal neurovascular axis and esthetic lines. Different authors have added terms such as "mini", "standard" and "expanded" to the technical variations of the facial translocation approach during recent decades in order to improve communication and comparison between them [1, 11, 12]. Complementary craniotomies or craniectomies are added to these approaches as necessary to assist radical block resections of tumors [13].

21.5.3.1 Mini Facial Translocation (Central)

This approach is used for tumors affecting the medial orbital wall, sphenoid and ethmoid sinus, and inferior clivus. The approach aims to achieve lateral displacement of the ipsilateral nasal bone and ipsilateral nasal process of the maxilla with its attached medial canthal ligament, lacrimal duct and skin. The skin incision passes along the lateral aspect of the nose and the infe-

rior aspect of the eyebrow with a triangular design at the level of the medial canthal ligament. Premolding of the miniplates before undertaking the osteotomies at the glabellar region and nasal process of the maxilla just medial to the infraorbital nerve foramen, allows quick and accurate replacement during the reconstruction phase. Titanium miniplates are usually used, but the use of resorbable plates can also be considered.

21.5.3.2 Minifacial Translocation (Lateral)

This approach is used for tumors located in the infratemporal fossa. The craniofacial anatomy is opened through a skin incision that runs from the inner canthus horizontally to the preauricular area and then vertically in front of the ear. The condyle and coronoid process of the mandible, zygomatic arch and malar eminence are laterally displaced or temporarily removed. Additional steps may include isolation of the intrapetrous carotid artery, dissection of the lateral wall of the orbit and a cavernous sinus approach. Again preplating and repositioning the fixations after reassembling the bone fragments is recommended.

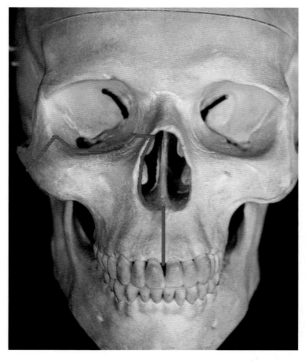

Fig. 21.4 Standard hemifacial translocation. Schema showing the osteotomies

21.5.3.3 Standard Hemifacial Translocation

This approach is illustrated in Figs. 21.4 and 21.5. It is
an excellent approach to the anterolateral regions of the
skull base, especially for lesions that extend from the
nasopharynx to the infratemporal fossa [1, 8]. A temporary tarsorrhaphy is advocated. The skin incision
starts at the lateral canthus and continues by the inferior
fornix of the lower eyelid through the medial canthus.
It can be extended to the preauricular area laterally. The
incision extends inferiorly lateral to the nose and includes an upper lip split. Intraorally, a vertical incision
is made in the vestibular sulcus and a paramedial
palatal incision is made extending to the ipsilateral
retrotuberosity area. While preserving the attachments
of the facial soft tissues to the underlying skeleton, the
osseous structures subjacent to the incision are exposed
including part of the zygoma, the infraorbital rim and

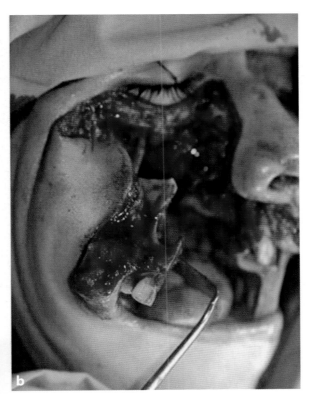

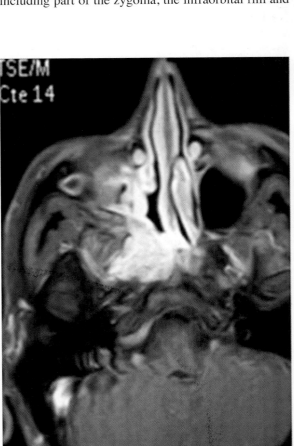

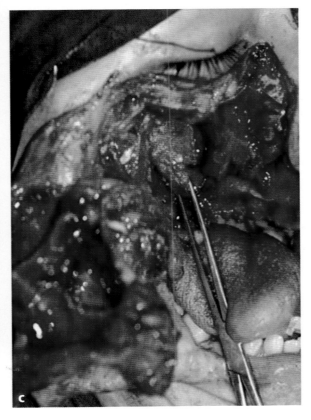

Fig. 21.5 Angiofibroma of the cavum, right side. **a** Axial MR
image. **b** Unilateral facial maxillocheek flap. **c** Wide and safe
exposure of the tumor

the nasomaxillary area, extending inferiorly as far as the alveolar process. Suarez et al. [14] described the replacement of the facial incisions by a midfacial degloving approach to avoid the sequela of facial scarring with the facial translocation procedure.

Once the facial skeleton has been exposed, the osteotomies are designed and the fixation plates are placed and removed ("preplating") before performing the bone cuts. The midfacial skeleton can be mobilized pedicled to the hemifacial soft tissues according to the different levels of the osteotomies (superiorly to the Le Fort I level, or at the levels for the hemi-Le Fort II or Le Fort III including a midpalatal split). The anterior frontal branch of the facial nerve (1.5–2 cm beyond the lateral canthus) can be used as an anatomical reference as a fulcrum to rotate the maxilla and its overlying skin laterally and inferiorly. The infraorbital nerve is electively sectioned along the floor of the orbit [15]. At the end of the procedure the nerve should be repaired. After excision of the lesion, the midfacial unit is replaced and the plates are placed again in order to fix the osseous structures in their previous position.

21.5.3.4 Extended Facial Translocation (Medial)

This approach incorporates the standard translocation unit plus the nose and the medial half of the opposite face (Fig. 21.6). It can be designed superior to the Le Fort I level in order to rotate the nasoethmoidomaxillary skeleton maintaining the alveolar process in its position or including the ipsilateral alveolar process and palate in the mobilized unit. A paranasal incision is placed on the contralateral side in order to expose the ipsilateral infratemporal fossa and central and paracentral skull base bilaterally including the optic nerves and both precavernous internal carotid arteries [16]. Bony fixation using preshaped miniplates again provides exact and stable reconstruction of the facial skeleton and the reestablishment of the occlusal plane if the whole upper maxilla is included in the osteotomy. Lacrimal structures must be maintained with temporary bilateral lacrimal silicone stents.

21.5.3.5 Extended Facial Translocation (Medial and Inferior)

This approach is used for exposure of the upper cervical regions and the parapharyngeal space associated with mandibular splitting. Transmandibular approaches are discussed in the Chapter 22.

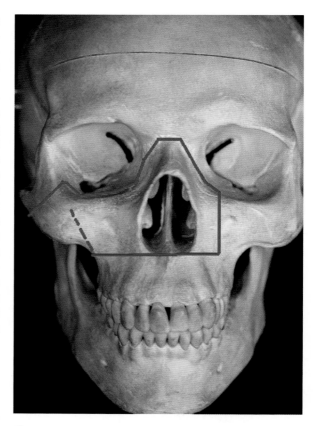

Fig. 21.6 Medial extended facial translocation. Schema showing the osteotomies

21.5.3.6 Extended Facial Translocation (Posterior)

This approach incorporates the ear, temporal bone and posterior fossa in the surgical field by extending the skin incision of the standard translocation posteriorly, just above the external ear. The incision then curves inferiorly over the occipital bone to the neck.

21.5.3.7 Bilateral Facial Translocation

This approach joins the bilateral standard translocation with or without a palatal split. The skin incision is extended bilaterally from the outer canthus to the contralateral outer canthus with a unilateral extension through the paranasal area and the upper lip. Osteotomies are performed bilaterally according to the same principles referred to concerning the standard hemifacial technique (Fig. 21.7). This extremely wide

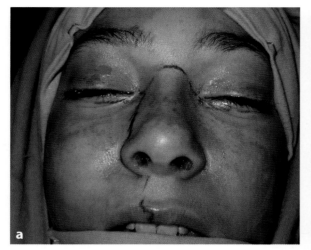

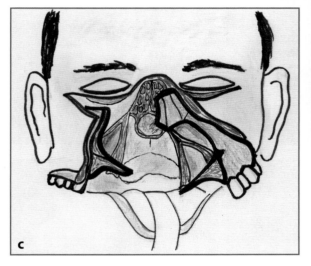

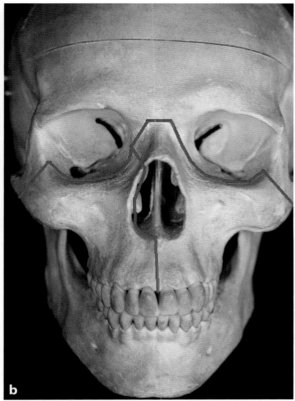

Fig. 21.7 Bilateral facial translocation. **a** Incision lines. The skin incision is extended bilaterally from the outer canthus to the contralateral outer canthus with a unilateral extension through the paranasal area and the upper lip. **b** Schema showing the osteotomies, which are performed bilaterally. **c** Displacement of facial units after osteotomies allowing wide exposure of the surgical field

approach provides access to both the infratemporal fossae and the central and paracentral skull base, the full clivus, and both internal carotid arteries, allowing excision of large lesions located in this area [1, 17] (Fig. 21.8). With the palatal split we can approach C2–C3, and C3–C4 by adding a mandibular split.

In all cases, an intracranial approach can be combined with transfacial access if indicated [1, 18].

21.6 Reconstruction

After resection of a lesion at the skull base, correct reconstruction is essential in order to achieve a good esthetic and functional result and to minimize complica-

tions. The basic principles of reconstruction in this area include:

- Repair of the dura, if necessary.
- Separation of the intradural compartment from the upper aerodigestive tract and obliteration of the dead space.
- Evaluation of bone defects and their repair if indicated.
- Repositioning of the composite vascularized maxillofacial units.

If the dura is damaged or resected, it must be repaired according to general neurosurgical techniques. Locoregional flaps such as the pericranial flap, based on the supraorbital and supratrochlear vessels, are methods of choice to reinforce the repair covering as a bar-

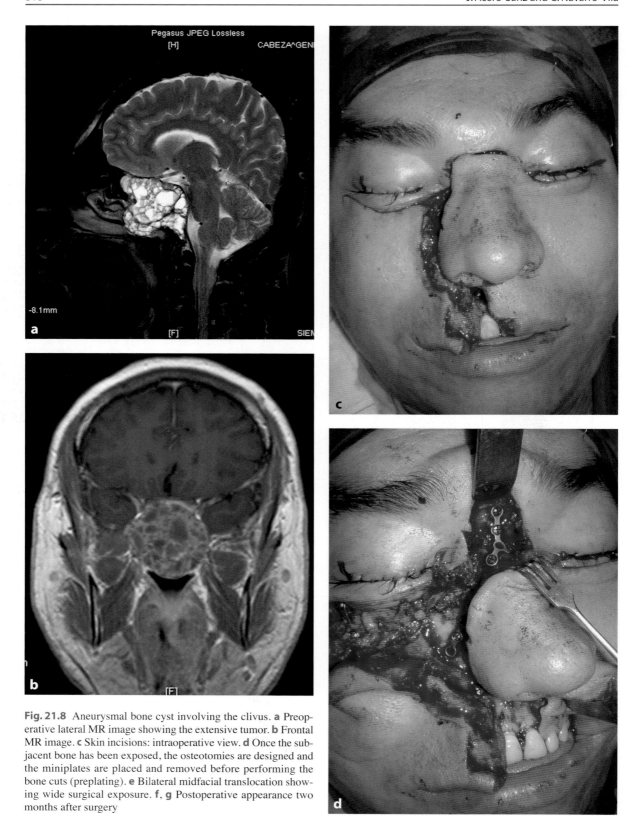

Fig. 21.8 Aneurysmal bone cyst involving the clivus. **a** Preoperative lateral MR image showing the extensive tumor. **b** Frontal MR image. **c** Skin incisions: intraoperative view. **d** Once the subjacent bone has been exposed, the osteotomies are designed and the miniplates are placed and removed before performing the bone cuts (preplating). **e** Bilateral midfacial translocation showing wide surgical exposure. **f, g** Postoperative appearance two months after surgery

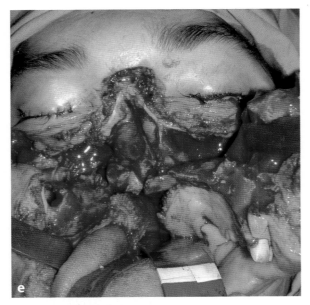

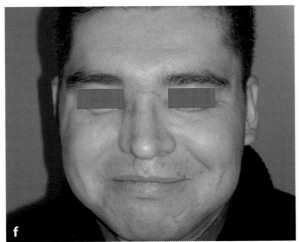

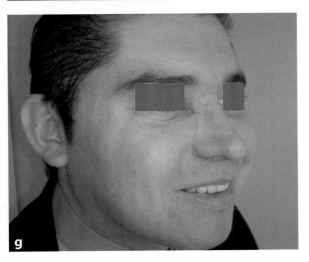

rier the defect in the cranial base. Careful closure of the mucosal layer of the nasopharynx and the palate is also important. If there are bone defects in the skull base, a good dural repair reinforced with a pericranial flap may be enough. For defects causing distortion of facial harmony, such as frontal defects or large orbital defects which can also impair visual function, repair with split calvarial bone grafts and/or titanium mesh can provide support for the globe and an adequate orbital volume. The approach may be varied for the treatment of a malignant tumor if part of the bone that would be translocated in the standard approach needs to be included in the resection. In this situation, the bone is repaired according to the methods referred to [1, 4, 6].

Postsurgical deep space needs to be avoided. If a pericranial or galeal flap is not enough for this purpose, the choice after a large resection is the transfer of a temporalis muscle flap or a microvascular flap to repair the defect. A temporalis muscle pedicled flap is based on the deep temporal arteries. It was described by Golovine for orbital repair after exenteration [19], and is a safe and simple flap that can cover the dura or obliterate the orbit or paranasal sinuses, but it has some disadvantages including a short arc of rotation and limited volume.

Large complex defects after resection associated with midfacial translocation approach can be reconstructed before repositioning of the mobilized structures using a free microvascular flap. A rectus abdominis flap, the latissimus dorsi and the greater omentum can be used to provide a vascularized barrier and restore the volume after large resections. Composite osseocutaneous flaps, such as the scapular flap, can provide a big volume of soft tissue combined with a bone fragment for complex tridimensional reconstructions.

Finally, as mentioned in section 21.5 Surgical Technique, the translocated maxillofacial segments pedicled to the soft tissues are repositioned and fixed three-dimensionally with micro- and miniplates if previously preplated, leading to reestablishment of the previous facial anatomy. Skin incisions are sutured over the repositioned facial skeleton.

21.7 Complications and Disadvantages

As well as advantages, the transfacial approaches also have disadvantages and potential complications. The need for temporary tracheostomy, submental intubation or postoperative endotracheal intubation for supplementary airway management needs to be considered in order to avoid postsurgical complications related to airway obstruction. Contamination of the surgical field due to exposure of the oral and nasopharyngeal cavity and paranasal sinuses may be associated with an increased risk of postoperative infection of the surgical wound and meningitis. Cerebrospinal fluid leakage may be associated with failure of wound closure, and requires adequate treatment. Precise reconstruction according to the basic principles of reconstruction reviewed in this chapter providing adequate separation of the intradural compartment from the airway and eliminating the postsurgical dead space is very important to prevent CSF leakage and infections [1, 6, 20].

The surgical technique in the transfacial approach needs facial incisions which have the potential to develop nonesthetic scars [17], although the incisions are placed in anatomical lines of separation of facial units. Lesions of structures including the teeth, facial bones, mucosal lining of the upper airway, soft and hard palate or tongue, are also associated with the procedure. Oronasal fistula can result after poor scarring of the mucosa of the palate. An adequate technique can prevent this complication. There are also potential risks related to the location of neurovascular structures such as the upper cervical and petrous segments of the internal carotid artery or the cranial nerves [1].

Temporary dysphagia, temporomandibular joint click and transient tongue weakness have been reported following mandibular swing procedures while midfacial swing is frequently associated with epiphora, postoperative diplopia (probably caused by temporary extraocular dysfunction) and facial swelling. Temporary postoperative lower eyelid suspension may prevent the development of ectropion. Complications related to failure of the osteosynthesis such as poor consolidation or misalignment of the bony segments can occur but severe complications are exceptional [6]. Hao et al. have reported a morbidity rate of 31% after resection of tumors of the paranasal sinuses and skull base via the midfacial translocation approach, including one case of blindness. The complication rate is higher in those with malignant tumors [4]. Crust formation is a postoperative complication in some patients, especially after postoperative radiotherapy. Free nonvascularized bone grafts are not recommended in those with previous or planned radiation therapy.

References

1. Janecka IP, Tiedemann K (1997) Skull base surgery: anatomy, biology and technology. Lippincott-Raven, Philadelphia
2. Jackson IT, Hide TA (1982) A systematic approach to tumours of the base of the skull. J Maxillofac Surg 10:92–98
3. Spencer KR, Nastri AL, Wiesenfeld D (2003) Selected midfacial access procedures to the skull base. J Clin Neurosci 10:340–345
4. Hao S, Pan WL, Chang CN, Hsu YS (2003) The use of the facial translocation technique in the management of tumors of the paranasal sinuses and skull base. Otolaryngol Head Neck Surg 128:571–575
5. Kaplan MJ, Fischbein NJ, Harsh GR (2005) Anterior skull base surgery. Otolaryngol Clin North Am 38:107–131
6. Moreira-Gonzalez A, Pieper DR, Balaguer-Cambra J et al (2005) Skull base tumors: a comprehensive review of transfacial swing osteotomy approaches. Plast Reconstr Surg 115:711–720
7. Clauser L, Vinci R, Curioni C (2000) Dismantling and reassembling of the facial skeleton in tumor surgery of the craniomaxillofacial area. History, surgical anatomy, and notes of surgical technique: Part 1. J Craniofac Surg 11:318–325
8. Hernandez-Altemir F (1986) Transfacial access to the retromaxillary area. J Maxillofac Surg 14:165–170
9. Krause F, Heymann E (1915) Tratado de las Operaciones Quirurgicas. Editorial Calleja, Madrid
10. Hernandez-Altemir F (1986) The submental route for endotracheal intubation. J Maxillofac Surg 14:64–65
11. Janecka I (1995) Classification of facial translocation approach to the skull base. Otolaryngol Head Neck Surg 112:579–585
12. Salyer KE, Bardach J (2004) Atlas de Cirugia Craneofacial y de Hendiduras, Vol I. Lippincott-Raven, Philadelphia. Edicion Español: Actualidades Medico Odontologicas Latinoamerica CA, Caracas
13. Torrens M, Al-Mefty O, Kobayashi S (1997) Operative skull base surgery. Churchill Livingstone, London
14. Suarez C, Llorente J, Munoz C, García L (2004) Facial translocation approach in the management of central skull base and infratemporal tumors. Laryngoscope 114:1047–1051
15. Ducic Y (2000) Preservation of the integrity of the infraorbital nerve in facial translocation. Laryngoscope 110:1415–1417
16. Movassaghi K, Janecka I (2005) Optic nerve decompression via midfacial translocation approach. Ann Plast Surg 54:331–335
17. Forar B, Derowe A, Cohen J et al (2001) Surgical approaches to juvenile nasopharyngeal angiofibroma. Oper Techn Otolaryngol Head Neck Surg 12:214–218
18. Martinez-Lage JL, Acero-Sanz J, Alvarez I, Carrillo R (1986) Fibroma osificante gigante. Abordaje combinado transcraneano y transfacial. Rev Iberoamericana Cirugia Oral Maxillofacial 8:61–68
19. Cuesta-Gil M, Concejo C, Acero J et al (2004) Repair of large orbito-cutaneous defects by combining two classical flaps. J Craniomaxillofac Surg 32:21–27
20. Gluckman JL, Gapany M (1995) Complications of surgery for neoplasms of the oral cavity, pharynx and cervical esophagus. In: Weissler MC, Pillsbury HC (eds) Complications of head and neck surgery. Thieme, New York

Transmandibular Approaches

22

Valentino Valentini, Andrea Cassoni, Andrea Battisti,
Paolo Gennaro and Giorgio Iannetti

22.1 Introduction

Lesions involving the middle cranial base, its underlying volumes, and the first cervical vertebrae can be adequately managed surgically by means of a series of different approaches. These have the following basic prerequisites: to supply adequate surgical light, to identify and preserve the neurovascular structures adjacent to the lesion, to restore an adequate barrier between the neurocranium and the upper aerodigestive tracts, and to preserve both the functionality and the appearance of the patient.

The approaches comprise a heterogeneous set of surgical techniques. No clear classification has yet been established. As a consequence, the terminology used to describe them is often confusing.

Despite this complexity, there are basically four ways by which the lesions (of the lateral sectors of the infratemporal fossa and/or the middle cranial base) can be resected: transtemporal, infratemporal, intracranial, and transfacial. These approaches, depending on the size and location of the lesion, may be used jointly resulting in so-called combined approaches.

Transmandibular approaches, the main topic of this chapter, tend to merge substantially with each of the four above approaches, although transmandibular means literally an approach involving exposure of the lesion by more or less substantial mobilization of the mandible portions, and consequently a transfacial approach.

However, in surgery, when the middle cranial base is entered laterally, it is impossible to obtain complete exposure only by mobilizing the mandible. Therefore, it is necessary to osteotomize and remove other bone structures such as, for example, the zygomatic arch and/or the temporal squama. Therefore, in the literature, approaches that should be indicated as transmandibular, are identified by their authors with the most varied names, sometimes creating confusion.

As mentioned above, transmandibular approaches can be classified as single approaches (when the approach obtained by mobilizing the mandible is exclusively transfacial) or as combined approaches (if the lesion is approached by combining mobilization of the mandible with that of other bone structures such as the zygoma or the temporal squama).

In addition, approaches can also be categorized as anterior or lateral, depending on whether the initial incision is carried out anteriorly in the mental region or submandibular region or laterally in the preauricular region and extended below along the anterior margin of the sternocleidomastoid muscle.

22.2 History

The first description of a mandibular osteotomy dating back to 1836 is that of Roux [1] who performed a median osteotomy to approach intraoral tumors with large dimensions and excessively rear positions, therefore requiring an unfavorable transoral approach. Subsequently, in 1844, Sedillot [2] described a modification of the latter approach substituting Roux's vertical osteotomy with an angular osteotomy which allowed the

G. Iannetti (✉)
Division of Maxillofacial Surgery
"Sapienza" University of Rome, Italy

bone stumps to draw nearer in a better way. As for the mandible, these first approaches were characterized by preservation. Indeed, at the end of the operation, the integrity was always preserved by means of gold plates fixed with sutures.

However, in 1861, Billroth stated that radical surgery might be obtained only and exclusively by surgically removing both the lesion and the nearby mandible portion. From that moment on, partial mandibulectomy became a genuine dogma casting a shadow on the mandibulotomic techniques based on mandible preservation.

In an article published in 1956, Conley [3] described demolishing techniques. This article is significant for lateral transmandibular surgery and describes a hemimandibulectomy carried out to remove lesions in the pterygoid area and infratemporal fossa. This highly demolishing approach remained unchanged for more than a century, until 1971 when Marchetta et al. reported the superfluousness of mandibulectomy if the lesion had not encroached upon the periosteum or invaded bones directly.

Mandibulotomic techniques developed in a new direction. The first significant development occurred at the beginning of the 1980s. These developments were based on mandibular preservation. Thus, in 1981, Spiro et al. reported their work on "mandibular swing" [4] which represents an ideal continuation of the approach described by Roux in the early 19th century. Many other authors besides Spiro et al. have contributed to developing anterior transmandibular approaches. Among these authors there were leading figures including Jackson and Hide [5, 6] McGregor and MacDonald [7], Biller et al. [8] and DeMonte et al. [9].

On the other hand, there were many other authors who contributed to lateral transmandibular surgery proposing less aggressive techniques than the one described by Conley.

Among these, Obwegeser [10] was the first to suggest a series of lateral mandibular osteotomies to ease the approach to the infratemporal fossa. He was followed by Pogrel and Kaplan [11] who described an approach based on a horizontal step osteotomy performed right above the lingula to preserve the lower alveolar nerve.

Another approach is that described by Attia et al. [12] who combined a horizontal osteotomy above the lingula with a parasymphyseal osteotomy with an upper reflection of the mandibular segment included between the osteotomies and an incision of the oral mucosa along the alveololingual sulcus.

22.3 Surgical Techniques

22.3.1 Anterior Approaches

22.3.1.1 Mandibular Swing

This approach is recommended to reach lesions occupying the parapharyngeal space, pterygomandibular space, and infratemporal fossa, but only lesions that are medial to the internal carotid artery and do not extend beyond the floor of the middle cranial fossa, and also when there is involvement of all extra- and intracranial structures of the cranial base lying along the midline of the latter. This approach is not recommended when the mandible is involved.

It is important to consider how this approach can ensure a simultaneous neck dissection, if necessary. First the lower lip is incised along the midline and and the incision is extended down below to encircle the chin (Fig. 22.1). Then, continuing on the neck, in the submandibular region, the incision is continued horizontally to the level of the mandibular angle. Then a second incision is performed, this time endo-orally, along the gingival fornix starting from the lower labial frenulum to the homolateral mandibular angle. In the midpoint of the exposed mandible, the periosteum is incised verti-

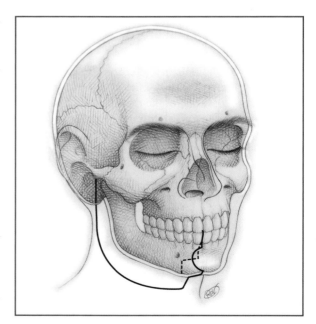

Fig. 22.1 Anterior single transmandibular approach; skin incision with lip-splitting, and mandibulotomy

cally and lifted to expose 2 cm of bone. The mental nerve is identified and preserved. Deep submandibular dissection is then performed through the platysma muscle in order to stage a superior base myocutaneous flap. Dissection is continued below the platysma and the superficial layer of the deep cervical fascia. The marginal branch of the facial nerve is identified and preserved. At this point, the submandibular space is at the level of the submandibular gland and mylohyoid muscle. Before continuing with the mandibular osteotomy, plates are molded and holes are made for screws (preplating) in order to achieve the best repositioning of the bone stumps at the end of the procedure.

Then, with a small saw a median osteotomy is carried out, passing through the two front incisors, or alternatively the medial incisor must be extracted and the osteotomy carried out through the alveolus of the extracted tooth. It is also possible to perform a paramedian osteotomy between the lateral incisor and the canine tooth. While the mandible is retracted laterally, an incision is performed along the lateral buccal pelvis to the retromolar region. This region is linked to the submandibular dissection to ease the lateral displacement of the mandible. In order to close at the end of the procedure, it is important to leave on the mandible lingual face an adequate mucosa cuff and mylohyoid muscle. To further improve the lateral movement of the mandible and enhance surgical light, the lingual nerve can be dissected. In some cases when the approach is not perfectly adequate, the lingual nerve can be sectioned so that it can be reanastomosed at the end of the procedure. The approach to the parapharyngeal space, infratemporal fossa and cranial base is obtained by sectioning the medial pterygoid muscle and the sphenomandibular ligament. The styloid process is identified and the insertions of the stylohyoid, stylopharyngeal and styloglossus muscles are disinserted.

For tumors extending towards the midline of the cranial base, it is possible to widen the operating field by performing an intraoral incision along the palate and pterygoid laminae about 1 cm medial to the gingival margin. A hemipalatal flap can then be lifted sacrificing the major palatine artery and the nerves on the side of the dissection. Once the level of the parapharyngeal space is reached by blunt dissection, it is necessary to create a surgical space behind the middle and upper constrictor muscles and above the hypoglossal nerve. The dissection must be extended between the paravertebral fascia and the constrictor muscle in order to emphasize the styloglossus and stylopharyngeal muscles together with the glossopharyngeal nerve. Following incising

these structures, retraction towards the opposite side of the oropharynx will provide a wider dissection plan.

To detach the rhinopharynx from the cranial base without damaging the mucosa and muscles, the eustachian tube and both palatine muscles must be interrupted. Once the cranial base is detached, the rhinopharynx too must be moved contralaterally in order to expose the upper cervical spine, the clivus, and the central portion of the cranial base.

Several reports of the use of the mandibular swing approach can be recommended [8, 9, 13, 14].

22.3.1.2 Transmandibular Approach Without Lip-Splitting

This technique [15] was introduced in order to carry out a neck dissection en bloc with tumor removal. It is based on two skin incisions, a vertical one extending from the mastoid to the clavicle, and a horizontal one in the submandibular region perpendicular to the first (Fig. 22.2a). For bilateral neck dissection, the same incisions are performed bilaterally. Once the mandibular region is reached, it is possible to isolate and preserve the marginal branch of the facial nerve, either by directly visualizing it or by previously finding, ligating and overturning the facial vessels at the level of the submandibular lodge. The periosteum of the external face of the mandible is incised and detached from the bone, but only when the periosteum is not contaminated by the tumor. In edentulous patients a transoral incision is placed along the mucosa of the alveolar arch or, in those with dental elements still present, along the gingival fornix. If the tumor has spread laterally to involve the cheek mucosa, the incision is placed with an appropriate safety margin. In this way, a tunnel is created below the healthy tissue.

If the masseter muscle is not contaminated by the neoplasia, it can be preserved and detached from the ascending branch of the mandible reaching the sigmoid incisure or further (only if the condyle must be resected as well). The cheek soft tissues, the masseter muscle, and the parotid gland, reflected at the top and laterally, determine a perfect exposure of the hemimandible. Mandibular osteotomies are carried out in the desired position. Usually, one osteotomy is carried out at the level of the mental foramen, and the other is performed just below the sigmoid incisure (Fig. 22.2b). These osteotomies, combined with the osteotomy of the pterygoid lamina, allow the infratemporal fossa to be managed easily.

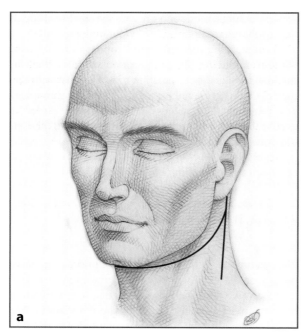

avoiding the vasculonervous bundle which, at this level, enters the hemimandible. Then, the latter is split. The osteotomy (Fig. 22.3) is performed with a drill or a reciprocating saw and the procedure is concluded with thin osteotomes starting from the medial cortex above the lingula along the anterior margin of the branch lateral to the second or third molar and reaching the lateral cortex. The same procedure is carried out contralaterally. The mandible is thus diverted to the bottom. At the end of the procedure, bone segments must be brought close and fixed with moldable titanium plates or with transcortical screws.

In order to make sure that the mandibular condyles are repositioned in their original place, preplating is possible. This is done if plates are used for fixing the mandible or for condylar reference when transcortical screws are used. This technique, modified from orthognathic surgery, provides good exposure of the cranovertebral joint beginning with exposure of C1, C2,

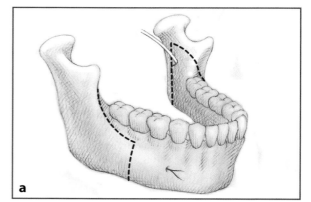

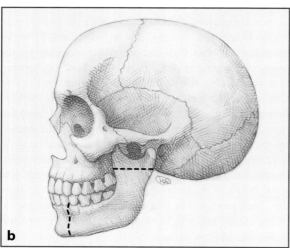

Fig. 22.2 Anterior transmandibular approach without lip-splitting. **a** Skin incision. **b** Parasymphyseal and horizontal mandibulotomies, below the sigmoid incisure

22.3.1.3 Bisagittal Transmandibular Approach

This approach has been reviewed by Vishteh et al. [16].

The mucosa is incised at the level of the retromolar trigone along the external oblique line of the right mandible. By detaching the subperiosteum, the mandibular branch and body can be exposed and the retractors positioned. The lingula is identified medially

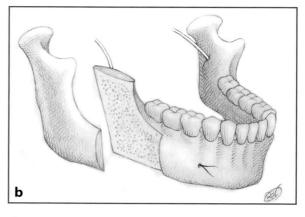

Fig. 22.3 Bilateral sagittal split osteotomy. **a** Dashed lines mark the mandibular osteotomies. **b** The mandible is spletted preserving V3

and the C2–C3 intervertebral disc, and in some cases, also most of the body of C3. The advantage of this technique is that it is less invasive than mandibular swing and it leaves no visible scars since the incisions are endooral. The only drawback is the possibility of damaging the lower alveolar nerve or the lingual nerve.

22.3.2 Lateral approaches

22.3.2.1 Transmandibular Approach According to Conley

The approach described by Conley in 1956 [3] involves a vertical skin incision from the labial commissure to the submandibular region continued horizontally to the homolateral mandibular angle. At this level, the incision is linked with a second incision, a preauricular pretragal and hemicoronal homolateral incision (Fig. 22.4).

Thus, two skin flaps are prepared: an upper flap enabling exposure of the temporal bone, the zygoma, and the parotid gland (the latter is isolated preserving the facial nerve in its context), and a lower flap enabling adequate exposure of the mandible, upper hyoid space, and oropharynx (Fig. 22.4b). Subsequently, the zygomatic

arch is osteotomized, and thus removed (Fig. 22.4c). Next, the temporal squama of the temporal muscle is disinserted, this time keeping its insertion at the level of the coronoid and allowing it to be overturned below. Then, the mandibular body is osteotomized and the condylar head of the glenoid cavity disinserted. At this point, complete exposure of the structures present in the upper hyoid space, the oral pelvis, the pharynx, the infratemporal fossa and the middle cranial base has been obtained.

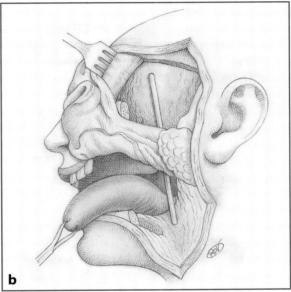

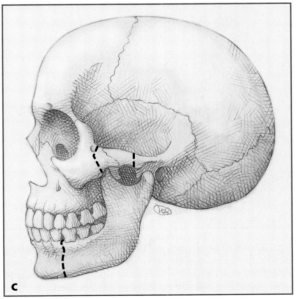

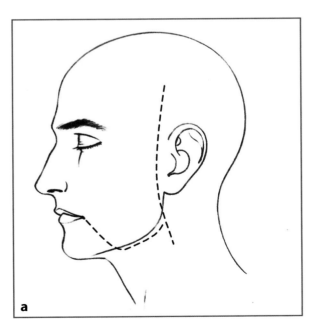

Fig. 22.4 Conley's lateral transmandibular approach. **a** Skin incision. **b** Intraoperative view; note preservation of the parotid gland. **c** Parasymphyseal and zygomatic arch osteotomies

22.3.2.2 Transmandibular Approach According to Obwegeser

This approach was originally described by Obwegeser in 1985 [10]. It consists of a pretragal preauricular incision extended posterosuperiorly following the curvature of the helix for about 2.5 cm. From this point, it is continued upward, posterior to the hairline. It is continued parallel stopping just above the external angle of the homolateral orbit (Fig. 22.5a). A skin flap is prepared allowing the temporal muscle to be exposed. At this point, the orbital margin and zygoma become visible within the operating field. Therefore, in order to expose the upper half of the mandible branch, the zygomatic arch and bone are osteotomized (Fig. 22.5b, c). These are then downturned, keeping them pedicled to the masseter muscle. In order to obtain the largest oral opening, a bite block is first placed. The coronoid process is then mobilized and rotated upwards, since it is connected to the temporal muscle.

The next step is ligation of the internal maxillary artery as well as the section of the pterygoid muscles. Except for the maxillary nerve (V2) and the main branches of the mandibular nerve, there are now no important structures between the eye of the operator and the tuberosity of the maxillary. If a malignant tumor has been found preoperatively to extend backward to the internal carotid, instead of removing just the coronoid, the mandibular branch can be mobilized by means of an osteotomy performed horizontally above the spine of Spix. Subsequently, the branch on the temporal bone is overturned after disarticulating the condylar head. When the third branch of the trigeminal cannot be preserved, an

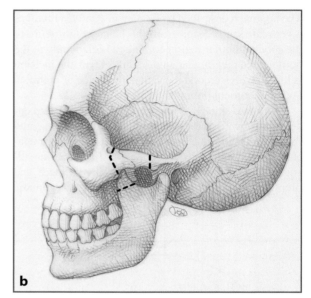

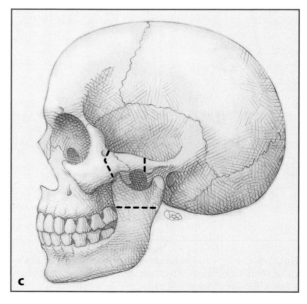

Fig. 22.5 Obwegeser's lateral transmandibular approach. **a** Skin incision. **b** Zygomatic arch and subcoronoid osteotomies. **c** Variation for a wider exposure: horizontal subsigmoidal instead of subcoronoid osteotomy; the condyle is disarticulated

oblique osteotomy can be performed at the level of the mandibular angle, sectioning V3 shortly after it enters the mandibular canal, thereby mobilizing a greater portion of the mandible to the advantage of a brighter surgical field. Moreover, manipulating the temporomandibular joint can be avoided by simply making an additional incision above the condylar head. This way, the mandible branch can be mobilized respecting the joint.

If only the condyle is mobilized but the approach gained is inadequate, the mandible branch can be removed with or without the condyle and kept in Ringer's solution. The mandible branch is then repositioned at the end of the procedure following the above instructions. At this stage of the dissection, the middle cranial base can be entered.

22.3.2.3 Transmandibular Approach with Double Mandibular Osteotomy and Additional Coronoidectomy

This approach is discussed by Lazaridis and Antoniades [17, 18].

The skin incision envisaged for this type of approach is extended from the helix root, along the preauricular fold, and protracted below encircling the ear lobe up to above the apex of the mastoid. Then, it is bent down and forward along the neck in the submandibular region as far as the mental symphysis. The skin flap is prepared, and then mobilized by rotating it anteriorly, thereby exposing the parotid gland, the sternocleidomastoid muscle, the great auricular nerve, and the cartilage of the external auditory canal. The great auricular nerve and the external jugular vein are then isolated and preserved so that the lower pole of the parotid gland is freed, and the posterior belly of the digastric muscle is exposed near its insertion to the mastoid. The fascia between the parotid gland and the cartilaginous portion of the external auditory canal is dissected and the parotid lobe is moved anteriorly to emphasize the cartilaginous pointer. Thereby the main trunk of the facial nerve is identified and demarcated by standard methods, thus improving its control during the procedure.

The submandibular skin flap is then prepared and rotated below towards the hyoid bone and above towards the mental symphysis. The plane below the platysma muscle must be followed and the marginal mandibular nerve of the facial nerve preserved.

At this point, mandibular osteotomies are carried out. The first is performed at the symphysis level anterior to the mental foramen between the canine and the first premolar to preserve the lower alveolar nerve. The second is carried out from the mandibular angle to the sigmoid incisure, after disinserting the masseter muscle. This submasseter dissection avoids damage to the facial nerve branches.

The next osteotomy is carried out at the base of the condyle to preserve the sensitivity of the mandible and lower lip. Finally, a coronoidectomy is performed to improve mandible mobility. The osteotomized mandibular segment can now be freed from the periosteum on the lingual side and rotated superiorly, thus paving the way for the approach to the deep parotid lobe, the eustachian tube, and the cranial base.

After removing the lesion, the mandible is repositioned and fixed using titanium plates, thus restoring the patient's regular occlusion. A draine is then placed and suturing is carried out by planes.

In another version of this technique, a vertical subsigmoid osteotomy is performed instead of the condylectomy.

22.3.2.4 Transmandibular Approach with Twofold Vertical Branch and Parasymphyseal Osteotomy

This approach is discussed by Lazaridis and Antoniades [18] and Smith et al. [19].

The patient is supine with the neck extended and head rotated towards the contralateral side. The incision is place along the cutaneous folds of the neck from the mastoid process to the chin. After separating the subcutis, a skin flap is lifted to the subplatysmatic subfacial plane, identifying and preserving the marginal nerve. Once the carotid fascia is exposed, the internal jugular vein, the internal and external carotid arteries, and the hypoglossal, accessory and vagus nerves are identified and preserved. The periosteum is incised on the lower margin of the mandible. The mandibular branch is approached through dissection of the masseter muscle from its insertion at the mandibular angle to the sigmoid incisure, thereby avoiding damage to the facial nerve.

The antilingular prominence on the lateral surface of the mandible, which is considered to indicate the position of the lingual nerve where the lower alveolar nerve penetrates the mandibular canal, is identified. The vertical subsigmoid osteotomy is delineated to lie posterior to the lingula in order to preserve the sensitivity of the mandible and lip (Fig. 22.6). The position

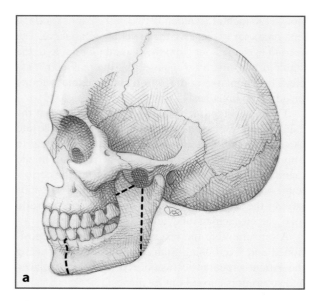

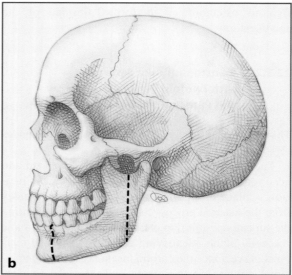

Fig. 22.6 a Smith's approach: vertical ramus and parasymphyseal osteotomies. **b** Lazaridis' modified Smith's approach: double mandibular osteotomy, vertical ramus and parasymphyseal, is combined with a subcoronoid osteotomy to improve mandibular mobility

of the mental nerve is traced by accurately dissecting the periosteum at the level of its exit from the mental foramen. Consequently, a second osteotomy is demarcated anterior to the mental foramen, between the canine and the first molar. Before concluding the osteotomy, the titanium plates should be molded (preplating) in order to restore the patient's physiolog-

ical occlusion. Once the osteotomy sites have been marked on the bone, the osteotomies are started using an oscillating saw or a thin bone cutter. The resulting mandibular segment is moved above and behind, where the bone part connected to the condyle is shifted posteriorly by levering up on the temporomandibular joint. Once the lesion has been removed, the mandibular segments are brought back together and fixed with the previously molded titanium plates.

22.3.3 Combined Approaches

22.3.3.1 Lateral Combined Transmandibular Approach

This approach, described by Sekhar et al. in 1987 [20], begins with a hemicoronal homolateral incision at the lesion. The incision is extended to the preauricular and pretragal region and extended inferiorly on the neck along the anterior margin of the sternocleidomastoid muscle (Fig. 22.7a). This is one of the author's favorite approaches. It can be performed using various approaches: single, lateral transfacial, or combined anterolateral transfacial, when dealing with a large number of lesions not involving, or worse, not encroaching on the middle cranial base but massively occupying the infratemporal fossa.

The transcranial–facial combined approach in most cases enables the removal en bloc of intra- and extracranial neoplastic lesions that are widely spread. This approach also allows the internal carotid artery to be mobilized, and, if necessary, substituted. A cervicofacial skin flap is separated from the temporal fascia, the fatty tissue, and the deep fascia of the neck. It is then rotated forward. The main trunk of the facial nerve and its major branches are then identified starting from the stylomastoid foramen to the parotid gland. These nerves are preserved leaving as much tissue as possible around them. To avoid traction on the facial nerve, when the mandible is dislocated, it is necessary to separate the parotid gland from the underlying masseter fascia, where the nerve passes.

At this point, once the facial nerve is safe, the zygomatic arch is osteotomized anteriorly and posteriorly, so it can be temporarily removed (Fig. 22.7b). Then the temporal muscle and fascia are mobilized and the insertion at the level of the temporal crest incised so that they can be lifted from the temporal fossa. In some cases that involve the orbit, the upper and lateral orbit walls may also be osteotomized and temporarily removed to approach the orbit. The mandibular condyle and the temporomandibular joint capsule are then dislocated anteroinferiorly, after disconnecting the insertions of the stylomandibular and sphenomandibular tendons from the mandible. To gain more space, or if reconstruction with a free muscle flap is planned, the mandibular condyle may also be removed (Fig. 22.7b). Condylar dislocation or removal is essential to have complete control of the infratemporal fossa and the anatomical structures present in it, including the lower portion of the middle cranial base. Having done that, the neck is dissected to expose the internal carotid artery, the internal jugular vein, and cranial nerves X, XI, and XII.

The next surgical step consists of preparing a small frontotemporal bone flap. Two osteotomies are performed with an oscillating saw. The first is medial to and the other posterior to the glenoid fossa. The entire bone flap is removed together with the root of the zygomatic arch and the glenoid fossa. Then the dura of the middle cranial fossa is separated from the bone in order to expose the arcuate eminence, the middle meningeal artery, V3, and the major superficial petrous nerve. The meningeal artery must be coagulated and sectioned, whereas the major superficial petrous nerve is dissected to avoid traction on the geniculate ganglion. The great wing of the sphenoid is removed, and the oval foramen emphasized laterally and anteriorly, the round foramen medially, and the upper orbital fissure inferiorly.

The second branch of the trigeminal will now be easily visible in the pterygopalatine fossa, and V3 will be exposed from its original point to its branching into the infratemporal fossa. The upper orbital fissure and the optic nerve canal can be decompressed by removing the orbital plate from the frontal and the small wing of the sphenoid bone. At the level of the middle cranial base floor, the bone portion medial to the glenoid fossa must be removed. The bone component of the eustachian tube and the tensor muscles of the tympanum are then exposed and sectioned. In this phase, great care must be taken not to damage the internal carotid artery.

The genu of the intrabone portion of the internal carotid artery lies medial to the eustachian tube, covered by a thin layer of bone. Here exposure of the artery is started following its passage below and above. Care must be taken when removing the posterosuperior bone portion at the genu of the internal carotid artery since this is where the cochlea and the geniculate ganglion of the facial nerve are located. Furthermore, particular accuracy is needed when mobilizing the carotid canal

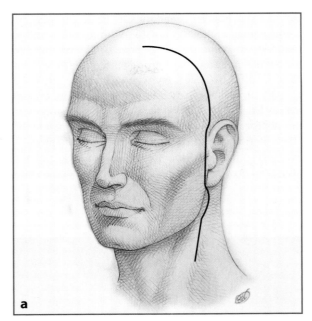

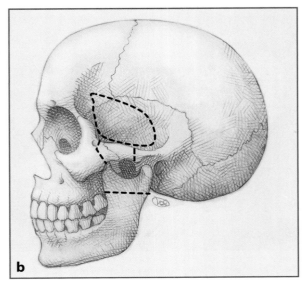

Fig. 22.7 Approach of Sekhar et al. **a** Coronal incision extended to the neck. **b** Osteotomy lines: the frontotemporal osteotomy is optional for middle skull base removal

artery to avoid damage to V3, which can be removed if it is infiltrated.

The mobilized artery must be moved forwards to protect it from possible damage. By removing the petrous bone medial to the carotid canal, as well as the apex region posterosuperiorly to the horizontal segment of the petrosal tract of the internal carotid, the petro-cervical synchondrosis and the clivus are exposed. As a consequence, they are visible within the operating field. At this point, the clivus bone can be removed to expose the dura from the petrosal apex of the great foramen. Caution is necessary when removing the bone near the occipital condyle to avoid damaging cranial nerves IX, X, XI, XII and the jugular bulb. Moreover, this approach allows removal of the superior part of the atlas anterior arch and the apex of the odontoid process. With the removal of the sphenoid at the base of the pterygoid process and medial to V2, the sphenoid sinus

can be exposed. The sphenoid lateral wall can be completely removed with this approach. However, in order to ensure optimal exposure, V2 may be sectioned and then reanastomosed at the end of the procedure.

This approach can be performed either sacrificing or preserving the parotid gland. For the latter, the facial nerve branches are identified and dissected so there is a better view of the infratemporal fossa, even at the expense of greater stress on the facial nerve.

Figure 22.8 shows surgical planning and intraoperative photographs of this approach.

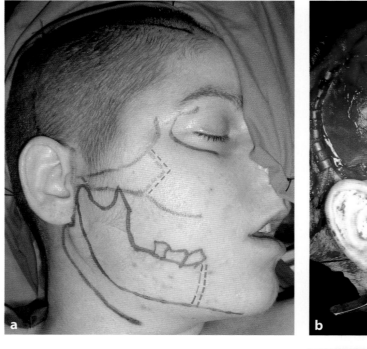

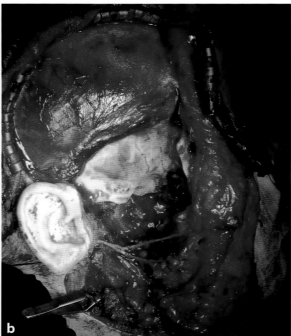

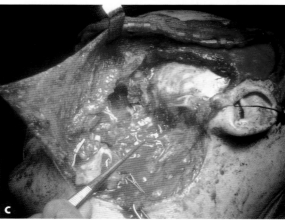

Fig. 22.8 a Surgical plan for the approach of Sekhar et al.; zygomatic and mandibular osteotomies are marked in green. **b** Intraoperative view: the parotid gland was sacrificed but the facial nerve was preserved; after soft tissue dissection and bone removal the middle skull base is widely exposed. **c** Under-view of the middle skull base

22.3.4 *Mandibular Subluxation*

Mandibular subluxation can be mono- or bilateral, depending on whether just the temporomandibular joint homolateral to the lesion is subluxed or both joints are subluxed. To maintain the mandible in its position, it might be useful to previously place an orthodontic arch. If such an arch is not available, the subluxed mandible can be stabilized by fixing it to the lower dental elements, or in edentulous patients by means of mandibular wiring suspending it to the anterior nasal spine. In the first case, on the lesional side, a metal wire is fastened by means of a steel ring to the first or second lower premolar. A second wire is similarly fastened on the opposite side to the first or second contralateral premolar. In edentulous patients or those suffering from paradontopathy, a metal wire is positioned on the lesional side around the mandibular body. Then the second wire is fastened to the lower nasal spine.

If the mandible is subluxed, 10 to 20 minutes are needed to obtain complete subluxation. The metal wires placed are interwoven to gain stabilization. In patients with an orthodontic arch, stabilization is obtained by means of elastic or steel wires fixed to the upper arch.

References

1. Butlin HT (1985) Diseases of the tongue. Clinical manuals for practitioners and students of medicine. Cassell, London, p 331
2. Sedillot A (1844) Paper presented to Academie des Sciences, 1844. Gaz d'Hopital, vol 17, p 83
3. Conley JJ (1956) The surgical approach to the pterygoid area. Ann Surg 144:39–43
4. Spiro RH, Gerold FP, Strong EW (1981) Mandibular "swing" approach for oral and oropharyngeal tumors. Head Neck Surg 3:371–378
5. Jackson IT, Hide TA (1982) A systematic approach to tumours of the base of the skull. J Maxillofac Surg 10:92–98
6. Jackson IT (1985) Craniofacial approach to tumors of the head and neck. Clin Plast Surg 12:375–388
7. McGregor IA, MacDonald DG (1983) Mandibular osteotomy in the surgical approach to the oral cavity. Head Neck Surg 5:457–462
8. Biller HF, Shuger JM, Krepsi YP (1981) A new technique for wide-field exposure of the base of the skull. Arch Otolaryngol 107:698–702
9. DeMonte F, Diaz E Jr, Callender D, Suk I (2001) Transmandibular, circumglossal, retropharyngeal approach for chordomas of the clivus and upper cervical spine. Technical note. Neurosurg Focus 10:E10
10. Obwegeser HL (1985) Temporal approach to the TMJ, the orbit and the retromaxillary-infracranial region. Head Neck Surg 7:185–199
11. Pogrel MA, Kaplan MJ (1986) Surgical approach to the pterygomaxillary region. J Oral Maxillofac Surg 44:183–187
12. Attia EL, Bentley KC, Head T, Mulder D (1984) A new external approach to the pterygomaxillary fossa and parapharyngeal space. Head Neck Surg 6:884–891
13. Krespi YP, Sisson GA (1984) Transmandibular exposure of the skull base. Am J Surg 148:534–538
14. Moreira-Gonzalez A, Pieper DR, Cambra JB et al (2005) Skull base tumors: a comprehensive review of transfacial swing osteotomy approaches. Plast Reconstr Surg 115:711–720
15. Cantù G, Bimbi G, Colombo S et al (2006) Lip-splitting in transmandibular resections: is it really necessary? Oral Oncol 42:619–624
16. Vishteh AG, Beals SP, Joganic EF et al (1999) Bilateral sagittal split mandibular osteotomies as an adjunct to the transoral approach to the anterior craniovertebral junction. Technical note. J Neurosurg 90(2 Suppl):267–270
17. Lazaridis N, Antoniades K (2003) Double mandibular osteotomy with coronoidectomy for tumours in the parapharyngeal space. Br J Oral Maxillofac Surg 41:142–146
18. Lazaridis N, Antoniades K (2008) Condylotomy or vertical subsigmoid osteotomy with a mandibulotomy anterior to the mental foramen for improved access to the parapharyngeal space tumors. J Oral Maxillofac Surg 66:597–606
19. Smith GI, Brennan PA, Webb AA, Ilankovan V (2003) Vertical ramus osteotomy combined with a parasymphyseal mandibulotomy for improved access to the parapharyngeal space. Head Neck 25:1000–1003
20. Sekhar LN, Schramm VL Jr, Jones NF (1987) Subtemporal-preauricular infratemporal fossa approach to large lateral and posterior cranial base neoplasms. J Neurosurg 67:488–499

Roberto Brusati, Federico Biglioli and Pietro Mortini

23.1 Introduction

Breakthrough of the cranial base because of chronic infections, fistulae, previous trauma or craniofacial resections without proper reconstruction leads to a high risk of life-threatening complications such as meningitis, brain abscess, cerebrospinal fluid leakage, vascular injury and neurological injury [1, 2]. Other complications such as osteomyelitis, ocular dystopia and distortion of facial morphology may occur if proper reconstruction is omitted. These complications may also delay the start of planned postoperative radiation treatment or chemotherapy.

In order to reduce the incidence of these problems, accurate planning of reconstruction is mandatory. The key point is to separate the endocranial contents from the pharynx and external environment by means of well vascularized tissue. The use of local flaps such as the pericranium, galea and temporal muscle is the first choice in most cases. If these flaps are not available due to previous surgery or radiotherapy, or because the amount of material is insufficient to adequately obliterate the residual spaces, microvascular flaps must be transferred to the cranial base. These are more reliable than pedicled flaps and their versatility ensures that different tissue components reach the cranial base. This is the reason for the enormous spread of microvascular reconstructions of the cranial base during the last 15 years.

Significant bone loss may lead to encephalocele through the anterior cranial base or may lead to ocular dystopia and facial disfigurement. In such cases, bone reconstruction must be accomplished. The best way is by harvesting and modeling bone grafts. Alloplastic materials may be considered under certain circumstances.

23.2 History

Removal of craniofacial tumors and other pathologies of the skull base often leads to huge losses of substance. Exposure of the dura mater and its partial removal is the reason for the high incidence of infection extending to the brain through the defect of the cranial base.

The first goal is to ensure dural closure primarily by simple suturing to separate at least the intradural spaces from the extradural ones. If this is not possible, the use of skin grafts has been proposed. Ketcham et al. [3] first reported the inadequacy of skin grafts in ensuring dural closure. These authors found a high percentage of patients with postoperative liquorrhea, a predisposing condition for ascending infections. Also, nonvascularized tissue may easily be colonized by bacteria, becoming a medium for their growth instead of antagonizing it. So the use of grafts directly exposed to the pharynx without any vascular diaphragm between the intracranial and extracranial spaces ends up as a factor leading to infections.

Later, the first attempts were made to separate the dura, repaired or simply exposed, from the extracranial spaces by means of vascularized local flaps [4]. In this way bacteria-laden secretions from the sinuses, nasal cavity and mouth could be properly isolated and countered by immune factors conveyed by the blood system. The recognition of the importance of vascularization

F. Biglioli (✉)
Dept of Maxillo-Facial Surgery
San Paolo Hospital, University of Milan, Italy

P. Cappabianca et al. (eds.), *Cranial, Craniofacial and Skull Base Surgery.*
© Springer-Verlag Italia 2010

was a great input to this surgery, leading to a high level of control of potentially lethal infections.

Still, there are situations where the use of local flaps was not possible. These are mainly when previous surgery, scars or radiotherapy have damaged the vascularity of the flaps. In other cases regional flaps that would be suitable have already been used and are no longer available for reconstruction. Finally, some losses of substance are simply too large to be filled by a local flap.

The development and wide use of myocutaneous pedicled flaps seemed to be the answer to these problems. Pectoralis major, latissimus dorsi and trapezius flaps became quickly popular due to their well-known reliability and ease of harvesting. Unfortunately, while the vascular supply to these flaps is guaranteed when they are utilized in nearby regions, more distal dissection of the flap in order to reach the cranial base frequently leads to partial necrosis of the flap. This is clearly indicated by the studies of Taylor and Palmer [5], who demonstrated that a flap extended as far as its third angiosome is less reliable. The practical consequence is that the distal part of the flap, the one reaching the cranial base, is the part that necrotizes in the event of partial flap loss, leaving the patient without effective reconstruction [6]. Other problems with pedicled flaps reaching the cranial base include detachment of the flap itself due to its weight, and retraction caused by scarring. In addition to this, reconstructions often have to be made in two steps: setting the flap and detachment/modeling of the flap 30–50 days later. This period of time is hard for patients, who are forced into an uncomfortable position and require a long hospitalization time. Failure of reconstruction after some weeks leads to a psychologically difficult situation both for the patient and the surgeon.

Finally, the advent of microvascular reconstruction gave rise to a new era with a higher reliability of reconstruction, and the ability to solve the problem of reconstructing the cranial base when local flaps are not feasible [7]. Technically, a watertight seal is easier to obtain with free flaps than with pedicled ones, because those have a cumbersome muscular pedicle.

23.3 Grafts

Grafts for reconstructing the anterior cranial base are mainly used in two different situations: when defects of the dura cannot be repaired directly and when bone loss would cause distortion of the facial morphology or

alter the position of the eyeball. More rare is the indication to reconstruct the lamina cribra to prevent postoperative encephalocele; this type of reconstruction is used when the entire lamina is resected.

In the early days of cranial-base surgery, only the need to repair lacerations of the dura mater or losses of substance was recognized. So dural repair was accomplished by direct suturing or, when large areas of dura

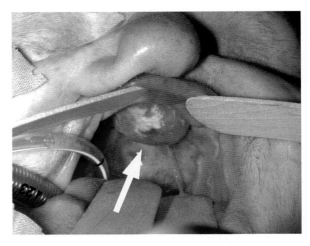

Fig. 23.1 Cocaine-addicted patient with resorption of the maxilla, soft palate, nasal bone and septum, lamina cribra and left papyracea, the frontal bone and the left eyeball. The patient developed an encephalocele (*arrow*) and was treated by local flap transposition during a first operation and by joining two temporal flaps on the midline during a second operation. Finally the situation was addressed utilizing a fasciocutaneous forearm microvascular flap

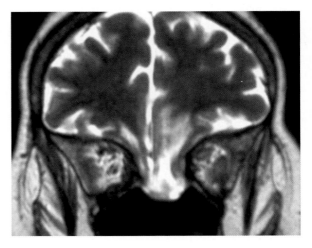

Fig. 23.2 MR image of the encephalocele

had been resected, patches of different tissues were used to cover the defects. These mainly comprised the pericranium, fascia lata, or bovine pericardium. The need for a watertight closure of the dura mater became universally recognized, but its description is beyond the scope of this chapter.

Once the dura is repaired or is simply exposed through the cranial base, even a small defect in the cranial base should be repaired to provide a better seal to prevent cerebrospinal fluid leakage and to separate bacteria-laden spaces from the sterile intracranial compartment. Initially a simple graft, without any vascularization, was employed. The tissue generally chosen was pericranium, a piece of temporalis muscle, fascia temporalis, fascia lata, fat, or skin. Sometimes a temporary nasal packing was added to stick the graft in place until healing occurred. All these practices might increase the risk of infection and necrosis of the tissues transposed as a nonvascularized environment without the possibility for pus to drain are conditions that favor ascending infections and liquorrhea.

Because of extensive bacterial colonization of the pharynx, grafts should be used in cranial base reconstruction only when external contaminated environments have not been opened or when a good simultaneous vascular seal is guaranteed by a vascular flap. These considerations apply not only to soft tissue grafts but also to reconstruction of bony structures. The argument is widely discussed in the literature, some authors being strongly in favor of bone reconstruction [8] while others judge it to be unnecessary in most circumstances [9]. Others stress the risk of infection of bone grafts and secondary osteitis if radiotherapy is to follow surgery [10]. However, when bone grafts are adequately covered by well-vascularized tissue, all these risks are limited.

The precise restoration of the anatomy of the regions involved in surgery is fundamental for the restoration of integrity both in terms of morphology and functionality.

Complete removal of the lamina cribra may lead to herniation of the cranial contents (Figs. 23.1 to 23.10). A soft tissue flap together with a dense grid of thick stitches can isolate the brain from the pharynx with subsequent formation of a strong scar. This may be sufficient for moderate defects, but has a high risk of encephalocele formation if the entire loss of the structure occurs, predisposing to potentially life-threatening ascending infections. In these circumstances, reconstruction is indicated.

Gross defects of the orbital roof also lead to deficits of the endoorbital structures. The usual consequences

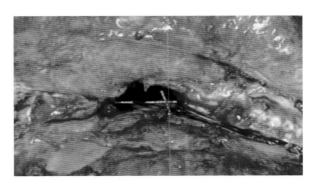

Fig. 23.3 The communication between anterior cranial fossa and the pharynx once the encephalocele had been reduced

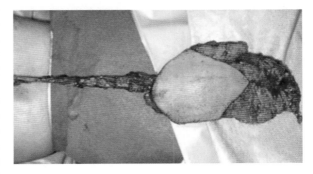

Fig. 23.4 The forearm free flap harvested

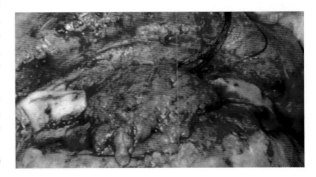

Fig. 23.5 The forearm free flap set in place to fill the defect and separate the intracranial and extracranial spaces

are bulbar dystopia, diplopia, transmission of cerebral pulses, and ophthalmoplegia because of scarring of the extrinsic ocular musculature. The anterior two-thirds of the orbital roof comprises the frontal bone and the posterior third the lesser wing of the sphenoid. The posterior two-thirds of the lateral wall comprises the great

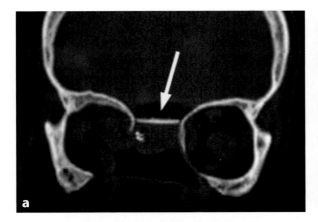

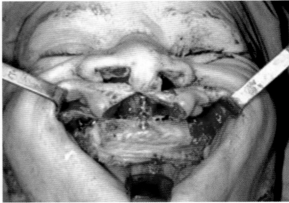

Fig. 23.7 During a following operation, the midface was reconstructed by placing a fibula free flap for the nose and a second fibula free flap for the maxilla and soft palate

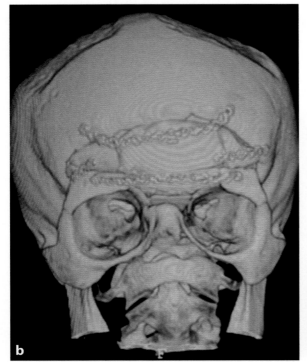

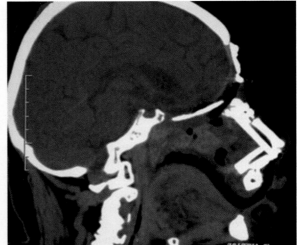

Fig. 23.6 Three months later, working in a sterile environment, the lamina cribra (**a** *arrow*) and the front (**b**) were reconstructed using calvarial grafts

Fig. 23.8 Postoperative CT image

wing of the sphenoid. These structures are fundamental to the separation of the orbital contents from the frontal lobes and the temporal lobes. Their removal entails negative effects on the eye with downward and forward bulbar dystopia, diplopia, transmission of cerebral pulses and occasional partial or complete ophthalmoplegia due to fibrosis of the oculomotor muscles. The orbital walls must be reconstructed to avoid those sequelae. This is mandatory in cranial base surgery for benign neoplasms and malformations [11]. The role of bone reconstruction is more controversial in surgery for malignant tumors. This is because the complexity of the region to be reconstructed leads the surgeon "not to dare too much". In fact in such cases resection leads to

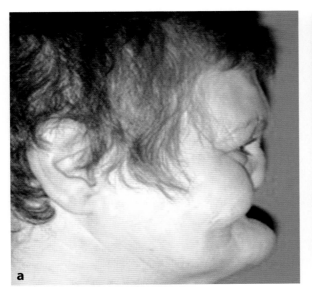
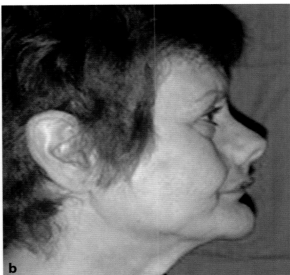

Fig. 23.9 The patient before (**a**) and after (**b**) midface reconstruction

loosing of a huge component of soft tissues. So it is more difficult to guarantee a perfectly hermetic coverage of the bone graft, a condition necessary to prevent infection and subsequent loss of the bone itself. The other reason is that radiotherapy is frequently indicated, and is a cause of secondary osteitis of the grafted bone that may lead to the necessity to remove it.

Bone loss may be replaced by numerous materials, bone graft being the first choice while alloplastic materials are used in selected cases [12]. The bone graft is preferably harvested from the internal cortex of the temporoparietal squamae in adults. This avoids a second surgical site to be worked on. If a greater quantity of bone is required, the ilium may be considered because it is pliable and therefore easier to model, and because of the great amount of bone available. This can be harvested as a single cortex graft, a bicortical piece or a piece including the iliac crest to produce, for example, a better reconstruction of the orbital rim. The bone can be harvested simultaneously while another team is working on the head. However, the use of the ilium involves a second surgical site with the associated morbidity.

Ribs are preferred in children, because it is generally very difficult to split the calvaria in this patient group, and the removal of bone from the ilium may disturb the growth of the pelvis. If more than one rib is necessary, they should not be contiguous and they can be taken with very little morbidity.

If a free flap is planned, one of the best multiple component donor sites is the lateral thoracic wall. In this case a latissimus dorsi free flap can be harvested when soft tissues are missing, and one or more ribs can be taken for bone reconstruction. The ribs are split in order to better curve the bone to mimic the orbital walls and to reduce the amount of bone taken. Other ribs can be shaped all in one to cover calvarial defects. Partial resorption of the split ribs may occur over the years, though this has not been documented among our patients. However, quick vascularization of the graft is

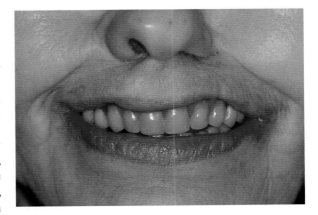

Fig. 23.10 Smiling after implantoprosthodontic rehabilitation

ensured by the porous structure of the ribs and their position surrounded by well-vascularized tissues.

Reconstruction of the roof of the orbit must proceed in anteroposterior direction as far as the bottom of the orbital cavity, leaving only a space to recreate the optic canal and superior orbital fissure. The correct position of the roof and of the orbital walls generally is better recreated by comparison with the other side (when this has not also been resected). So a bilateral exposure of the region is generally preferable to optimize the reconstructive results. The upper third of the face must be free of cover when preparing the surgical field. Thus the eyeball position can be checked at the end of orbital reconstruction, and this will allow the correct position of the eyeball to be easily maintained, and most ocular complications are limited.

The stability of reconstruction is ensured by recreating precisely the anatomy of the roof and fixing the bone graft to the buttress of the lateral and medial walls using mini- and microplates and screws. Modeling calvarial grafts may be more challenging due to their low plasticity compared to rib grafts. Nevertheless, it is possible to obtain similar results utilizing calvaria to those obtained using the ribs. The time for neovascularization is definitely longer, and indeed may take more than a year. This must be taken into account when radiotherapy may be the next therapeutic option. In fact nonvascularized bone is more likely to be damaged by radiation.

Many alloplastic materials such as titanium mesh, hydroxyapatite, bone cement, plastic and acrylic materials have been proposed as substitutes for bone grafts. The use of these materials generally allows saving of surgical time while reducing morbidity at the donor site. Prefabricated and computer-generated materials have recently been described [13]. A clear indication is secondary reconstruction of larger areas of substance loss or reconstruction of esthetically challenging regions such as the supraorbital rim, where a good profile is easily achieved using this methodology. The use of alloplastic materials also avoids the harvesting of large amounts of bone.

The main risk in the use of alloplastic materials is postoperative infection that invariably leads to loss of the reconstruction. Later extrusion of the reconstructive materials is rare if they are well covered by vascularized soft tissues.

The lamina cribra is a structure often affected by trauma, osteotomies, and resections. Its partial loss or monolateral removal seldom needs to be reconstructed by bone [14]. Generally the interposition of a vascularized local flap or microvascular flap is sufficient to prevent most local complications. When the entire lamina

is missing, the risk of brain prolapse through the anterior cranial base is too high and bony reconstruction is mandatory. Isolation of bone from the source of bacterial contamination is accomplished by interposition of vascularized tissue and cranialization of the frontal sinuses when these are opened. If preexisting infection is present or there is incomplete separation from the pharynx by the flap, bone reconstruction should be delayed for a few months. Generally a single layer of internal cortical cortex is enough to fill the defect.

When part of the frontal bone is missing, there may be a consequent esthetic deficit. The best way to restore its integrity is to use bone grafts split from the parietal calvaria. If the defect covers the entire frontal bone or more, alloplastic materials are preferred to avoid huge morbidity at the donor site or the necessity to choose a second site such as the iliac region. The best way to restore the integrity of the frontal bone is by utilizing an alloplastic graft premodeled by computer on the basis of a CT scan [15].

23.4 Local flaps

Local flaps are the workhorse of reconstruction of the anterior cranial base. The most utilized flap is the pericranium. Others are the galeal, galeopericranial and temporalis muscle flaps and, more recently, nasal or nasopharyngeal mucosal flaps harvested endoscopically. Since their routine use in craniofacial reconstruction, the rate of infections, cerebrospinal fluid leaks and neurologic complications has fallen [16].

Pericranial flaps can be positioned easily over the anterior cranial base and adapted to the loss of substance because of their optimal pliability. Healing is rapid and guaranteed by their vascular supply. If a thicker flap is required, the galea is considered. This tissue is immediately subdermal, being continuous laterally with the superficial temporalis fascia and the subcutaneous muscular aponeurotic system. Anteriorly it includes the frontalis muscles. The main vascular supplies are the anterior branches of the superficial temporal artery, the supraorbital artery and the supratrochlear artery. Both the supraorbital and the supratrochlear arteries ramify into a superficial and a deep plexus at their emergence from the bony foramina. Galeopericranial flaps are based on the superficial plexus, while pericranial flaps are based on the deep plexus [17].

Based on their vascular anatomy, galeal flaps may be harvested with a frontal or lateral pedicle based on the superficial temporal artery. When a lateral pedicle is chosen, the flap is best harvested with a bilateral pedicle if its length crosses the midline, because vascular anastomoses are few there. In this case the galea is rotated down and forward as a visor to cover the defect. Pericranial flaps are generally based on the anterior pedicle when this is not interrupted by cancer resection or preexisting scars. In this is the case, a lateral vascular pedicle is chosen. Finally, a galeopericranial flap can be harvested. This is best vascularized and must include both layers at least proximal to the hilum of the vessels.

While pericranial flaps with good vascularization seldom give rise to complications, galeal flaps may lead to a few. In fact, the vascularization is generally optimal but the thin layer of skin may lead to esthetic deficits especially in the frontal region. This is more evident if there are irregularities in the plane under the skin. Also the thin skin of the forehead repositioned at the end of surgery is more likely to ulcerate. This relative delicacy of the skin after galea flap harvesting must be taken into consideration when planning a frontal reconstruction with alloplastic materials. An ulcer over them would invariably lead to the removal of the hard tissue reconstruction.

Other problems include alopecia because a lesion involving the hair bulbs. Scalp necrosis is a severe complication but extremely rare. This is more likely to occur if a deficit of vascularization of the skin was present before surgery and underestimated, for example in the case of an irradiated field. Finally, if the higher branches of the facial nerve are damaged during harvesting of a flap, the frontalis muscles loose function resulting in drooping of the eyebrows. This deficit is less visible when bilateral; it is very unpleasing when it occurs only on one side.

The temporalis muscle flap is a good choice for anterolateral skull-base defects with a small/medium loss of substance [18]. Its use as a flap was first described by Golovine in 1898 [19]. Huge defects may not be fully covered by the muscle. Sometimes part of the muscle is resected together with the tumor, so the remaining part is too small to be considered for reconstruction of the region.

The temporalis muscle is assessed by asking the patient to clench the teeth during physical examination. Its thickness is variable, and is generally four to five times that of the galea. It may be really useful for coverage of the orbit following exenteration of the eye. The arc of rotation of the flap is limited. It may be increased by sectioning the coronoid process of the mandible but, even so, the flap cannot be extended beyond the midline of the anterior cranial base by more than 1 or 2 cm.

Covering defects of the entire skull lamina cribra may require two temporal muscle flaps joined in the midline of the cranial base. This is a second choice compared to the advancement of a pericranial or a galeopericranial flap. The principal vascular pedicle comprises the deep temporal arteries arising from the internal maxillary artery, a terminal branch of the external carotid artery. If the main pedicle is interrupted, the flap may be harvested relying on the middle temporal artery which originates from the external carotid artery [5].

Local deficits must be taken into consideration when utilizing a temporal flap for reconstruction. In fact, if all the muscle is used the region remains sunken and esthetically poor. A filling prosthesis may be positioned in place of the muscle at the same stage, but carries the adjunctive risk of infection. This is a little lower if the prosthesis is placed secondarily. When less muscle is required for reconstruction, generally the anterior half of it is turned to repair the deficit, while the posterior half is translated anteriorly to cover the esthetic deficit.

A typical complication of temporalis flap harvesting is a lesion of the frontal branch of the facial nerve. That is located just underneath the temporoparietal fascia, approximately 2 cm from the lateral aspect of the eyebrow. Its deficit is clearly visible with unpleasing drooping of the eyebrow and lack of frontalis muscle function. Local pain and secondary reduction of mouth opening may be seen on follow-up. While pain is generally difficult to be cured, mouth opening may be treated with functional therapy and rarely by surgery.

Nasal and nasopharyngeal mucosal flaps harvested and positioned endoscopically have gained importance in recent years, together with the spread of endoscopy in cranial base surgery [20]. The development of new instrumentation and imaging technology has given a great boost to this specific field. At the beginning non-vascularized pieces of tissue were transposed to the cranial base to seal defects in order to prevent rhinorrhea for small defects, with a success rate of 95%. Recently vascularized mucoperiosteal and mucoperichondrial flaps based on the nasoseptal artery system have been described. All the considerations discussed above concerning the safety of reconstruction of the cranial base with local flaps perfectly apply for these flaps. The complication rate is extremely low, with the evident added advantage of low morbidity and the avoidance of an open approach. This is true especially for conditions treated completely by endoscopy such as some tumors and secondary liquorrhea. If an open approach is chosen, via a coronal incision for example, a classical local flap seems more reasonable.

23.5 Locoregional flaps

Locoregional pedicled flaps have mostly been abandoned in cranial base reconstruction as their reliability is less than that of free flaps. Their current indication is for patients with a high risk of complications following microsurgery. Such patients include the elderly, diabetic and vasculopathic patients, and generally subjects in poor general condition. Locoregional flaps mainly utilized for cranial base reconstructions are pectoralis major, lower trapezius and latissimus dorsi myocutaneous flaps [21, 22].

All these flaps are less reliable than microvascular flaps as their distal vascular supply is doubtful and this is the part of the flap that reaches the cranial base. Also their weight is not negligible and detachment of the flap with a residual fistula is a serious complication [23].

In anterior cranial base reconstruction, it is more difficult for a locoregional pedicled flap to reach the receiving surgical field than in lateral cranial base reconstruction. In such cases a two-stage reconstruction is sometimes required. The first operation leaves the pedicle dangling to allow the flap to reach the defect; during the second operation the pedicle is cut and the flap better adapted to the receiving surgical field. Even in cases treated with a single-stage operation, the cumbersome pedicle may have to be thinned in a second operation. Another problem is the difficulty harvesting the flap at the same time as the resection, which may lead to an increasing in the operative time.

Finally, the morbidity following the harvest of locoregional flaps is negligible only for the pectoralis major, being considerable for the lower trapezius and the latissimus dorsi. For of all these reasons, locoregional flaps are utilized only in selected cases, and are a second choice for reconstructing the anterior cranial base.

23.6 Microvascular flaps

Microvascular flaps comprise tissues harvested from a donor site where their main vascular pedicles are sectioned and successively anastomosed to receiving vessels adjacent to the region where the flaps are transposed. This has many advantages:

- The best tissue is chosen for reconstruction. This has to be compared to the limited type of tissue available with local flaps.
- Different tissues may be harvested and compounded together in the same chimera flap. For example, the vascularized rib and skin of the abdomen may be included in the rectus abdominis muscle free flap transfer. The possibility of working with different tissues, and the ease of placement improves a factor often neglected: the esthetics of the operated region.
- A wide variety of tissues may be harvested and transferred at one time.
- Donor sites with lower morbidity can be chosen.
- Optimally vascularized tissues are transferred to regions where sometimes the local tissue conditions (and therefore also local flap conditions) have deteriorated because of radiotherapy, previous surgery, etc.
- Distant receiving vessels may be reached by the vascular pedicle when local receiving vessels are not present or in bad condition.
- Double team working allows contemporaneous harvesting of the flap and demolition/operation of the cranial base thus reducing the operation time. This is not possible when utilizing local or locoregional flaps.
- The reliability of free flaps is 92–98%, similar to that of local flaps, but with a reduced cerebrospinal fluid leakage rate of 3–10% in craniofacial surgery [24]. These minimal percentages have been found since the introduction of free flap surgery for craniofacial reconstructions. The reason is because large vascularized flaps provide better separation and coverage of dead spaces.

While complications with local flaps are mainly correlated with late wound breakdown problems, complications with free flaps are more likely to happen in a primarily acute surgical context [25].

Most utilized free flaps are the fasciocutaneous forearm, the fasciocutaneous anterolateral tight, the musculus and musculocutaneous rectus abdominis and latissimus dorsi [7, 26–28]. All of those have their particular characteristics and they are utilized according to their features and personal experience.

The fasciocutaneous forearm flap is 5–20 mm thick with a medium area coverage (15×15 cm at the most). These characteristics make the flap ideal for surface lining of the skin or pharyngeal mucosa. Its pedicle is particularly long (15–30 cm depending on the height of the patient and type of harvesting). This allows receiving vessels of the neck to be reached if the superficial temporal artery and vein are not suitable.

The fasciocutaneous anterolateral tight flap is 8–30 mm thick with an area coverage that may be as large as 15×30 cm. This allows the repair of a very large surface [29]. Dead spaces may also be filled by bending the flap. Its very low morbidity and low esthetic impact at the donor site are the reasons for the wide use of this flap over recent years. The pedicle is 10–13 cm long, enough to reach the receiving vessels of the neck only if the flap is to be placed with the vascular pedicle beginning not higher than the central third of the face. If the placement is higher, anastomoses should be accomplished on temporal or facial vessels.

The rectus abdominis flap is one of the most popular free flaps in cranial base reconstruction [30]. This is because its high vascular flow makes it extremely reliable. The possibility to include the subcutis of the abdomen makes it very bulky (depending obviously on how fat the person is), and it therefore can be adapted to cover large dead spaces. One or more vascularized ribs may also be included in the flap to reconstruct, for example, the orbital walls. The pedicle is 10–12 cm long and may be elongated by a further 5 cm by tracing it inside the muscle. Morbidity is not negligible.

The latissimus dorsi free flap is also very popular in cranial base reconstruction. As in rectus abdominis, the vascular flow through the flap is high and this is a good guarantee against failure. The vascular pedicle is 12–14 cm long and may be elongated by a further 6–8 cm by dissecting it intraparenchymally and harvesting a strip of muscle together with the pedicle. This allows cervical vessels to be reached easily to perform large anastomoses. In fact the diameter of the artery and vein of the pedicle is between 2.5 and 6 mm.

Different types of tissue may be taken from the same surgical donor site (Figs. 23.11 to 23.16). The skin pad overlying the muscle may be harvested up to 50×30 cm. Multiple rib grafts may be picked up while the thoracodorsal nerve together with its distal branches may be used to reconstruct the facial nerve when this is included in the resection. Morbidity in generally quite low and discomfort for the patient does not last more than three weeks.

Some specific details must be known when performing microsurgical craniofacial reconstruction.

Although tunneling of the pedicle is chosen by some authors to reach distant vessels, we consider it too risky because inadvertent twisting may block blood flow and lead to flap loss. Also there may be a risk of postoperative hematoma because of compression of the vein of the pedicle in the tunnel. In order to avoid those complications an anterior skin flap may be elevated in the cervicofacial region to reach cervical vessels without tunneling. The skin incision is as for a face-lift, extending inferiorly in a natural skin crease of the neck. With this procedure the whole course of the pedicle is in view, so twisting can be identified and hemostasis guaranteed.

The receiving vessels are a key point in the success of microvascular reconstruction. Generally the superficial temporal vessels are the nearest to the flap. It is extremely important to avoid damage to these vessels when executing the coronal incision. In many secondary operations these are found to have been previously cut.

The vessel dimensions are important. In particular the superficial temporal vein may have a diameter significantly smaller than the vein of the flap pedicle. This leads to stasis of the vein flow negatively affecting the blood flow of the whole flap. If this is the case, any trick must be used to plan a vein anastomosis on larger vessels in the neck region.

The second nearest receiving vessels are generally the facial vessels. These may easily be found at the inferior mandibular border or just below it, immediately anterior to the masseter muscle. The vein is normally a little larger than the superficial temporal vein.

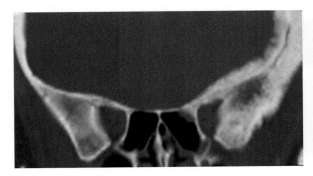

Fig. 23.11 CT image of an en plaque meningioma invading the sphenoid wing

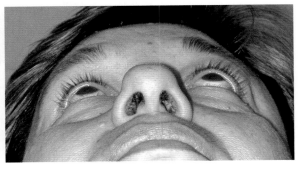

Fig. 23.12 Left exophthalmos due to reduced orbital volume because of the tumor

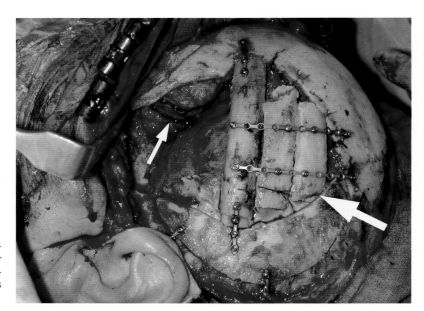

Fig. 23.13 The orbital walls reconstructed with split rib grafts (*smaller arrow*). The temporal bone reconstructed with full-thickness rib grafts (*larger arrow*)

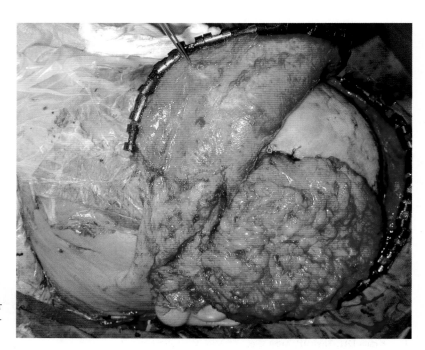

Fig. 23.14 A latissimus dorsi muscular and adipose flap placed to cover the encephalon and the bone grafts

If it is possible for the pedicle to reach the neck region to accomplish the anastomosis, this is the best option since numerous arteries and veins are then eligible for the anastomosis. An advantageous venous drainage may be guaranteed by a terminolateral anastomosis with the internal jugular vein. This maintains its main flow with a negative pump effect on the venous drainage of the flap. The arterial receiving vessels most utilized in the neck are the superior thyroid, facial, lingual and terminal segment of the external carotid ar-

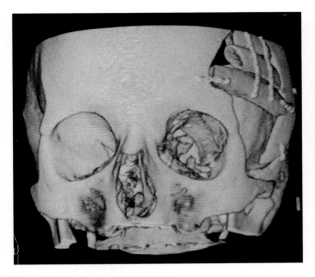

Fig. 23.15 Postoperative 3-D CT image

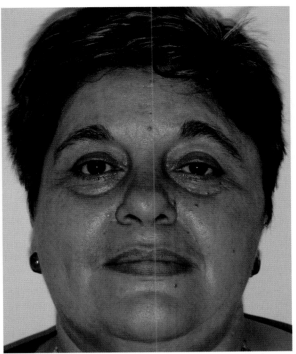

Fig. 23.16 Appearance of the patient 1 year after surgery

tery. The choice of vessel depends on the vascular requirements of the flap (muscular and large flaps require greater blood flow), the geometry of the receiving vessels and pedicle course, and the comfort of working.

Flaps have the highest risk of vascular impairment during the first 48 hours and this decreases during the following 7–10 days. So monitoring blood flow through the flap is fundamental to avoiding flap loss, an eventuality that may be potentially life-threatening in cranial base reconstruction.

Monitoring of the flap is still very controversial in the literature [31]. Most authors agree on the reliability of clinical investigation for visible flaps, flap color, dermographism and bleeding after puncture being the must important factors. Buried flaps must necessarily be monitored instrumentally. If there is any doubt about the vascularization of the flap, is mandatory to re-explore the surgical site immediately. In fact a period of only a few hours is available to save the flap before thrombosis of the microcirculation occurs and the flap is definitively lost. Specific antiaggregant and anticoagulant therapy, together with posture studied intraoperatively to avoid kinking of the pedicle and promote venous drainage, must be taken during the first 7–10 postoperative days.

References

1. Kraus DH, Shah JP, Arbit E et al (1994) Complications of the craniofacial resection for tumors involving the anterior skull base. Head Neck 16:307–312
2. Ganly I, Patel SG, Singh B et al (2005) Complications of craniofacial resection for malignant tumors of the skull base: report of an International Collaborative Study. Head Neck 27:445–451
3. Ketcham AS, Hoye RC, Van Buren JM (1966) Complications of intracranial facial resection for tumors of the paranasal sinuses. Am J Surg 112:591
4. Johns ME, Winn HR, McLean WC, Cantrell RW (1981) Pericranial flap for the closure of defects of craniofacial resection. Laryngoscope 91:952–959
5. Taylor GI, Palmer JH (1987) The vascular territories (angiosomes) of the body: experimental study and clinical applications. Br J Plast Surg 40:113–141
6. Janecka IP, Snyderman CH (1993) Regional flaps and craniofacial skeleton. In: Sekhar LN, Janecka IP (eds) Surgery of cranial base tumors. Raven Press, New York, pp 413–427
7. Chiu SE, Kraus D, Bui DT et al (2008) Anterior and middle cranial fossa skull base reconstruction using microvascular

free tissue techniques. Surgical complications and functional outcomes. Ann Plast Surg 60:514–520

8. Derome P (1988) The transbasal approach to tumours invading the base of the skull. In: Schmidek H, Sweet W (eds) Current techniques in operative neurosurgery. Grune and Stratton, New York, p 629

9. Cantù G, Riccio S, Bimbi G et al (2006) Craniofacial resection for malignant tumours involving the anterior skull base. Eur Arch Otorhinolaryngol 263:647–652

10. Hochman M (1995) Reconstruction of midfacial and anterior skull-base defects. Otolaryngol Clin North Am 28:1269–1277

11. Brusati R, Biglioli F, Mortini P et al (2000) Reconstruction of the orbital walls in surgery of the skull base for benign neoplasm. Int J Oral Maxillofac Surg 29:325–330

12. Greenberg BM, Schneider SJ (2005) Alloplastic reconstruction of large cranio-orbital defects: a comparative evaluation. Ann Plast Surg 55:43–51

13. Saringer W, Nöbauer-Huhmann I, Knosp E (2002) Cranioplasty with individual carbon fibre reinforced polymer (CFRP) medical grade implants based on CAD/CAM technique. Acta Neurochir 144:1193–1203

14. Georgantopoulou A, Hodgkinson PD, Gerber CJ (2003) Cranial-base surgery: a reconstructive algorithm. Br J Plast Surg 56:10–13

15. Scolozzi P, Martinez A, Jaques B (2007) Complex orbito-fronto-temporal reconstruction using computer-designed PEEK implant. J Craniofac Surg 18:224–228

16. Snyderman CH, Janecka IP, Sekhar LN et al (1990) Anterior cranial base reconstruction: role of galeal and pericranial flaps. Laryngoscope 100:607–614

17. Jackson IT, Adham MN, Marsh WR (1986) Use of galeal frontalis myofascial flap in craniofacial surgery. Plast Reconstr Surg 77:905–910

18. Raffaini M, Costa G (1994) The temporoparietal fascial flap in reconstruction of the cranio-maxillofacial area. J Craniomaxillofac Surg 22(5):261–267

19. Golovine SS (1898) Procede de cloture plastique de l'orbite apres l'exenteration. J Fr Ophtalmol 18:679–691

20. Hadad G, Bassagasteguy L, Carrai RL et al (2006) A novel reconstructive technique after endoscopic expanded endonasal approaches: vascular pedicle nasoseptal flap. Laryngoscope 116:1882–1886

21. Resto VA, McKenna MJ, Deschler DG (2007) Pectoralis major flap in composite lateral skull base defect reconstruction. Arch Otolaryngol Head Neck Surg 133:490–494

22. Chen W, Deng YF, Peng GG et al (2007) Extended vertical lower trapezius island myocutaneous flap for reconstruction of cranio-maxillofacial defects. Int J Oral Maxillofac Surg 36:165–170

23. Janecka IP, Sekhar LN (1989) Surgical management of cranial base tumours: a report on 91 patients. Oncology 3:69–74

24. Urken ML, Catalano PJ, Sen C et al (1993) Free tissue transfer for skull base reconstruction analysis of complications and a classification scheme for defining skull base defects. Arch Otolaryngol Head Neck Surg 119:1318–1325

25. Heth JA, Funk GF, Karnell LH et al (2002) Free tissue transfer and local flap complications in anterior and anterolateral skull base surgery. Head Neck 24:901–911

26. Cordeiro PG, Santamaria E (1997) The extended, pedicled rectus abdominis free tissue transfer for head and neck reconstruction. Ann Plast Surg 39:53

27. Joos U, Mann W, Gilsbach J (1998) Microsurgical treatment of midfacial tumours involving the skull base. J Craniomaxillofac Surg 26:226–234

28. Schliephake H, Schmelzeisen R, Samii M, Sollmann WP (1999) Microvascular reconstruction of the skull base: indications and procedures. J Oral Maxillofac Surg 57:233–239

29. Valentini V, Cassoni A, Marianetti TM et al (2008) Anterolateral thigh flap for the reconstruction of head and neck defects: alternative or replacement of the radial forearm flap? J Craniofac Surg 19:1148–1153

30. Yamada A, Harii K, Ueda K, Asato H (1992) Free rectus abdominis muscle reconstruction of the anterior skull base. Br J Plast Surg 45:302–306

31. Brix M, Muret P, Mac-Mary S et al (2006) Microdialysis of cutaneous free flaps to monitor results of maxillofacial surgery. Rev Stomatol Chir Maxillofac 107:31–37

Subject Index